PHYSICAL PRINCIPLES
of
ULTRASONIC
DIAGNOSIS

MEDICAL PHYSICS SERIES

CONSULTING EDITOR

J. M. A. Lenihan

Department of Clinical Physics and Bio-
engineering, Western Regional Hospital
Board, Glasgow, Scotland

Volume 1. P. N. T. WELLS. Physical Principles of Ultrasonic Diagnosis. 1969

PHYSICAL PRINCIPLES
of
ULTRASONIC
DIAGNOSIS

P. N. T. Wells
*University of Bristol and United Bristol
Hospitals, Bristol, England*

1969

Academic Press · London · New York

ACADEMIC PRESS INC. (LONDON) LTD
24-28 Oval Road
London NW1 7DX

U.S. Edition published by
ACADEMIC PRESS INC.
111 Fifth Avenue
New York, New York 10003

Library of Congress Catalog Card Number: 76-92398
Standard Book Number: 12-742950-6
Printed by photolithography in Great Britain by
T. & A. Constable Ltd., Edinburgh

PREFACE

In this book, I have tried to describe the basic physical principles of ultrasonics in medical diagnosis, and to review the techniques of its application. The purpose of the book is both to make rediscovery unnecessary, and also to form a foundation upon which new work may be based. No attempt has been made to dilute the contents, which are intended to cover every aspect of the subject without trespassing too far into the realm of clinical application. The rather unusual arrangement of the references has been chosen to enable the cited literature on each subject to be found as easily as possible.

This book lies in the limbo between three disciplines—physics, engineering and medicine—and specialists in one field are generally content to leave common problems to those in the others. I hope that those important exceptions to this general rule, the medical physicists and the bioengineers, will find that the book has at least partly achieved its aims.

The regrettable tendency to leave scientific matters to other people is particularly common amongst medical specialists. It is thanks to the few who do not share this attitude—and I myself have been unusually fortunate to work with many—that the techniques of ultrasound in medical diagnosis have developed at all. However, this progress has really been depressingly slow during the past fifteen years. I believe that this is because the subject is now so complex that it can no longer be advanced by the efforts of a few isolated individuals covering too wide a field in too little depth.

The potential rewards of research into ultrasonic diagnosis are immense, provided that this research can be made on an adequate scale. I hope that those who read this book will come to appreciate this. What is needed is the establishment of a few research units integrated within University hospitals, each with a staff of perhaps eight or ten people, at least one being medically qualified. The stream of clinical material being thus assured, adequate and independent finance and wise guidance are the only prerequisites for success.

August 1969   P. N. T. WELLS

ACKNOWLEDGEMENTS

I am indebted to Mr. M. Halliwell and to Mr. D. H. Follett, who read and criticized much of the first four chapters of this book. I am also especially grateful to Prof. K. T. Evans, Dr. C. F. McCarthy and Dr. F. G. M. Ross for permission to publish Figs. 4.38, 4.39, 4.40 and 4.46, parts of which were obtained during the course of clinical work carried out in collaboration between us.

So many individuals have contributed, wittingly or unwittingly, to the preparation of this book that it would be invidious to try to apportion my gratitude. I am grateful to them all, whether for encouragement, discussion, criticism, or just plain hard work. Those whom I can remember are listed here; to those inadvertently omitted, I apologize and offer my thanks.

Mr. T. G. Brown; Mr. M. A. Bullen; Mr. L. A. Cram; Prof. I. Donald; Mr. J. E. E. Fleming; Dr. H. F. Freundlich; Mr. A. J. Hall; Dr. D. Holt; Prof. D. E. Hughes; Mr. J. Angell James; Mrs. L. W. Lawes; Dr. J. M. A. Lenihan; the Librarians in Engineering, Medicine and Physics, University of Bristol; Mrs. Anita Rawcliffe; Prof. A. E. A. Read; Mr. J. Tomlinson; Dr. B. Watrasiewicz; and Mrs. Valerie Wells.

My own work on diagnostic ultrasonics has been made possible by grants and facilities, for which I am most grateful, made available by the Medical Research Council, the Department of Health and Social Security (Health), the Board of Governors of the United Bristol Hospitals, and Tenovus.

Figures 4.12, 4.26, 4.42, 4.43, 4.44, 4.45, 4.47 and 5.2 are reproduced by kind permission of the Editor of Ultrasonics.

Finally, it is a pleasure to acknowledge both the help and the courtesy of the staff of the Academic Press, without whose hard and patient work this book would not have been produced.

CONTENTS

Preface v

Acknowledgement vi

1. FUNDAMENTAL PHYSICS
   1.1 Wave Motion 1
   1.2 Velocity of Propagation 2
   1.3 Wavelength and Frequency 5
   1.4 Velocity in Biological Materials 5
   1.5 Intensity and the Decibel Notation 7
   1.6 Particle Pressure 9
   1.7 Characteristic Impedance 9
   1.8 Reflection and Refraction at Plane Surfaces . . . 10
   1.9 Reflection at Rough Interfaces and Small Obstacles . . 14
   1.10 Standing Waves 15
   1.11 Transmission through Layers 16
   1.12 The Doppler Effect 17
   1.13 Radiation Pressure 18
   1.14 Non-planar Waves 19
   1.15 Attenuation Mechanisms 19
   1.16 Absorption in Biological Materials 22
   1.17 Non-linear Effects with Waves of Finite Amplitude . . 26

2. THE TRANSDUCER
   2.1 Piezoelectricity 28
   2.2 Piezoelectric Constants 29
   2.3 Piezoelectric Transducers for Ultrasonic Diagnosis . . 30
   2.4 Resonance 33
   2.5 Q-factor 35
   2.6 Short Pulses 37
   2.7 Pulse Frequency Spectrum 43
   2.8 Mechanical Impedance Matching 46
   2.9 Electrical Impedance Matching 49
   2.10 Dynamic Range 51

3. THE ULTRASONIC FIELD
   3.1 Steady State Conditions 53
   3.2 Focussing Systems 58

3.3   Transient Conditions 63
3.4   Methods of Observation 65
3.5   Power Measurement 73

4. PULSE-ECHO TECHNIQUES
4.1   Introduction 77
4.2   Timing Circuits 96
4.3   The Transmitter 97
4.4   Radio Frequency Amplifiers 99
4.5   Video Amplifiers 123
4.6   Cathode Ray Tube Displays 134
4.7   Data Presentation Systems and Clinical Applications. . 141
4.8   Measurement of System Performance 188

5. DOPPLER TECHNIQUES
5.1   Transmission Techniques 193
5.2   Reflection Techniques 194
5.3   Transmitters and Receivers 200
5.4   Methods of Doppler Signal Analysis 204
5.5   Clinical Applications 206

6. MISCELLANEOUS TECHNIQUES
6.1   Introduction 210
6.2   Unscanned Transmission Techniques 210
6.3   Mechanically Scanned Transmission Techniques . . 211
6.4   Electrically Scanned Transmission Techniques . . 213
6.5   Ultrasonic Holography 217

7. THE POSSIBILITY OF HAZARD IN ULTRASONIC
   DIAGNOSIS
7.1   Introduction 222
7.2   Ultrasonic Field Parameters 222
7.3   Interactions of Ultrasonic Waves with Biological Tissues . 223
7.4   Conclusions 226

REFERENCES 227

GLOSSARY 253

MATHEMATICAL SYMBOLS 259

AUTHOR INDEX 267

SUBJECT INDEX 275

1. FUNDAMENTAL PHYSICS

1.1 WAVE MOTION

Ultrasonic energy travels through a medium in the form of a wave. In studying such waves, it is best to begin with the simplest type: this is a sinusoidal vibration which has only a single frequency component, and which occurs in an isotropic medium which is perfectly elastic. The energy is transmitted continuously, and the vibration is in simple harmonic motion; the particles of the medium in which the wave is travelling suffer periodic disturbances about their mean positions. A particle is an element of volume which is continuous with its surroundings, but small enough for quantities which are variable within the medium to be constant within the particle. The movement of the particles is resisted by elastic forces due to the molecular structure of the medium.

Wave motions can take a number of different modes. Medical ultrasonic diagnostic techniques are usually based on the propagation of longitudinal waves. Longitudinal sound waves can be propagated in all types of media, and occur when the particle motion is in the same direction as that of the flow of energy. In an infinite or fluid medium this kind of vibration is called a bulk wave; but when it occurs in a solid bar where stress along the direction of propagation alters the width of the bar, it is called a rod wave. Transverse waves occur when the particle motion is perpendicular to the direction of propagation. This kind of wave cannot be supported within a fluid, because fluids do not possess shear elasticity. Transverse waves are seldom of importance in diagnostic techniques. In addition, there are a number of other wave modes, a description of which is outside the scope of this book.

The discussion which follows applies to plane, non-spreading waves. The displacement amplitude u from the mean position of particles in simple harmonic motion, at any instant t, and at a fixed point along the direction of propagation of the wave where $u = 0$ when $t = 0$, is given by

$$u = u_0 \sin \omega t \qquad (1.1)$$

where $\quad u_0 =$ maximum displacement amplitude,

and $\quad \omega = 2\pi f$, where f is the frequency of the wave.

Velocity is equal to rate of change of position, and so it may be found by differentiating the particle displacement with respect to time.

Thus
$$v = \frac{\delta u}{\delta t} = u_0 \omega \cos \omega t \qquad (1.2)$$

Similarly, the acceleration a of the particle towards its mean position may be found by differentiating the particle velocity with respect to time.

Thus
$$a = \frac{\delta v}{\delta t} = -u_0 \omega^2 \sin \omega t \qquad (1.3)$$

The significance of the negative sign is that the particle is decelerating as it moves away from its mean position.

It can be seen from Equations (1.1), (1.2) and (1.3) that the phase of the particle velocity leads that of the particle displacement by a time interval corresponding to $\frac{\pi}{2}$ radians of phase-angle difference, whilst the acceleration is π out of phase with the displacement.

1.2 VELOCITY OF PROPAGATION

It is important to realize that, although energy is transmitted through the medium as the result of a wave motion, no net movement of the medium is required for this to occur.

Figure 1.1 shows how the particle displacement amplitude depends upon the distance x along the direction of propagation of the wave. In the situation illustrated, the time chosen is such that $u = 0$ when $x = 0$.

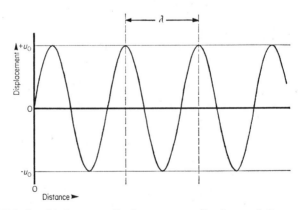

Fig. 1.1 Relationship between displacement amplitude u and distance x along the direction of propagation.

However, in general terms

$$u = u_0 \sin \left[\omega \left(t - \frac{x}{c} \right) \right] \qquad (1.4)$$

where $c =$ velocity of propagation of the wave,

and $\left[\omega \left(t - \frac{x}{c} \right) \right] =$ phase angle of the wave.

In reality, the whole of the curve in Fig. 1.1 is moving forward with a velocity c, which is measured by the distance which any particular part of the curve travels in unit time. For this reason, it is sometimes called a travelling or progressive wave. The phase of the wave indicates in what part of the vibrational cycle the wave happens to be at any particular instant of time. The transmission of the disturbance is not infinitely fast, because a delay occurs between the movements of neighbouring particles. The velocity of propagation is controlled by the density of the medium and its elasticity. The relationship depends upon the kind of material and the wave mode. It can be shown (Wood (1932), pp. 51–52) that, for longitudinal waves in fluids

$$c = \sqrt{\frac{K_a}{\rho}} \qquad (1.5)$$

where $K_a =$ adiabatic bulk modulus,

and $\rho =$ mean density of medium.

The adiabatic bulk modulus (which is the reciprocal of the adiabatic compressibility) is not the same as the isothermal bulk modulus K_i obtained by static measurements, although for most liquids the two quantities are almost equal.

Thus $K_a = \gamma K_i \qquad (1.6)$

where $\gamma =$ the ratio of specific heat at constant
                         pressure to that at constant volume.

In the case of longitudinal bulk waves in isotropic solids, the situation is complicated by the fact that the shear rigidity of the medium couples some of the energy of the longitudinal wave into a transverse mode (Wood (1932), p. 252). The appropriate modulus for calculating the velocity contains not only a term which depends upon the bulk modulus, but also one which depends upon the shear modulus. The formula quoted by Wood is—

$$c = \sqrt{\frac{K + \frac{4}{3}G}{\rho}} \qquad (1.7)$$

where $G =$ shear modulus.

The bulk and shear moduli are related to Young's modulus Y and Poisson's ratio σ as follows—

$$K = \sqrt{\frac{Y}{3(1 - 2\sigma)}}$$

and
$$G = \sqrt{\frac{Y}{2(1 + \sigma)}}$$

Substitution of these values in Equation (1.7) gives—

$$c = \sqrt{\frac{Y(1 - \sigma)}{(1 - 2\sigma)(1 + \sigma)\rho}} \tag{1.8}$$

The elastic constants are temperature-dependent, and so the velocity alters with temperature. The relationship can be quite complicated; for example, Fig. 1.2 shows the temperature variation of the velocity of ultrasound in distilled water at atmospheric pressure.

The velocities of ultrasound in some common non-biological materials are set out in Table 1.1. The values given correspond to temperatures within the range 17 to 25°C.

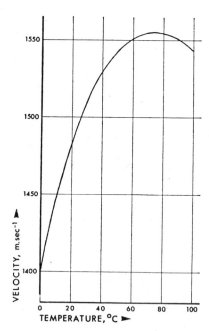

FIG. 1.2 Variation of propagation velocity with temperature in water. (Data of Greenspan and Tschiegg, 1959.)

TABLE 1.1

Propagation velocities of some common non-biological materials

Material	Velocity m sec^{-1}
Air at S.T.P.	331
Mercury	1450
Water	1480
Castor oil	1500
Polythene	2000
Perspex*	2680
Brass, mean value	4490
Aluminium	6400

* Trade name of Imperial Chemical Industries for polymethylmethacrylate.
From data quoted by Kaye and Laby (1959).

In some media, the velocity is partly dependent upon the frequency of the wave. This phenomenon is known as velocity dispersion. Velocity dispersion, when it does occur, is usually very small.

1.3 WAVELENGTH AND FREQUENCY

The distance between any two corresponding points on consecutive cycles, such as two successive wave crests in Fig. 1.1, is called the wavelength λ of the wave.

The time taken for the wave to move forward a distance equal to one wavelength is called the period T, and the number of waves or cycles which pass any given point in unit time is called the frequency f of the wave.

Hence
$$T = \frac{1}{f} \tag{1.9}$$

$$\lambda = cT \tag{1.10}$$

and
$$c = f\lambda \tag{1.11}$$

1.4 VELOCITY IN BIOLOGICAL MATERIALS

The velocity of ultrasound in biological materials exhibits only a small dispersion, which means that it is independent of frequency for most practical purposes. The velocity in one kind of soft tissue is almost the same as that in another. The velocity in bone is up to about three times faster than that in soft tissues.

A few articles have appeared in the literature in which results are given for measurements of velocity in biological materials. Biological tissues are complicated structures, and their elastic moduli are not easily measured. Therefore, the most reliable estimates of velocity in these materials are those made by direct measurements.

TABLE 1.2

Propagation velocities of some biological materials

Tissue	Mean velocity m sec^{-1}	s.e. of Mean velocity m sec^{-1}*	Source of data†
Fat	1450	6	d
Aqueous humour of eye	1500	—	e
Vitreous humour of eye	1520	—	e
Human tissue, mean value	1540	—	c
Brain	1541	11	c, d
Liver	1549	12	c, d, f
Kidney	1561	2	c, d, f
Spleen	1566	12	c, d, f
Blood	1570	—	a
Muscle	1585	3	c, d, f
Lens of eye	1620	—	e
Skull-bone	4080	—	b, g

* The standard error of the mean value of velocity gives an indication of the scatter of the data. If a much larger number of measurements had been available, the mean value of the velocity would have been likely to lie within the limits of ±2 s.e., with a probability of 0·95.

† Sources of data: a. Urick (1947), b. Theisman and Pfander (1949), c. Ludwig (1950), d. Frucht (1953), e. Begui (1954), f. Goldman and Richards (1954), g. Wells (1966a).

Table 1.2 gives some published data for various mammalian tissues, including those for man when available. The velocity depends upon the temperature of the specimen, and its physiological condition. The values given in the Table were obtained at temperatures within the range 20 to 37°C, and, wherever possible, they are for fresh materials. The frequencies at which the measurements were made lay within the range 0·8 to 12 MHz. In muscle, the measurements of Goldman and Richards (1954) show that the velocity is significantly slower along the axis of the fibres than across the fibres: but this difference in velocity is only about 0·4%. The value for the velocity in muscle given in the table is the mean of various data, and no account has been taken of the direction of propagation.

1.5 INTENSITY AND THE DECIBEL NOTATION

The energy e of a particle oscillating with simple harmonic motion is the sum of its potential energy e_p and its kinetic energy e_k. The potential energy is equal to the work done in distorting the particle from its position of static equilibrium within the medium; the kinetic energy is the energy possessed by the particle by virtue of its mass and velocity. When $u = u_0$, $e_k = 0$ and $e = e_p$; but when $u = 0$, $e_p = 0$ and $e = e_k$. Also, when $u = 0$, $v = v_0$ and, if m is the mass of the particle,

$$e = \tfrac{1}{2}mv_0^2$$

The total mass of particles per unit volume is equal to the mean density ρ of the medium. The corresponding total energy E of all the particles in unit volume is the energy density.

Hence $$E = \tfrac{1}{2}\rho v_0^2 \tag{1.12}$$

The energy travels through the medium with the wave velocity c. The energy which passes through unit area in unit time (which is the intensity I of the wave) is equal to the total energy contained in a column of unit area and length equal to $\left[\dfrac{c}{(\text{unit time})}\right]$.

Hence $$I = cE \tag{1.13}$$

and $$I = \tfrac{1}{2}\rho c v_0^2 \tag{1.14}$$

A convenient unit for the measurement of ultrasonic intensity is the Wcm^{-2}. However, the need often arises for the levels of two intensities (or, more fundamentally, of two powers) to be compared, as, for example, in the measurement of absorption. It may be an advantage to express this kind of ratio as a logarithm, because this affords a simple method of expressing numbers which extend over many orders of magnitude, and because the arithmetic product of two or more quantities is obtained by the addition of their logarithms. Two logarithmic units are in common use: they are the decibel (dB), and the neper. Historically, the neper is the older unit, and it frequently appears in the literature. However, the decibel is nowadays almost always used by electrical engineers, and it is used throughout this book. The units are defined as follows—

$$\text{Power level} = 10 \log_{10} \frac{P_2}{P_1} \text{ decibels} \tag{1.15}$$

$$= \log_e \frac{A_2}{A_1} \text{ nepers,}$$

TABLE 1.3

Power and amplitude ratios for various decibel levels

dB	Power ratio	Amplitude ratio
0·0	1·000	1·000
0·5	1·122	1·059
1·0	1·259	1·122
1·5	1·413	1·189
2·0	1·585	1·259
3·0	1·995	1·413
4·0	2·512	1·585
5·0	3·162	1·778
6·0	3·981	1·995
7·0	5·012	2·239
8·0	6·310	2·512
9·0	7·943	2·818
10	10·000	3·162
12	15·850	3·981
14	25·120	5·012
16	39·810	6·310
18	63·10	7·943
20	100·0	10·00
25	316·2	17·78
30	1,000	31·62
35	3,162	56·23
40	10,000	100·00
45	31,620	177·80
50	10^5	316·20
60	10^6	1,000
70	10^7	3,162
80	10^8	10,000
90	10^9	31,620
100	10^{10}	10^5
110	10^{11}	$3·162 \times 10^5$
120	10^{12}	10^6
130	10^{13}	$3·162 \times 10^6$

where P_1 and P_2 are the two powers, and A_1 and A_2 are the corresponding maximum wave amplitudes.

It is sometimes more convenient to measure the wave amplitude than the power, in which case the relationship for decibels becomes—

$$\text{Power level} = 20 \log_{10} \frac{A_2}{A_1} \text{ decibels} \qquad (1,16)$$

1 neper is equal to 8·686 dB.

The decibel levels corresponding to a wide range of power and amplitude ratios are set out in Table 1.3.

It is important to realize that it is meaningless to express a particular ultrasonic power, intensity or amplitude in terms of decibels, unless a reference level is also stated. Thus, for example, an intensity of 16 dB above 1 Wcm^{-2} is equal to 39·81 Wcm^{-2}.

The ultrasonic absorption coefficient α of a medium may be expressed in terms of dB cm^{-1}. This unit defines the decibel ratio of the intensities in the medium at any two points 1 cm apart, along the direction of propagation of a plane wave. If the absorption is proportional to some power of the frequency, say n, then $\dfrac{\alpha}{f^n}$ is a constant.

The half-power distance (the distance for half the energy to be absorbed) is almost exactly equal to the length of the path traversing which the intensity falls by 3 dB.

1.6 PARTICLE PRESSURE

The oscillations of the particles in the medium lead to the formation of regions of compression and rarefaction, relative to the mean pressure. The derivation of the relationship between pressure and the other parameters of the wave is rather complicated (Blitz (1963), pp. 10–14). It can be shown that, for plane progressive waves in a non-absorbent medium,

$$p = \rho c v = \rho c v_0 \sin \omega t \tag{1.17}$$

1.7 CHARACTERISTIC IMPEDANCE

The relationship between pressure, velocity and the quantity ρc (see Equation (1.17)) is analogous to that which exists in electricity between voltage, current and impedance, as described by Ohm's Law. For this reason, the quantity ρc is known as the characteristic impedance Z of the medium. The characteristic impedance is defined entirely in terms of constants of the medium; the unit in which it is measured is sometimes called the Rayl, after Lord Rayleigh. The quantity occurs in most forms of equations giving the intensity of the wave. The characteristic impedance ratio determines the reflection at interfaces between two media (see Section 1.8).

In electricity, the impedance of a circuit may be both resistive and reactive. In the case of plane waves in a non-absorbent medium, the characteristic impedance is a real quantity and the medium behaves as a pure resistance.

Table 1.4 gives approximate values of characteristic impedance for a variety of materials, both non-biological and biological. The figures given

TABLE 1.4

Characteristic impedances of some common materials

Material		Characteristic impedance c.g.s. Rayl × 10⁻⁵ (g. cm⁻² sec⁻¹) × 10⁻⁵
Non-biological	Air at S.T.P.	0·0004
	Castor oil	1·43
	Water	1·48
	Polythene	1·84
	Araldite*	3·00
	Perspex	3·20
	Aluminium	18·0
	Mercury	19·7
	Brass	38·0
Biological	Fat	1·38
	Aqueous humour of eye	1·50
	Vitreous humour of eye	1·52
	Brain	1·58
	Blood	1·61
	Kidney	1·62
	Human tissue, mean value	1·63
	Spleen	1·64
	Liver	1·65
	Muscle	1·70
	Lens of eye	1·84
	Skull-bone	7·80

* Araldite is a trade name of CIBA (A.R.L.) Ltd.
Data of Kossoff (1966), for casting resin D, hardener 951: other values calculated from data in Tables 1.1 and 1.2.

were calculated from the commonly accepted values of density. The imaginary component of the characteristic impedance is negligible for biological materials (Ludwig, 1950).

1.8 REFLECTION AND REFRACTION AT PLANE SURFACES

When a plane wave meets the boundary between two different media, it may be partially reflected. The reflected wave is returned in the negative direction through the incident medium, at the same velocity as it approached the boundary. The transmitted wave continues to move in the positive direction, but at the velocity corresponding to propagation in the medium beyond the boundary. Just as in optics, the geometrical laws of reflection apply, and the angles of incidence and reflection are equal in the same plane. However, if the ultrasonic wavelength is comparable with the linear dimensions of the reflecting object, the geometrical laws cease to apply, and diffraction occurs. This situation is mentioned again in Section 1.9; in the meanwhile, it will be assumed the wavelength is small compared with the dimensions of the reflector, and that the reflection is of a specular nature.

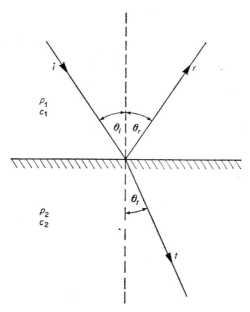

FIG. 1.3 Directions of incident, reflected and transmitted waves at a plane surface.

In Fig. 1.3, the suffixes i, r and t refer to the incident, reflected and transmitted waves, and 1 and 2, to the incident and transmitting media. As in optics—

$$\theta_i = \theta_r \tag{1.18}$$

By Snell's Law—

$$\frac{\sin \theta_i}{\sin \theta_t} = \frac{c_1}{c_2} \tag{1.19}$$

For equilibrium, the total pressure on each side of the interface must be equal, and the particle velocity on each side of the interface must be continuous. These conditions are satisfied when—

$$p_i + p_r = p_t \tag{1.20}$$

and

$$v_i \cos \theta_i - v_r \cos \theta_r = v_t \cos \theta_t \tag{1.21}$$

The negative sign in Equation (1.21) indicates that the direction of the reflected wave is reversed.

But

$$p = \rho c v \qquad \text{(see Equation (1.17))}$$

Therefore
$$\frac{p_i}{Z_1} \cos \theta_i - \frac{p_r}{Z_1} \cos \theta_i = \frac{p_t}{Z_2} \cos \theta_t$$

The simultaneous solutions to these equations are given by—

$$\frac{p_r}{p_i} = \frac{Z_2 \cos \theta_i - Z_1 \cos \theta_t}{Z_2 \cos \theta_i + Z_1 \cos \theta_t} \qquad (1.22)$$

and
$$\frac{p_t}{p_i} = \frac{2Z_2 \cos \theta_i}{Z_2 \cos \theta_i + Z_1 \cos \theta_t} \qquad (1.23)$$

The quantities $\frac{p_r}{p_i}$ and $\frac{p_t}{p_i}$ are known as the pressure reflectivity and transmissivity of the interface.

At normal incidence, $\theta_i = \theta_t = 0$ and Equations (1.22) and (1.23) become—

$$\frac{p_r}{p_i} = \frac{Z_2 - Z_1}{Z_2 + Z_1} \qquad (1.24)$$

and
$$\frac{p_t}{p_i} = \frac{2Z_2}{Z_2 + Z_1} \qquad (1.25)$$

If $Z_1 = Z_2$, $\frac{p_r}{p_i} = 0$ and there is no reflected wave.

If $Z_2 > Z_1$, the reflected pressure wave is in phase with the incident wave; but if $Z_2 < Z_1$, the reflected pressure wave is π radians out of phase with the incident wave.

The quantities $\frac{I_r}{I_i}$ and $\frac{I_t}{I_i}$ are known as the intensity reflection coefficient α_r and the intensity transmission coefficient α_t of the boundary.

$$p_0 = \rho c v_0 \qquad \text{(from Equation (1.17))}$$

and
$$I = \tfrac{1}{2}\rho c v_0^2 \qquad \text{(see Equation (1.14))}$$

Therefore
$$I = \frac{1}{2} \frac{p_0^2}{\rho c}$$

Substitution of this expression for I in Equations (1.22) and (1.23) gives

$$\alpha_r = \left(\frac{Z_2 \cos \theta_i - Z_1 \cos \theta_t}{Z_2 \cos \theta_i + Z_1 \cos \theta_t}\right)^2 \qquad (1.26)$$

and
$$\alpha_t = \frac{4Z_2 Z_1 \cos^2 \theta_i}{(Z_2 \cos \theta_i + Z_1 \cos \theta_t)^2} \qquad (1.27)$$

TABLE 1.5

Reflection of longitudinal waves normally incident on the plane boundary between two media, expressed in decibels below the level from a perfect reflector

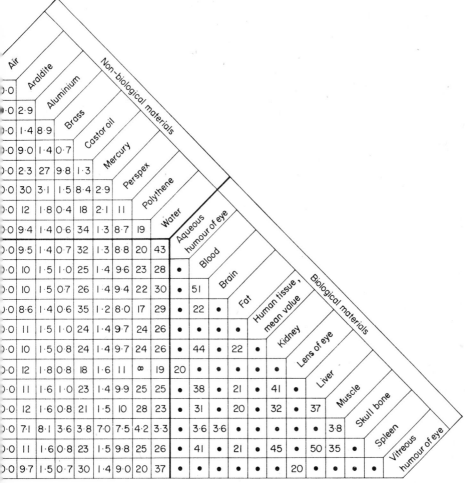

	Air	Araldite	Aluminium	Brass	Castor oil	Mercury	Perspex	Polythene	Water	Aqueous humour of eye	Blood	Brain	Fat	Human tissue, mean value	Kidney	Lens of eye	Liver	Muscle	Skull bone	Spleen
Araldite	0·0																			
Aluminium	0·0	2·9																		
Brass	0·0	1·4	8·9																	
Castor oil	0·0	9·0	1·4	0·7																
Mercury	0·0	2·3	27	9·8	1·3															
Perspex	0·0	30	3·1	1·5	8·4	2·9														
Polythene	0·0	12	1·8	0·4	18	2·1	11													
Water	0·0	9·4	1·4	0·6	34	1·3	8·7	19												
Aqueous humour of eye	0·0	9·5	1·4	0·7	32	1·3	8·8	20	43											
Blood	0·0	10	1·5	1·0	25	1·4	9·6	23	28	•										
Brain	0·0	10	1·5	0·7	26	1·4	9·4	22	30	•	51									
Fat	0·0	8·6	1·4	0·6	35	1·2	8·0	17	29	•	22	•								
Human tissue, mean value	0·0	11	1·5	1·0	24	1·4	9·7	24	26	•	•	•	•							
Kidney	0·0	10	1·5	0·8	24	1·4	9·7	24	26	•	44	•	22	•						
Lens of eye	0·0	12	1·8	0·8	18	1·6	11	∞	19	20	•	•	•	•	•					
Liver	0·0	11	1·6	1·0	23	1·4	9·9	25	25	•	38	•	21	•	41	•				
Muscle	0·0	12	1·6	0·8	21	1·5	10	28	23	•	31	•	20	•	32	•	37			
Skull bone	0·0	7·1	8·1	3·6	3·8	7·0	7·5	4·2	3·3	•	3·6	3·6	•	•	•	•	•	3·8		
Spleen	0·0	11	1·6	0·8	23	1·5	9·8	25	26	•	41	•	21	•	45	•	50	35	•	
Vitreous humour of eye	0·0	9·7	1·5	0·7	30	1·4	9·0	20	37	•	•	•	•	•	•	•	20	•	•	•

Non-biological materials

Biological materials

● Indicates that the corresponding boundary is unlikely to be of practical interest

At normal incidence, $\theta_i = \theta_t = 0$, and Equations (1.26) and (1.27) become—

$$\alpha_r = \left(\frac{Z_2 - Z_1}{Z_2 + Z_1}\right)^2 \tag{1.28}$$

and
$$\alpha_t = \frac{4Z_2 Z_1}{(Z_2 + Z_1)^2} \tag{1.29}$$

Values for normal incidence intensity reflection at the boundaries between various media (calculated from Equation (1.28) and the data in Table 1.4) are given in Table 1.5. The results are expressed in decibels below the level from a perfect reflector. This facilitates the comparison of one reflectivity with another. Thus, for example, the reflection from a water–fat interface is 29 dB below that from a perfect reflector, whilst that from a water–muscle interface is 23 dB below the same reference level. It follows that the reflection from a water–fat interface is 6 dB below that from a water–muscle interface. It is most important to realize that the data given in Table 1.5 apply only in the case of normal incidence on an extensive flat boundary, and that the values will differ for other angles of incidence, and for surfaces which are not flat.

In certain circumstances, oblique incidence is accompanied by energy conversion from one wave mode to another. This may occur, for example, when a longitudinal wave in a liquid meets the boundary with a solid. At normal incidence, a longitudinal wave is propagated in the solid. However, at oblique incidence, a distortion of the surface of the solid occurs which is due to the existence of both shear and compressional forces. The shear forces in the solid cannot be balanced by opposing forces in the liquid, because the liquid is non-viscous. Therefore, both transverse and longitudinal waves are propagated in the solid. The transverse wave velocity is lower than that of the longitudinal wave, and so the transverse wave is transmitted at a less oblique angle than the longitudinal wave.

1.9 REFLECTION AT ROUGH INTERFACES AND SMALL OBSTACLES

A plane wave incident on a rough surface between two media of differing characteristic impedance appears as a specular reflection with an additional scattered field. The theoretical aspects of the phenomenon is very complicated. For example, LaCasce (1961) has discussed the conflicting theories of Lord Rayleigh and Yu. P. Lysanov for the special case of a perfectly reflecting interface of sinusoidal profile. The theoretical problem of the reflection from an irregular or rough surface is enormously more difficult.

If the obstacle in the ultrasonic beam has dimensions which are smaller than, or comparable with, the wavelength of ultrasound, diffraction occurs and the waves change their direction of motion and bend around the obstacle. In the case of a very small obstacle, it can be shown (Rayleigh (1878), pp. 135–138) that, for a given characteristic impedance ratio, the amplitude of the scattered waves varies inversely as the square of the wavelength of the incident wave. Therefore, the intensity of the wave which returns towards the source varies inversely as the fourth power of the wavelength. However, if the obstacle has linear dimensions which are of the same order as the wavelength the pressure of the wave reflected in any particular direction depends upon the characteristic impedance ratio, and the orientation and shape of the obstacle. For example, Tamarkin (1949) has studied the scattering from cylindrical obstacles with a diameter to wavelength ratio of about ten. In this situation, the scattering mechanism is in the transition zone between the geometrical region and the region of Rayleigh scattering, and the process is primarily diffractive.

1.10 STANDING WAVES

When the paths of two waves of equal frequency, travelling in different directions, cross each other, they interfere to form a standing, or stationary, wave pattern. This is because, where the particle displacements are in phase, they add together, and where they are out of phase, they subtract one from the other. The simplest case is that of a wave normally incident on a reflecting surface, suffering interference with the reflected wave. There is no flow of energy along the axis of a standing wave system. However, there is a flow of energy if a travelling wave is superimposed on a standing wave: this occurs, for example, when a surface is not a perfect reflector. If the standing wave is considered alone, there are certain points, called nodes, at which the particle displacement is always zero; these are spaced at half wavelength intervals. Half-way between each node, the peak particle displacement has a maximum value, and an antinode is said to occur.

In practice, standing waves seldom occur in the absence of travelling waves. Therefore, the minimum particle displacement amplitude usually has some finite value. In a non-absorbent medium, the standing wave ratio SWR is defined as the ratio of the pressure amplitude at an antinode to that at a node. The relationship is—

$$\text{SWR} = \frac{p_{0_i} + p_{0_r}}{p_{0_i} - p_{0_r}} \tag{1.30}$$

The standing wave ratio is unity when $p_{0_r} = 0$, which occurs when there is no reflection at the boundary.

1.11 TRANSMISSION THROUGH LAYERS

If a wave is transmitted through three media separated by plane parallel surfaces, partial reflection may take place at each boundary. This leads to the establishment of standing wave systems in the first and second media. The standing wave in the second medium controls the reflection into the first medium, and the transmission into the third. The situation is very complicated at oblique incidence. However, at normal incidence, it can be shown (Kinsler and Frey (1962), p. 138) that the power transmission coefficient α_t is given, for lossless media, by—

$$\alpha_t = \frac{4Z_3 Z_1}{(Z_3 + Z_1)^2 \cos^2 k_2 l_2 + \left(Z_2 + \dfrac{Z_3 Z_1}{Z_2}\right)^2 \sin^2 k_2 l_2} \tag{1.31}$$

where $k_2 = \dfrac{2\pi}{\lambda}$, the wavelength constant of the second medium

and $l_2 =$ thickness of second medium.

The values of α_t corresponding to some conditions of special interest are given in Table 1.6. If the thickness l_2 is either very much less than a quarter wavelength, or an integral number of half wavelengths, transmission is

TABLE 1.6

**Transmission coefficients of layers of special thicknesses.
(For explanation, see Section 1.11)**

Thickness l_2	Value of $k_2 l_2$	Transmission coefficient α_t
$\ll \dfrac{\lambda_2}{4}$	$\ll \dfrac{\pi}{2}$	$\dfrac{4Z_1 Z_3}{(Z_1 + Z_3)^2}$
$n\dfrac{\lambda_2}{2}$	$n\pi$	$\dfrac{4Z_1 Z_3}{(Z_1 + Z_3)^2}$
$(2n - 1)\dfrac{\lambda_2}{4}$	$(2n - 1)\dfrac{\pi}{2}$	$\dfrac{4Z_1 Z_3}{\left(Z_2 + \dfrac{Z_1 Z_3}{Z_2}\right)^2}$

independent of the properties of the second medium. In the case when l_2 is very small, the approximation is that the cosine term in Equation (1.31) tends to unity, and the sine term, to zero. However, if Z_2 is very small compared with Z_1 and Z_3 (for example, if the second medium is a thin layer of gas trapped between two solid media), then $\dfrac{Z_1 Z_3}{Z_2}$ becomes very large and the term containing the sine function is no longer negligible.

If the thickness of the second medium is an odd integral number of quarter wavelengths, α_t becomes unity when $Z_2 = \sqrt{Z_1 Z_3}$. Therefore, it is possible to obtain complete transmission from one medium to another of different characteristic impedance, by the use of a suitable thickness of an intermediate medium whose characteristic impedance is the geometric mean of the other two. It is important to appreciate that this phenomenon is frequency selective, for it occurs only when the thickness of the intervening medium is an odd integral number of quarter wavelengths.

1.12 THE DOPPLER EFFECT

The apparent frequency of a constant frequency source is dependent both on the motion of the source and that of the receiver. For example, if the receiver is approaching the source, it will encounter more waves in unit time than if it remains stationary: thus, there is a change in the apparent wavelength.

If all the velocities act along the same straight line, it can be shown (Stephens and Bate (1950), pp. 146–149) that the apparent frequency f_r at the receiver is given by—

$$f_r = \left(\frac{c - v_r}{c - v_s}\right) f$$

where $v_r =$ velocity of the receiver away from the source,

$v_s =$ velocity of the source in the same direction as v_r,

and $f =$ the frequency of the source.

This equation can be rearranged to give the value of $f_D = (f_r - f)$, the Doppler shift frequency, thus—

$$f_D = \left(\frac{c - v_r}{c - v_s} - 1\right) f \tag{1.32}$$

The Doppler effect is sometimes used to study the movements of reflecting interfaces. When both the source and the receiver are stationary, the reflecting interface alters the direction of the waves in such a way that they appear to originate from a virtual source at a distance from the receiver equal to the total distance travelled by the waves. Thus the effect is the same as if the source and the receiver were moving apart with identical velocities, equal to that of the reflector. Therefore, the change in frequency f_D at the receiver is given by

$$f_D = -\left(\frac{2v_i}{c + v_i}\right) f \tag{1.33}$$

where $v_i =$ velocity of reflecting interface away from the source.

If a wave is transmitted through a medium which itself moves with a velocity v_m along the direction of propagation, the apparent frequency at the receiver is the same as the frequency of the source. However, there is a shift of the effective velocity from the propagation velocity, by an amount equal to v_m.

In cases where the various velocities do not all act along the same straight line, the appropriate velocity vectors should be used for calculating the Doppler shift.

1.13 RADIATION PRESSURE

A wave exerts a static pressure on any interface where there is an alteration in characteristic impedance, and on any medium in which absorption occurs. This static pressure is quite distinct from the oscillating particle pressure of the wave. The theoretical aspect of the matter has received considerable attention and its mechanism is still, to some extent, a subject of speculation. However, it has long been accepted that the radiation pressure is equal to the mean energy density of the ultrasonic wave, and it is independent of the frequency (Wood (1932), pp. 430–431). The mean energy density of a continuous wave of constant amplitude is equal to the intensity divided by the propagation velocity (see Section 1.5). The pressure on a perfect absorber is equal to the energy density, whereas that on a perfect reflector is twice the energy density. This is because a single momentum change occurs at an absorber, whilst two momentum changes occur at a reflector. The momentum theory of radiation pressure has been reviewed by Borgnis (1953). Thus, in the case of complete absorption of a finite beam of plane waves,

$$F = \frac{P}{c} \qquad (1.34)$$

where $F =$ force due to radiation pressure,

and $P =$ ultrasonic power.

The same relationship applies for a pulsed ultrasonic beam, provided that P is taken as the time average of the ultrasonic power.

Seegall (1961) has shown experimentally that the radiation pressure may be amplified by a factor of at least 80 when resonant standing waves occur.

One of the most popular explanations of the radiation pressure effect is by analogy to the effect of the application of an alternating electric voltage to a non-linear load, which results in the appearance of both a.c. and d.c. components (Hueter and Bolt (1955), pp. 43–48, and Blitz (1963), pp. 16–17). In the case of a vibrational wave, the non-linear element is the density of the propagating medium.

Another theory of the radiation pressure phenomenon, due to Larmor, is explained, for example, by Stephens and Bate (1950), pp. 419–421. In this theory, the reflecting surface is moved normally to meet the incident waves, and so the reflected waves have a shorter wavelength than the incident train, due to the Doppler effect (see Section 1.12). Therefore the reflected waves are compressed into a smaller space, and so the energy density is increased. This energy increase is due to the moving reflector doing work against the waves.

1.14 NON-PLANAR WAVES

The previous discussions have been concerned with the behaviour of plane, non-spreading waves. Such a wave can be represented in terms of a single space variable: the wave front retains the same shape throughout space, and varies only in scale. However, in many situations, the shape of the wave-front is non-uniform, and the plane wave relationships no longer apply. The error introduced by considering such waves to be planar depends upon the degree of deviation from wave-front uniformity.

The spherical wave is the simplest form of non-planar wave. Such a wave is generated by a source which is very small compared with the wavelength of the ultrasound (see Section 3.1.a), and the wave-front is in the form of a spherical surface. At large distances from the source, where the radius of the spherical surface is much larger than the wavelength, the wavefront is essentially plane over distances comparable with the wavelength.

The shape of an ultrasonic field may be computed by considering that the wavefront of a disturbance is at any instant the envelope of an infinite number of secondary spherical waves proceeding from every point on the wavefront at some preceeding instant. This important theorem, known as Huygen's principle, is mentioned again in Section 3.1.

1.15 ATTENUATION MECHANISMS

The intensity of a wave of ultrasound travelling through a medium may be attenuated by any of several different mechanisms. One of the mechanisms is the result of deviation from a parallel beam, so that the energy per unit area is reduced. This attenuation may be calculated from geometrical considerations. For a uniform beam of ultrasound, the intensity is inversely proportional to the area of the beam cross-section. In the case of a converging beam, such as occurs in a focussing system, the intensity of the beam is increased towards the focus.

Another attenuation mechanism is due to scattering by elastic discontinuities within the medium. A discontinuity acts as a reflecting surface, the size of which in relation to the wavelength of the ultrasound determines its effect as a scatterer (see Section 1.9). The energy which is scattered no longer moves in the original direction of propagation, and so attenuation of the beam occurs.

These two effects are not really absorption mechanisms, for none of the ultrasonic energy is converted from its vibrational form. True absorption mechanisms involve energy conversion, and the most important of these mechanisms are explained in the following paragraphs.

Elastic hysteresis, which describes the situation which occurs when an adiabatic stress and the strain which it produces are not in a linear relationship, gives rise to a non-viscous mechanism in which the dissipation of energy is proportional to the strain, rather than to the rate of change of strain. The energy loss is constant for each stress cycle, independent of the period, and so hysteretic absorption is directly proportional to the wave frequency.

Absorption in fluids is determined mainly by viscosity and heat conduction (Hueter and Bolt (1955) p. 402). The classical analysis of the phenomenon is based on the fact that the viscosity of the medium tends to oppose the vibrational motion of the particles, and some of this energy is converted into heat. If heat conduction is significant, thermal energy may also move in space. The times necessary for viscous stresses to be equalized, or for heat conduction to occur from high to low pressure regions of the ultrasonic field, control the lag between the pressure and density of the medium. This kind of phase relationship can be accounted for by assuming, for example, that the adiabatic compressibility is a complex quantity. The time lags account for the energy absorption. For a constant mass of fluid, the volume is inversely proportional to the density. If the alternating pressure is plotted against the volume, the result is a loop. The area of the loop is equal to the work done per cycle, and this is zero only when the pressure and the density are in phase. When they are not in phase, work is done on the fluid: this work appears as heat, and absorption occurs. In the case of a liquid, this kind of absorption is due mainly to viscosity.

Another mechanism by which absorption can occur arises because energy can exist in a system in various forms, such as molecular vibrational energy, lattice vibrational energy, translational energy, and so on. When an ultrasonic wave passes through a medium, there is an increase in energy in one or more of these forms. All the different forms in which the energy can be stored are coupled together in various ways. Consider, for example, a small element of volume of a liquid supporting an ultrasonic wave. During the compressive part of the wave, a temperature rise might occur in the translational energy of the molecules in the element. If none of this energy flowed into another form, then, when decompression occurred, the increased translational energy would be returned to the vibrational energy of the wave, and no absorption would have occurred. However, it always happens that some of the translational energy flows into another form during the compression half-cycle. This process is not instantaneous, and so, during decompression, some of the energy returns out of phase. This results in absorption: Litovitz (1959). The mechanism is known as relaxation. Relaxation differs from absorption due to, for example, heat conduction, in that energy does not move through space with finite velocity under the action of a temperature gradient, but it is stored internally, only to be released out of phase.

The magnitude of relaxational absorption is determined by the time constant of the relaxation process. At low frequencies, the phase delay in energy transfer is negligible, and absorption is small. The absorption increases with increasing frequency, up to a maximum value when the shared energy is in anti-phase; above this frequency, the absorption falls because there is less time available for energy to flow from one form to another. Typically, maximum absorption due to relaxation occurs at frequencies around 2 to 5 MHz. There is a further absorption peak at a frequency around 1000 MHz, due to a resonance phenomenon which occurs when the energy exchange is coupled only in a restricted frequency range.

It should be realized that ultrasonic absorption may be due to the combined effects of several different mechanisms, although in certain situations one particular mechanism may predominate. Therefore, disagreement is frequently found between the measured absorption of, for example, a liquid, and the value calculated from classical considerations

TABLE 1.7

Absorption coefficients of some common non-biological materials

Material	α at 1 MHz dB cm^{-1}	Approximate frequency dependence† of α
Mercury	0·00048	f^2
Water	0·0022	f^2
Aluminium	0·018	f
Castor oil	0·95	f^2
Perspex	2·0	f
Polythene	4·7	$f^{1·1}$
Araldite*	6	f
Air at STP	12	f^2

* Data of Kossoff (1966), for casting resin D, hardener 951; other data quoted by Kaye and Laby (1959).
† Frequency dependence is for frequencies below about 10 MHz.

based on viscosity. Indeed, it was this kind of observation which led to the development of the relaxation theory.

Table 1.7 gives the values of the absorption coefficients of some common non-biological materials.

1.16 ABSORPTION IN BIOLOGICAL MATERIALS

The mechanisms by which ultrasound is absorbed by biological materials are rather complicated. No general theory of absorption seems to be possible, but occasional references appear in the literature to the specific mechanisms of absorption by non-biological materials, when these have some resemblance to the biological situation. Thus, Fry (1952) demonstrated that relaxation mechanisms (see Section 1.14) can yield a linear frequency dependence of the ultrasonic absorption coefficient if a spectrum of relaxation frequencies is assumed. Again, Fry and Dunn (1962) pointed out the similarity of the absorption coefficients of soft tissues to those of viscous oils. Heat conduction is a relatively unimportant mechanism contributing to absorption in biological systems. Most tissues are able to support shear waves, but these decay rapidly: this effect is sometimes important at interfaces where mode conversion occurs (Section 1.8).

Kossoff (1966) quoted the condition that the absorption coefficient may be considered to be a real quantity if $\frac{\alpha c}{2\pi f} \ll 0.1$, where α is in dBcm^{-1}, c in m.sec^{-1}, and f in Hz. This condition is satisfied by biological materials, at least in the lower megahertz frequency range.

Unfortunately, there is a wide variation between the results of the few investigators who have published their data. There are a number of reasons for these disagreements. Each investigator has his own individual preferences by way of apparatus and experimental technique. There is no doubt that there are errors in some results due to the existence of resonant standing waves in the measuring system: Dunn and Fry (1961) have mentioned this difficulty. The majority of measurements have been made using pulse techniques in order to avoid the establishment of resonant standing waves. However, the frequency spectrum of the pulse depends not only upon its fundamental frequency, but also upon its shape and duration (see Section 2.7), and so it is often difficult to relate the measurement of absorption to any particular frequency. Another problem is that some tissues are anisotropic. Thus, the absorption rate exhibits directional variations in muscle, where the fibres lies approximately parallel to one another: Hueter (1948) found a two-to-one difference in absorption in striated muscle between measurements made with the ultrasound directed across and along the muscle bundles.

The physiological condition of the specimen is important. In the case of post-mortem material, the absorption often changes quite soon after death, and this rate of change is determined to some extent by the conditions of storage. Dunn (1965) quoted data of Hueter which showed that the absorption coefficient of liver, measured at frequencies in the range 1 to 6 MHz, remains almost constant until about nine hours after death, and then decreases during the next ten hours. This decrease in absorption coefficient varies from approximately a factor of eight at 1·4 MHz to less than a factor of two at about 6 MHz. The measurements were made at 25°C, but the tissue was maintained at 10°C between measurements.

The absorption rate depends upon the temperature of the specimen on which the measurements are made. Dunn (1962) reported a positive temperature coefficient of absorption for the spinal cord of young mice within the range 2 to 45°C. This observation tends to exclude viscosity as a principal cause of absorption in this tissue, since viscosity decreases with increasing temperature. In contrast, however, Carstensen, *et al.* (1953) found that the temperature coefficient of absorption was negative in the case of blood, for the frequency range 1 to 3 MHz, and for temperatures between 10 and 40°C.

Several attempts have been made to collect together all the relevant data on absorption, and to present it in a coherent form. Goldman and Hueter (1956, 1957) and Dunn (1965) have done this. The absorption coefficient α for soft tissues is approximately proportional to frequency and usually lies in the range 0·5 to 3·5 dB cm^{-1} MHz^{-1}. The implication of an absorption rate which is directly proportional to frequency is that there is a constant loss per cycle. This indicates a broad spectrum of time constants in the loss mechanisms. However, some tissues (for example, liver and fat, see Figs 1.4.a and 1.4.b) exhibit a minimum value of $\frac{\alpha}{f}$ in the frequency range 1 to 4 MHz.

The absorption in blood has been quite thoroughly investigated by Carstensen *et al.* (1953) and Carstensen and Schwann (1959a and 1959b). Accurate results can be obtained for blood, on account of its homogeneity and the similarity of different samples. $\frac{\alpha}{f}$ increases with frequency (see Fig. 1.4.c), and the absorption seems to be determined largely by the protein content, both in the plasma and within the cells. However, the presence of intact cells in suspension contributes to the absorption. This is thought to result from a viscous interaction between the fluid and the cells, which fail to follow the oscillatory motion set up by the wave, because of their greater density.

The absorption rate in bone differs considerably from that in soft tissues. The results of Hueter's (1952) measurements on skull bone (see Fig. 1.4.d) indicate that the absorption is roughly proportional to the square of the frequency, up to about 2 MHz; above this frequency, there seems to be a lower power frequency dependence. The absorption coefficient, about 13 dB cm^{-1} at 1 MHz, is an order of magnitude greater than that of soft tissues. The absorption mechanisms are certainly more complicated than

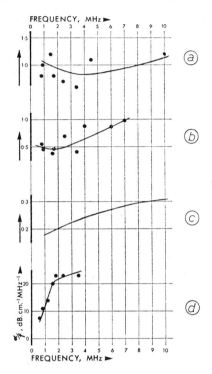

Fig. 1.4 Variation of $\frac{\alpha}{f}$ with frequency in some biological materials. (a) Liver: (data of Hueter, 1948; Colombati and Petralia, 1950; and Hueter, T. F. and Cohen, M. S., quoted by Goldman and Hueter, 1956). (b) Fat: (data of Pohlman, 1939; Colombati and Petralia, 1950; and Schwann, H. P. and Carstensen, E. L., quoted by Goldman and Hueter, 1956, 1957). (c) Blood: (data of Carstensen, Li and Schwann, 1953). (d) Skull bone: (data of Hueter, 1952).

those in soft tissues, and scattering and conversion to shear waves of short range are likely to be important factors. It may be that the change in frequency dependence at about 2 MHz occurs because Rayleigh-type scattering (see Section 1.9) ceases to be important at higher frequencies.

Absorption in lung tissue containing air has been determined by Dunn and Fry (1961). Freshly excised specimens of tissue from dog were used, and calculations from the results of transmission measurements made at a frequency of 1 MHz, and a temperature of 35°C, yielded a value for the absorption coefficient of 41 dB cm^{-1}. This high rate of absorption may be due to the radiation of energy by pulsating gaseous structures in the lung tissue, and, if this is the case, calculation indicates that the frequency for minimum absorption may be a little higher than 1 MHz.

Probably it is a result of the complexity of the problems involved that the data available on experimentally determined absorption coefficients are rather meagre. What few results there are have been obtained not only with tissues from man, but also with those from a wide variety of animals. This contributes to the scatter of the data.

TABLE 1.8

Values of α/f of some biological materials

Tissue	Mean α/f dB.cm^{-1}.MHz^{-1}*	s.e. of mean α/f dB.cm^{-1}.MHz^{-1}†	Frequency range MHz*	Source of data‡
Aqueous or vitreous humour of eye	0·10	—	6–30	h, m
Blood	0·18	—	1·0	g
Fat	0·63	0·073	0·8–7·0	a, c, j
Medulla oblongata, along fibres	0·80	0·071	1·7–3·4	c
Brain	0·85	0·056	0·9–3·4	c, d
Liver	0·94	1·058	0·3–3·4	b, c, e, i
Kidney	1·0	0·04	0·3–4·5	b, e
Spinal cord	1·0	—	1·0	l
Medulla oblongata, across fibres	1·2	0·05	1·7–3·4	c
Muscle, along fibres	1·3	0·07	0·8–4·5	b, c
Heart muscle	1·8	0·10	0·3–4·5	b, e
Lens of eye	2·0	—	3·3–13	h, m
Muscle, across fibres	3·3	0·35	0·8–4·5	b
Skull-bone	20	—	1·6	f
Lung	41	—	1·0	k

* Where a single frequency appears in the frequency range column, α/f may not be a constant. In such cases, the value given for α/f corresponds to the frequency stated in the frequency range column. (See text, Section 1.16.)

† The standard error of the mean value of α/f gives an indication of the scatter of the data. If a much larger number of measurements had been available, and if the absorption coefficient is proportional to frequency within the range under consideration, then the mean value of α/f would have been likely to lie within the limits of ±2 s.e., with a probability of 0·95.

‡ Sources of data: a. Pohlman (1939), b. Hueter (1948), c. Colombati and Petralia (1950), d. Hueter and Bolt (1951), e. Esche (1952), f. Hueter (1952), g. Carstensen, Li and Schwann (1953), h. Begui (1954), i. Hueter, T. F. and Cohen, M. S. quoted by Goldman and Hueter (1956), j. Schwann, H. P. and Carstensen, E. L. quoted by Goldman and Hueter (1956, 1957), k. Dunn and Fry (1961), l. Dunn (1962), m. Filipćzynski, Etienne, Lypacewicz and Salkowski (1967).

Table 1.8 has been prepared from some of the best results available, and may be used to obtain approximate values for the absorption coefficients of some common tissues. Where a single frequency appears in the frequency range column, this indicates the only frequency at which measurements were available for inclusion in the Table, and the corresponding value of $\frac{\alpha}{f}$ may not be even approximately constant.

It has already been mentioned that some tissues have an absorption coefficient which is not directly proportional to the frequency. In view of the wide scatter of the data, this may be the case for some of the tissues listed with values for a range of frequencies in Table 1.8. For example, $\frac{\alpha}{f}$ is shown plotted against frequency, in Fig. 1.4.a for liver, and in Fig. 1.4.b for fat. However, it is not possible to draw any firm conclusions from these graphs.

There is no doubt that the results of experimental measurements of greater precision than those currently available would be valuable in helping to elucidate the absorption mechanism.

1.17 NON-LINEAR EFFECTS WITH WAVES OF FINITE AMPLITUDE

The linear wave equation, which forms the theoretical basis for much of the earlier part of this chapter, is strictly applicable only in the case of a wave of infinitesimally small amplitude. If the wave amplitude is finite, the waveform becomes distorted by the generation and growth of harmonics during the course of propagation; the process is slowed down in lossy media by the dissipative processes. The matter has been discussed, for example, by Zarembo and Krasil'nikov (1959). In a lossy medium, a finite amplitude wave which is initially sinusoidal can either become close to a sawtooth in shape, with a front thickness of much less than $\frac{\lambda}{2}$, or be so absorbed that the non-linearities produce no significant effect. The behaviour of a wave depends upon its energy density and the absorption characteristics of the medium.

An important consequence of the breakdown of the linear wave equation at finite amplitudes is that the absorption coefficient of a medium may differ from the value measured at very small amplitudes. Near to a source radiating finite amplitude sinusoidal waves, α is close to that for small amplitudes; beyond this region, α has a maximum value; but at larger distances, where absorption has so reduced the wave amplitude that the waveform returns to the sinusoid, α again tends to the value for small amplitudes. For example, Fox (1950) demonstrated that the absorption coefficient of water at a frequency of 10 MHz is independent of intensity below about 0·04 Wcm^{-2}, but is increased by a factor of five at an intensity of about 5 Wcm^{-2}. It had been originally supposed that this effect might be due to cavitation, but Fox (1950) was unable to demonstrate any striking relationship between the quantity of dissolved gas and absorption in water, nor did he find any sudden change in the magnitude of the effect as the intensity was increased, such as might have been expected at the onset of cavitation. However, Fox and Wallace (1954) were able to show that a theory based on considerations of the non-linear elastic properties of the medium is able to satisfy the experimental data. This theory has been further tested by Ryan *et al.* (1962).

The situation is rather more complicated in the case of finite amplitude waves of a frequency similar to that of the relaxation frequency of the propagating medium (see Section 1.15). It seems likely that intensity-dependent absorption in such media is associated with irreversible processes, the effect of which increases with increasing amplitude. This theory is supported by the statement of Zarembo and Krasil'nikov (1959) that the finite wave amplitude absorption coefficients of certain polymers are time-dependent.

Dunn (1962) has measured the effect of intensity on the absorption coefficient of the spinal cord of the young mouse. At a frequency of 1 MHz, the absorption coefficient is independent of intensity within the range 5 to 200 Wcm^{-2}. Presumably, the same value of α applies at intensities below 5 Wcm^{-2}. It seems reasonable to assume that other soft tissues, possessing similar values of $\dfrac{\alpha}{f}$, also have values of α which are, for most practical purposes, independent of intensity at levels which are not sufficiently high to cause irreversible damage.

2. THE TRANSDUCER

2.1 PIEZOELECTRICITY

Certain materials have the property that the application of an electric voltage causes a mechanical deformation. This characteristic is known as the direct piezoelectric (pressure-electric) effect. The magnitude of the mechanical deformation is directly proportional to the applied voltage, for deformations within the elastic limits of the material. Similarly, the application of a mechanical stress to a piezoelectric material causes a voltage to appear across the material, in direct proportion to the applied stress. This characteristic is known as the converse piezoelectric effect.

Piezoelectric materials belong to a large group of devices, known as transducers, which are capable of converting one form of energy into another.

The piezoelectric effect can only occur in materials which lack a centre of symmetry. Therefore, piezoelectric materials are anisotropic. The electric charges bound within the ionic lattice of the material can interact with an applied electric field, to produce a mechanical effect. Thus, piezoelectricity provides a coupling between electric and dielectric phenomena.

Certain naturally occurring crystals, such as quartz and tourmaline, are piezoelectric by virtue of their ionic charge distributions. The same characteristic is found in many artificially grown crystals, such as those of ammonium dihydrogen phosphate, lithium sulphate and lead niobate.

Another group of artificial materials, known as polarized polycrystalline ferroelectrics, possess strong piezoelectric properties. Polarization of a ferroelectric material is carried out by heating it, preferably to a temperature just above the Curie point, and then allowing it to cool slowly in the presence of a strong electric field, typically $20 \, \text{kV. cm}^{-1}$, applied in the direction in which the piezoelectric effect is required. This process tends to align the individual charge domains along the direction of the polarizing field, in a manner analogous to the magnetization of a material by the application of a strong magnetic field. This similarity is the reason why the piezoelectric ceramics are known as ferroelectrics.

Barium titanate was the first artificial ferroelectric material to become available commercially. The characteristics of barium titanate are improved by the addition of small quantities of chemicals such as lead and calcium titanates, which give more stable dielectric properties and a wider range of operating temperature. However, an important development was the discovery by Jaffe *et al.* (1955) of very strong piezoelectric effects in polarized lead titanate zirconate solid solutions. These solid solutions possess a sufficiently large ferroelectric moment and high Curie temperature to permit variations in chemical composition or thermal treatment which can result in improvements in certain physical properties whilst retaining substantial piezoelectric effects. The details of most of these processes are guarded by industrial secrecy, but some information has been given by, for example, Berlincourt *et al.* (1960), Berlincourt, Jaffe *et al.* (1960), Crawford (1961), and Brown *et al.* (1962).

2.2 PIEZOELECTRIC CONSTANTS

There are a number of coefficients which describe the relationship between the mechanical and electrical behaviour of piezoelectric materials. The theory becomes rather complicated if anything more than a superficial treatment is attempted. Piezoelectricity is quite fully described elsewhere by, for example, Mason (1950). For simplicity, only the coefficients which are most important in the application of ultrasonics to diagnosis are explained in the following sub-sections.

2.2.a Piezoelectric Coefficients

The strain produced in a transducer by the application of unit electric field is called the piezoelectric coefficient d. Therefore, the d coefficient is often called the transmitting constant of the transducer. Alternatively, the d coefficient may be defined by the converse relationship of the charge density output per unit applied stress under short-circuit conditions.

The piezoelectric coefficient g is defined as the electric field produced under open-circuit conditions per unit applied stress. The g coefficient is often called the receiving constant of the transducer, because receiving amplifiers are generally voltage sensitive, rather than charge sensitive.

2.2.b Dielectric Constant

The dielectric constant ϵ of a transducer has the same meaning as in electrostatics. However, its value depends upon the degree of mechanical freedom of the transducer. Two values are generally given in the literature. For one, the transducer is clamped so that it cannot move in response to an applied field (a situation which is very difficult to achieve in practice): this value is designated as ϵ^S. For the other, the transducer is free to move without restriction, and the value is designated as ϵ^T.

The piezoelectric coefficients d and g are related to the appropriate dielectric constant thus—

$$d = g\epsilon^T. \tag{2.1}$$

2.2.c Electromechanical Coupling Coefficient

The ability of a transducer to convert electricity from one form to another is measured by its electromechanical coupling coefficient k, defined by—

$$k^2 = \frac{\text{stored mechanical energy}}{\text{total stored energy}}$$

The quantity k^2 is not the same as the efficiency of the transducer. If the transducer is lossless, some of the absorbed energy is converted, either from the electrical to the mechanical form or vice versa, and all the energy is absorbed, either dielectrically or elastically. The electromechanical coupling factor describes how the total energy is shared for storage. The efficiency of the transducer depends on the total losses of the conversion process, and describes how much of the total energy is lost as heat.

The electromechanical coupling and piezoelectric coefficients are related by the equation—

$$k^2 s^E = dg \qquad (2.2)$$

where $s =$ elastic compliance of the transducer.

The elastic compliance depends upon the electrical loading of the transducer. Two values are generally given in the literature: these are s^E, for constant electric field, and s^D, for constant charge density.

The dependence of the dielectric and elastic constants on the electrical loading of the transducer is controlled by the electromechanical coupling coefficient.

Thus $\epsilon^S = (1 - k^2)\epsilon^T \qquad (2.3)$

and $s^D = (1 - k^2)s^E \qquad (2.4)$

Thus, the quantity k^2 is the fractional decrease in the permittivity or the compliance of the transducer due to the piezoelectric effect.

2.3 PIEZOELECTRIC TRANSDUCERS FOR ULTRASONIC DIAGNOSIS

Narrow beams of ultrasonic radiation are almost always used in ultrasonic diagnosis. Such a beam is often best generated by a disc of piezoelectric material electrically excited by means of two electrodes, one on each parallel surface: the disc resonates at a frequency at which its thickness is an odd integral number of half wavelengths (see Section 2.4).

A stress applied to a solid in any direction can be resolved into three tensile stress components and three shear stress components, respectively along and about the x, y and z axes. Piezoelectric coefficients are usually described in terms of a standard tensor notation, which enables the effect along one axis to be expressed: (see Mason (1950) pp. 440–451, for a description of tensor theory and application). Figure 2.1 shows the co-ordinate system which is generally used. A double subscript describes each coefficient. In the case of the piezoelectric coefficients (see Section 2.2.a), the first subscript is the electrical direction, and the second is the mechanical direction. Subscripts 1, 2 and 3 apply to tensile stresses and strains, and 4, 5 and 6, to shear stresses and strains. Thus, d_{11} is the piezoelectric coefficient

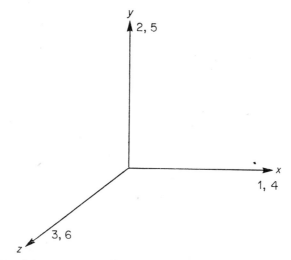

FIG. 2.1 x, y, z, co-ordinate system used in tensor notation.

which relates voltage to tensile strain along the x-axis; d_{14} relates voltage to shear strain along the x-axis; and d_{31} relates voltage along the z axis to tensile strain along the x-axis.

Thickness expanding quartz transducers are of the X-cut variety (Mason (1950), p. 83). The corresponding piezoelectric transmitting and receiving coefficients are accordingly designated as d_{11} and g_{11}. However, it happens that the convention for piezoelectric ceramics is equivalent to polarization and expansion along the z-axis for thickness expanding discs, and the appropriate transmitting and receiving constants are d_{33} and g_{33}.

The mechanical and electrical constants of quartz and two typical lead titanate zirconate thickness expanding disc transducers are given in Table 2.1.

It can be seen from Equation (2.1) that, for a given value of g, the value of d is large if the dielectric constant is large, and vice versa. Thus, although quartz has a value of g which is equal to about twice that of the lead titanate zirconates, its d value is relatively low because its dielectric constant is so

TABLE 2.1

Principal electromechanical properties of some common transducer materials

	Quartz, X-cut (see note i)	*PZT-4 (see note ii)	*PZT-5 (see note ii)
Tensor subscript for thickness expanding disc	11	33	33
Transmitting constant d m.volt^{-1}	$2 \cdot 31 \times 10^{-12}$	289×10^{-12}	374×10^{-12}
Receiving constant g volt m. newton^{-1}	$5 \cdot 78 \times 10^{-2}$	$2 \cdot 61 \times 10^{-2}$	$2 \cdot 48 \times 10^{-2}$
Coupling coefficient k	$0 \cdot 095$	$0 \cdot 70$	$0 \cdot 705$
Elastic compliance at constant field s^E m^{2}newton^{-1}	$12 \cdot 8 \times 10^{-12}$	$15 \cdot 5 \times 10^{-12}$	$18 \cdot 8 \times 10^{-12}$
Free dielectric constant ϵ^T farad m^{-1}	$4 \cdot 00 \times 10^{-11}$	1150×10^{-11}	1500×10^{-11}
Wave velocity m.sec^{-1}	5740	4000	3780
Density g. cm^{-3}	$2 \cdot 65$	$7 \cdot 5$	$7 \cdot 75$
Acoustic impedance c.g.s. Rayl	$1 \cdot 52 \times 10^6$	$3 \cdot 00 \times 10^6$	$2 \cdot 93 \times 10^6$
Mechanical Q	>25,000	500	75
Curie temperature, °C	573	328	365

* PZT is a registered trade name of the Brush Clevite Co. Ltd.
 (i) Data quoted by Cady (1946), Mason (1950), and from Bechman (1958).
 (ii) Data extracted from Bulletin 66011/B (1967): Brush Clevite Co. Ltd.

small. A large value of d is desirable for the generation of ultrasonics, and a large value of g, for detection. However, a large value of dielectric constant is also desirable in a detector, because this minimizes the shunting effect of the capacitance of the connecting cable. For this reason, although quartz has a large g value, better sensitivity as a receiver is usually obtained in practice with lead titanate zirconate.

The elastic compliance does not differ markedly between different transducer materials. Therefore, it can be seen from Equation (2.2) that the electromechanical coupling coefficient k depend upon the product dg. If a transducer is to operate both as a transmitter and as a receiver, it is desirable for both d and g to be large. Generally, the best combined sensitivity (largest value of dg) is obtained with the transducer with the largest value of k.

The choice of the best transducer material depends upon the particular application for which it is intended. Of the two lead titanate zirconates listed in Table 2.1, both have a similar piezoelectric performance, but the mechanical Q-factor (see Section 2.5) of PZT-4 is much greater than that of

PZT-5. Therefore PZT-4 is best suited for use as a transmitter, and PZT-5 best fits the requirements for use as a receiver of short pulses, or as a combined transmitter-receiver. Another factor which may affect the choice of material is the alteration of characteristics with time; the characteristics of PZT-5 change much less with age than those of PZT-4 (Crawford, 1961).

The lead titanate zirconates are superior to quartz as transducer materials in almost every practical respect at frequencies below about 15 MHz. However, for fundamental operation at higher frequencies (see Section 2.4), quartz is the most widely used transducer, despite its low piezoelectric coupling. This is because of its excellent mechanical properties, and because its low permittivity can often become an advantage.

In some situations, it is best to use separate transducers as transmitter and receiver. Walker and Lumb (1964) have shown that the overall sensitivity using lead titanate zirconate as the transmitter and lithium sulphate as the receiver is almost 600 times greater than that which can be obtained using quartz as a transmitter-receiver. A disadvantage of lithium sulphate is that it is very hygroscopic, and complete waterproofing of the crystal is often necessary. Another factor which may cause difficulty is its rather low permittivity compared with the ceramics.

The electrical connections to a transducer are made by means of electrodes. In the case of a transducer with a low permittivity, the electrical requirements for the electrodes are not stringent. However, with a high dielectric constant, very close contact between the electrodes and the transducer is necessary. For this reason, electrodes usually consist of a layer of metal which is evaporated, sputtered or fired on to the transducer. Commonly used metals for this purpose are silver and gold.

2.4 RESONANCE

Figure 2.2 represents a disc transducer, of characteristic impedance Z_t, mounted between loading and backing media, of characteristic impedances Z_l and Z_b respectively. If a sinusoidal voltage is applied to the transducer, the piezoelectric effect will cause the transducer to alter its thickness in sympathy with the applied voltage. The movements of the faces of the transducer radiate energy into the loading and backing media, the quantity of energy radiated by each face being determined by the characteristic impedances at the boundary between the transducer and the medium, as described in Section 1.8. Therefore, some of the vibrational energy is reflected back into the transducer at each face, except in the unusual circumstance when the corresponding characteristic impedance ratio is unity.

The energy reflected at each face of the transducer travels back across the transducer towards the opposite face. Meanwhile, if sinusoidal excitation is employed, the instantaneous value of the voltage applied to the transducer is changing, so that when the energy reflected within the transducer arrives at the opposite face, a new stress situation exists due to the piezoelectric effect. The total stress is equal to the sum of the piezoelectric stress and the stress due to the reflected wave. The phase relationship between these stresses depends upon the thickness and the propagation velocity of the transducer, and the frequency of the applied voltage. If the thickness of the transducer is exactly half a wavelength, the stresses reinforce each other, and

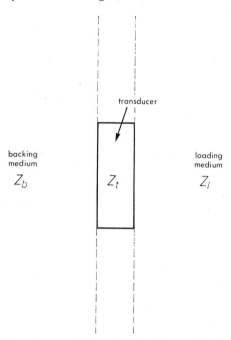

FIG. 2.2 Transducer radiating into loading and backing media.

the transducer resonates with maximum displacement amplitude at its faces. However, the stresses are in opposition if the transducer is of wavelength thickness, and the displacement amplitude is then a minimum.

The frequency which corresponds to a half wavelength thickness is called the fundamental resonant frequency of the transducer. The transducer will also resonate when driven at frequencies at which its thickness is an odd integral number of half wavelengths. A transducer which is being driven at three times its fundamental frequency is said to be operating at its third harmonic, and so on.

Similar considerations apply in the case of a transducer acting as a receiver. Maximum sensitivity occurs at resonance, when the frequency of the mechanical stress corresponds to an odd integral number of half wavelengths of transducer thickness.

If the transducer is driven, electrically or mechanically, at a frequency at which its thickness corresponds to an integral number of wavelengths, the stress waves due to the drive and those due to the internal reflections are in antiphase at the transducer faces. Therefore, the transducer has a minimum sensitivity at these frequencies.

Maximum efficiency for power generation is generally obtained by the use of a transducer of half wavelength thickness, arranged in a mounting system in which $Z_b \ll Z_t$. In practice, the backing medium is usually air. Almost complete reflection then occurs at the back face of the transducer, so that maximum power is available for transmission into the load.

The thickness of a half wavelength transducer at a given frequency is directly proportional to the propagation velocity in the transducer. Calculations based on the data given in Table 2.1 yield, for a fundamental 1 MHz transducer, thicknesses of 0·29 cm for quartz, 0·20 cm for PZT-4, and 0·19 cm for PZT-5. The thickness is inversely proportional to the frequency.

2.5 Q-FACTOR

The quality factor Q of a transducer determines its frequency characteristic. Transducers with a high Q-factor have an output which is more critically dependent upon frequency than those with a low Q, as shown in Figs 2.3.a

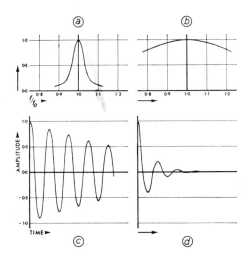

FIG. 2.3 Effect of Q-factor on circuit characteristics.

(a) High-Q ⎫
(b) Low-Q ⎬ frequency response curves.

(c) High-Q ⎫
(d) Low-Q ⎬ decrement curves.

$Q = 20$ for (a) and (c); $Q = 2$ for (b) and (d).

and 2.3.b. The value of the Q-factor can be obtained from this kind of graph by the relationship—

$$Q = \frac{f_0}{f_2 - f_1} \tag{2.5}$$

where f_0 = frequency for maximum amplitude,

f_1 = frequency below resonance for a reduction in amplitude of 3 dB,

and f_2 = frequency above resonance for a reduction in amplitude of 3 dB.

Figures 2.3.a. and 2.3.b are drawn for Q values of 20 and 2 respectively. The decrement of free vibration in a high-Q system is characterized by a long time-constant, in comparison with that for a low-Q system: see Figs 2.3.c and 2.3.d. The relevant relationship is—

$$Q = 2\pi \left(\frac{\text{energy stored}}{\text{energy lost per cycle}} \right) \tag{2.6}$$

It can be shown (Millman and Taub (1956), pp. 52–53) that—

$$Q = \pi N \tag{2.7}$$

where N = number of cycles of oscillation for amplitude to decrease to $\frac{1}{e}$ of its initial value (e = 2·718).

Now, $\dfrac{A_0}{A_1} \times \dfrac{A_1}{A_2} \times \ldots \times \dfrac{A_{N-1}}{A_N} = e$

where $A_0, A_1, \ldots, A_{N-1}, A_N$ = amplitudes of successive cycles.

Hence, $\log_e \dfrac{A_0}{A_1} = \log_e \dfrac{A_1}{A_2} = \ldots = \log_e \dfrac{A_{N-1}}{A_N} = \dfrac{\log_e e}{N} = \dfrac{1}{N}$

Therefore $$Q = \frac{\pi}{\log_e \dfrac{A_0}{A_1}} \tag{2.8}$$

Figures 2.3.c and 2.3.d are for Q values of 20 and 2 respectively.

The quantity $\log_e \dfrac{A_0}{A_1}$ is called the logarithmic decrement of the system.

The mechanical Q is independent of the transducer dimensions, but proportional to the order of the harmonic (Hueter and Bolt (1955), p. 106).

Another aspect of the importance of the Q-factor of the transducer is its effect upon the electrical performance of the system. The mechanical and electrical Q-factors are related by the electromechanical coupling coefficient (Blitz (1963), p. 54). The electrical Q is a measure of the loss of the system as a transducing mechanism: transducers with high Q-factors are more efficient than those with low Q-factors.

A practical measure of the frequency characteristic of a transducer is its frequency bandwidth. This is determined by the combined effects of the mechanical and electrical Q-factors. In some applications, such as the generation and detection of short ultrasonic pulses (see Sections 2.6, 2.8 and 2.9), a wide frequency band is required. This can be achieved by lowering the mechanical Q of the transducer, for example by the use of a highly absorbent matched backing medium, and by lowering the electrical Q, by means of a suitable low shunting resistance.

2.6 SHORT PULSES

2.6.a Basic Principles

The understanding of the problems involved in the generation of short ultrasonic pulses is simplified if each radiating face of the transducer is considered as an individual source, separated from the other face by a delay line consisting of the transducer itself. This concept was first proposed by Cook (1956), and later developed by Jacobsen (1960). A treatment which gives results similar to those of Cook (1956) was developed independently by Ponomarev (1957). The analysis of the transient response of a transducer may be based on the assumption that, if an electrical step impulse is applied, four ultrasonic pulses are generated, two at each face. Of each of these two pairs of stress waves, one travels into the transducer, and the other travels into the loading or backing medium. The relative magnitudes of these pulses are determined by the characteristic impedances Z_t, Z_b and Z_l (see Fig. 2.2). The two pulses within the transducer travel backwards and forwards, and are reflected and transmitted at the transducer faces. The stress wave in either the loading or the backing medium may be computed from the progress of the pulses as they move through the system. This kind of analysis is not limited to the case of an electrical step impulse, but it can be extended to other forms of excitation, such as the transient impulse and the gated sine wave. The process is described in more detail in Section 2.6.b.

One of the commonest methods by which a short ultrasonic pulse may be generated is by the application of a transient electrical pulse to the transducer. This can be done, for example, by suddenly discharging a capacitor through the transducer by means of a thyratron or a mercury wetted relay. The thyratron is usually preferable, for it has no moving parts. A typical circuit is described in Section 4.3. As a result of the sudden application of the electrical pulse, the transducer rings at its fundamental resonant frequency: the duration of the radiated stress wave pulse depends upon the

Q-factor of the system. If the electrical pulse is short compared with the natural period of oscillation of the transducer, the amplitude of the second radiated stress wave is larger than that of the first, provided that the Q of the system permits this. The subsequent stress wave amplitudes decay exponentially at a rate determined by the system Q (see Section 2.5).

The observation of the pulse of stress waves presents some difficulties. A receiving transducer and oscilloscope of very wide frequency band are required in order to study the true shape of the pulse. Some suitable detectors for this purpose are described in Sections 3.3.b and 3.4. However, a much more convenient method, which has many practical applications, is to reflect the pulse back into the transducer from which it originated, and to use this transducer as a receiver. This double transducing process has a double restriction on bandwidth.

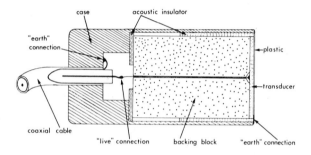

FIG. 2.4 Construction of a typical transducer probe for short pulse operation.

It has already been mentioned (see Section 2.5) that the mechanical Q of a transducer can be controlled by altering the characteristics of the backing medium. Figure 2.4 shows a typical form of construction for a probe for the generation and detection of short pulses. The backing material is chosen to have a similar characteristic impedance to that of the transducer, and to absorb as much as possible of the energy which enters it. Energy which enters, but which is not absorbed in the backing material may be reflected into the load after a delay determined by the dimensions and characteristics of the probe. This is one of the factors which determines the dynamic range of the device (see Section 2.10). Washington (1961) concluded the best compromise for the material of the transducer backing was obtained with a 2 to 1 (by weight) tungsten powder to Araldite mixture. The compromise is between pulse duration and sensitivity: the shorter the pulse, the lower the sensitivity. This is because a large fraction of the total ultrasonic energy is absorbed by the backing in a device which generates a short pulse in the load. Lutsch (1962) investigated the properties of solid mixtures of tungsten and rubber powders in epoxy resins, from the point of view of providing the best backing material for pulse transducers. He recommended that the ratio of resin to tungsten powder should be chosen to satisfy the impedance specification, which determines the pulse length, and that rubber powder should be added to increase the attenuation. Rubber powder has similar characteristic impedance to that of Araldite, but, for example, the addition of 5% by volume of rubber powder to a 10% by volume mixture of tungsten powder in Araldite increases the attenuation from 5·6 to 8·0 dB.cm^{-1} at 1 MHz. At this frequency, unloaded Araldite has an absorption coefficient of about 2·0 dB.cm^{-1}.

The acoustic insulator shown in Fig. 2.4 between the case of the probe and the transducer and backing block assembly minimizes the coupling of ultrasonic energy into the case. This would be undesirable because the case is often made of a low-loss material, such as a metal, and is likely to ring for some time in response to an ultrasonic transient. Ringing of the case would reduce the dynamic range of the device (see Section 2.10). Cork and rubber are suitable acoustic insulators.

The radiating face of the transducer may be protected by a thin film of material, such as a plastic like Araldite. The thickness of this film to some extent controls the performance of the device (see Section 2.8).

Figure 2.5 shows oscillograms of pulses, generated by the application of a fast electrical transient (about 0·05 μsec rise time) to 2 MHz transducers with various backing materials. The degree of damping provided in the transducer used to obtained Fig. 2.5.a was heavy, that in Fig. 2.5.c, light, and that in Fig. 2.5.b, an intermediate value. These oscillograms do not represent the real shapes of the corresponding ultrasonic stress waves, but they are the result of the double transducing process which has been previously described. Therefore, although the stress amplitudes of the third and subsequent half-cycles of the ultrasonic wave must be less than that of the second half-cycle (because of the form of excitation), nevertheless the observed pulse continues to build up for about six half cycles in the case of the lightly damped transducer. This is because of the restricted band-width of the transducer when acting as a receiver. This theory is supported by the experimental results of Cook (1956), who demonstrated that the propagated stress wave from a transducer excited by a fast transient pulse consists of a series of stress transients of short rise times, alternating in polarity and separated by a time interval equal to one half the fundamental period of the transducer.

Single stress waves of very short duration may be generated by exciting a thick slab of piezoelectric material by means of a very short electrical transient. As postulated by Cook (1956), each face acts as a separate source. The duration of the stress waves which are generated depends upon the duration of the electrical transient and the total equivalent inductance of the system. For each excitation, an exponentially decaying train of stress waves is radiated into the load. The waves are separated by time intervals deter-mined by the transit time (which may be made to be quite long) of a stress wave within the piezoelectric block. Details of some of the techniques involved have been given, for example, by Carome *et al.* (1964) and by Petersen and Rosen (1967).

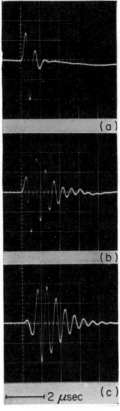

FIG. 2.5 Received voltage pulses with various degrees of transducer damping. (a) Heavy damping. (b) Intermediate damping. (c) Light damping.

It is possible to detect very fast stress waves in a similar manner, but confusion may arise if observation is attempted of several waves arriving spaced in time. If the wavetrain is sufficiently long, the later pulses are indistinguishable from secondary signals due to the earlier pulses travelling within the detector. In addition, the detector voltage is not a replica of the incident stress wave, but it is proportional to its time integral (Redwood, 1963; Carome *et al.* 1964). This is because the voltage across the detector is proportional to the space integral of the strain within it, and the space profile of the strain is of the same form as the time profile of the incident stress wave. Thus, a voltage replica of the stress wave may be obtained by differentiation of the voltage output from the detector.

An interesting method for the generation and detection of very short stress waves has been described by Van der Pauw (1966). The transducer is so arranged that it effectively has only one interface: the two electrodes lie side by side in the form of a comb on the radiating surface of a slab of ferroelectric material. Permanent polarization is achieved by the application of a high voltage between the electrodes at an appropriate temperature. Therefore, the polarization is of opposite sign at the two electrodes. The result is that both electrodes operate in phase when an exciting voltage is applied, so that two longitudinal waves are radiated in opposite directions perpendicular to the interface. The frequency-dependent effect which is due to the transit time between the two electrodes of a conventional transducer (Cook, 1956) does not occur in a planar transducer. However, the sensitivity of the device is about 10 dB lower than that of a conventional transducer, mainly because of its inhomogeneous polarization.

2.6.b Detailed Analysis

The mathematical analysis of the waveform of the stress wave generated by the application to the transducer of a given electrical voltage waveform is rather complicated. An extension of similar considerations applies to the case of a receiving transducer. The most thorough investigation seems to be due to Redwood (1961, 1963, 1964). For many practical applications, a graphical analysis described by Redwood (1963) will provide a sufficiently accurate result.

Redwood (1963) studied the specific case of a 1 cm diameter transducer of characteristic impedance 24×10^5 c.g.s. Rayl (barium titanate), radiating into a perfectly absorbent backing medium and a loading medium (water) of characteristic impedances 19×10^5 and $1\cdot5 \times 10^5$ c.g.s. Rayl respectively. The time of travel between the faces of the transducer was $0\cdot2$ μsec, corresponding to a fundamental resonant frequency of $2\cdot5$ MHz. Figure 2.6 shows the waveforms constructed by graphical analysis for this particular case. The exciting voltage waveform (Fig. 2.6.a) was observed by means of a wide-band oscilloscope. Figure 2.6.b, which represents the radiated stress wave, was constructed from the voltage waveform, taking into account the external radiation from the front face of the transducer, the internal radiation from the back face, and the reflection from the back face of the internal wave generated at the front face. Thus, the analysis is similar to that of Cook (1956), described in Section 2.6.a. The fourth and subsequent terms were not included in the graphical construction, because they are small in amplitude and their estimation is subject to cumulative error.

Figure 2.6.b was derived on the assumption that the voltage waveform is

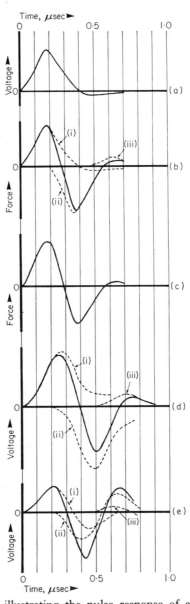

FIG. 2.6 Diagrams illustrating the pulse response of a 2·5 MHz transducer. (a) Exciting voltage waveform. (b) Propagated stress wave. (c) Propagated stress wave, modified by transducer time constant. (d) Integration by open circuit detector. (e) Effect of time constant in detection. (i), (ii) and (iii) correspond respectively to the contributions from the front face, the back face, and the front face by reflection from the back face. (Adapted from Figs. 4a, 4b, 6, 7b and 9 respectively of Redwood (1963).)

reproduced exactly as a stress waveform. However, the capacitive elements in the equivalent circuit of the transducer cannot be neglected in a rigorous analysis. Redwood (1963) calculated the effect of the transducer time constant on the radiated pulse. Figure 2.6.c shows the modified waveform. The overall effect on shape is quite small, and the time positions of the wave peaks and zeros are negligibly affected. Thus, for most practical purposes, the effect of this time constant may be neglected.

If the stress wave shown in Fig. 2.6.c is reflected back into the transducer, the output voltage depends upon the electrical load. With an open circuit transducer, the output voltage is proportional to the difference in the displacements of the surfaces, and the resultant voltage waveform is shown in Fig. 2.6.d. However, if the transducer is electrically loaded, the voltage waveform is modified by the introduction of a time constant in the equivalent circuit. Figure 2.6.e shows the voltage waveform generated by the transducer in response to the stress wave shown in Fig. 2.6.c, with the transducer terminated by 37Ω (two 75Ω resistive loads in parallel) and an additional shunt capacitance of 800 pF.

Redwood (1963) was able to verify the results of this analysis by experiment. For some measurements, a long block of piezoelectric ceramic was used as a non-resonant detector (see Section 2.6.a), and for others, the same transducer was used both to generate and to receive the pulses.

In principle, this method of analysis may be extended to other forms of electrical excitation and to the detection of other forms of stress wave. However, for conditions resulting from more complex excitations than the approximately half-sinusoid considered by Redwood (1963), graphical analysis becomes rather difficult.

Beveridge and Keith (1952) analysed the transient response of a transducer by consideration of an electrical transmission line having a steady-state response identical to that of the transducer, and having a transient response which could be calculated in a straightforward manner. This approach may be helpful in certain problems. However, it is usually found that the response to complex excitation is most easily investigated by direct measurement.

2.7 PULSE FREQUENCY SPECTRUM

The frequency associated with a continuous wave train of constant frequency has a single value: all the energy occurs at this single frequency. However, in a wave train which is discontinuous, the energy distribution is not monotonic, but it is spread over a frequency spectrum.

The analysis of the amplitude distribution of a wave train into its frequency spectrum is based on Fourier's theorem. In its simplest form, this states that any periodic variation which fulfills certain conditions regarding continuity may be considered as the sum of a number of sinusoids whose periods exhibit a simple relationship. In addition, the equivalent series of sinusoids is unique for any given periodic variation.

In the case of a pulse, graphical integration may be used to evaluate the amplitudes of the sine and cosine series for various values of frequency, as follows—

$$A_s(\omega) = \int_0^\infty F(t) \sin \omega t \, dt, \tag{2.9}$$

and $\quad A_c(\omega) = \int_0^\infty F(t) \cos \omega t \, dt, \tag{2.10}$

where $\quad A_s(\omega) =$ amplitude of the sine term corresponding

to the frequency $f = \dfrac{\omega}{2\pi}$,

$A_c(\omega) =$ amplitude of the cosine term corresponding

to the frequency $f = \dfrac{\omega}{2\pi}$,

and $\quad F(t) =$ instantaneous value of the pulse amplitude

corresponding to the frequency $f = \dfrac{\omega}{2\pi}$.

The overall amplitude of the spectrum $A(\omega)$ at any particular frequency $\dfrac{\omega}{2\pi}$ may be calculated from the corresponding values of $A_s(\omega)$ and $A_c(\omega)$, as follows—

$$A(\omega) = \sqrt{(A_s(\omega))^2 + (A_c(\omega))^2}. \tag{2.11}$$

Redwood (1963) calculated the frequency spectrum of the pulse shown in Fig. 2.6.c. The corresponding amplitude distribution, for a repetition frequency of 1000 per sec, is shown in Fig. 2.7. The frequency of maximum amplitude of the spectrum (1.9 MHz) is markedly shifted from the fundamental resonant frequency of the transducer (2·5 MHz). The pulse has a half-amplitude bandwidth of 2·5 MHz, and a half-power bandwidth of 1·8 MHz.

The frequency spectrum is of considerable importance in diagnostic systems employing pulsed ultrasonics. Pellam and Galt (1946) pointed out that the frequency spectrum is modified by transmission through a medium in which the absorption coefficient depends upon the frequency. If, as is usual, the absorption increases with increasing frequency, then the high frequency components of a pulse are attenuated more than those of low frequency, and there is a shift downwards of the centre frequency of the spectrum. Kolsky (1956) discussed this effect in some detail, and Redwood (1963) calculated, using the technique of Fourier synthesis, how a frequency dependent absorption alters the pulse shape. He concluded that large errors are possible in the measurement of absorption if the pulse has a broad spectrum, since its amplitude is maintained by the low frequency components. Accurate absorption measurements can only be achieved by the use of a narrow frequency spectrum, which in turn requires the use of a relatively large number of cycles. The corollary of this phenomenon, that

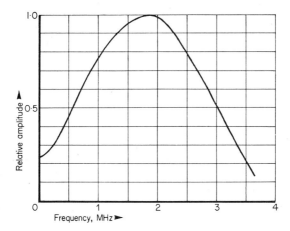

FIG. 2.7 Frequency amplitude spectrum of the pulse shown in Figure 2.6.c. (Adapted from Fig. 10 of Redwood, 1963).

the effective absorption coefficient of a medium depends upon the characteristics of the ultrasonic pulse, has important implications in diagnosis: see Section 4.1.b. Errors in velocity measurements are also possible, because of shifts in the time positions of the wave amplitude zeros due to pulse stretching, but these errors are not usually large, nor is their effect magnified by dispersion. The theory of the accuracy of the pulse method for measuring the absorption and velocity of ultrasound has been given in detail by Merkulova (1967).

The effect of absorption on the frequency spectrum is illustrated in Fig. 2.8. In this figure, curve (i) represents the same spectrum as that shown in Fig. 2.7, but redrawn with the amplitude expressed in decibels. The maximum amplitude occurs at 1·9 MHz, and is chosen to correspond to 0 dB in Fig. 2.8. This spectrum is that for zero dispersive absorption. Curves (ii)–(v) show how the spectrum is shifted to lower frequencies, and the amplitude is decreased, for a pulse travelling through increasingly dispersive absorbers. For example, if the propagating medium has an absorption coefficient of 1 dB.cm^{-1}.MHz^{-1}, which is quite typical for a biological soft tissue (see Table 1.8), then an absorption rate of 5 dB . MHz^{-1} is equivalent to a path length of 5 cm. in the medium, and so on. Thus, these curves also illustrate the effect on the frequency spectrum which occurs as the pulse travels various distances in a dispersive absorber.

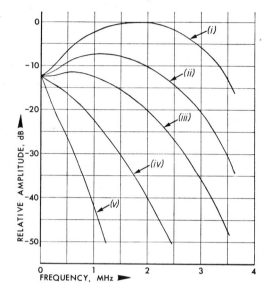

FIG. 2.8 Effect of dispersive absorption on pulse frequency spectrum. (i) No absorption (Figure 2.7 redrawn with decibel scale). (ii) Absorption 5 dB MHz^{-1}. (iii) Absorption 10 dB MHz^{-1}. (iv) Absorption 20 dB MHz^{-1}. (v) Absorption 40 dB MHz^{-1}

Similar effects have been observed in polycrystalline materials. Thus, Markham (1963) has investigated the effect of scattering losses in polycrystalline silver on the frequency spectrum of the ultrasonic pulse, and Serabian (1967) has studied the same effect in graphite. The theory and discussion presented by these authors may be found to be helpful in assessing the significance of dispersive absorption in diagnostic situations.

2.8 MECHANICAL IMPEDANCE MATCHING

The effects of matching the characteristic impedance of the transducer to the backing and loading media have been quite thoroughly investigated, particularly by Kossoff (1966). He used a rather sophisticated piezoelectric ceramic, PZT-7A, as the transducer, but his results are equally applicable to other transducer materials. His analysis is to some extent based on the earlier work of McSkimin (1955), who showed that the bandwidth of a transducer can be increased by the use of a matching layer of suitable thickness and characteristic impedance, included between the transducer and the load. Such a layer acts as a mechanical transformer which reflects an increased load into the transducer (see Section 1.11). Thus, the power is more efficiently absorbed by the load, and the system has a reduced loss. The matching layer is frequency selective, and optimization is based on a compromise between the efficiency of the system and bandwidth limitation due to the frequency selective components.

Various combinations of backing and matching are possible. Kossoff (1966) considered a 2 MHz transducer of 2·5 cm diameter, working into a water load, and presented his data mainly in the form of separate graphs of transmitting and receiving transducer voltage transfer functions, plotted against the fractional deviation from the open-circuit resonant frequency.

Walker and Lumb (1964) have described how the loop gain of a transducer system consisting of a transmitter and a receiver may be estimated. The reflection conditions in the definitions of loop gain and voltage transfer function as calculated by Kossoff (1966) are different, but the principles are the same. However, a simple calculation of loop gain or voltage transfer function requires a simple transmitter voltage waveform which has the same shape as the propagated stress wave. This condition is not satisfied in the case of a shock excited transducer, and the calculation becomes much more difficult. Shock excited systems are most easily investigated by direct measurement, using some kind of standard reflecting surface.

Kossoff's (1966) results have been recalculated for Fig. 2.9 to give the overall voltage transfer functions, and so correspond to the output voltages obtained after perfect reflection with zero loss of the ultrasonic wave generated by a given input voltage. The frequency response of the air-backed transducer has the narrowest bandwidth. The transducer with an unmatched tungsten powder in Araldite backing has a similar bandwidth to that of the unbacked transducer matched to the load, but it has an overall voltage transfer function corresponding to some 8 dB lower sensitivity. If poor sensitivity and some degree of ripple can be tolerated in the pass band, a transducer matched to both the load and backing has the widest band-width. A transducer which is matched to the backing but unmatched to the load has a similar bandwidth, but greater ripple and even lower sensitivity.

The tungsten powder in Araldite backing material used by Kossoff (1966) was made by adding 100 to 200 g of tungsten powder to 40 ml of Araldite (100 parts casting resin D and 50 parts polyamid 75), and centrifuging the mixture. The characteristic impedance varied from 6 to 16×10^5 c.g.s. Rayl. Kossoff (1966) quotes the value of the characteristic impedance of PZT-7A as $37·5 \times 10^5$ c.g.s. Rayl. Matching of the load (water, $Z = 1·48 \times 10^5$ c.g.s. Rayl) or the backing was accomplished by means of a quarter-wave layer of Araldite containing aluminium. This was prepared by mixing 1·5 parts by weight of aluminium powder with 1 part of Araldite

(100 parts casting resin D and 10 parts of hardener 351), which gave an impedance of $5 \cdot 5 \times 10^5$ c.g.s. Rayl.

Kossoff's (1966) analysis is based on a steady state situation. This is because the action of a matching layer depends upon the existence of an equilibrium standing wave system. The time required for the establishment of steady state conditions depends upon a number of factors, and in particular, upon the losses of the system: the greater the losses, the more

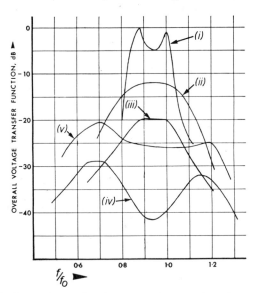

FIG. 2.9 Bandwidths of overall voltage transfer functions for various transducer systems. (f/f_0 = fractional frequency deviation.) (i) Air backed: unmatched to load. (ii) Air backed: matched to load. (iii) Tungsten powder in Araldite backed: unmatched to load. (iv) Matched to tungsten powder in Araldite backing: unmatched to load. (v) Matched to tungsten powder in Araldite backing: matched to load. (Adapted from Figs. 5, 6, 11, 12, 16, 19 and 20 of Kossoff, 1966).

rapidly does the transient situation approach that of the steady state. Therefore, although the steady state bandwidth can be improved by the techiques developed by Kossoff (1966), these improvements become less significant as the duration of the ultrasonic pulse is decreased.

Theoretical prediction of the bandwidth of a transducer is apt to be rather inaccurate, on account of the difficulties involved in estimating the magnitudes of the various factors which control the frequency response. Therefore, it is generally better to measure the frequency response of a particular transducer by an experimental method. Gericke (1966) has described an automatic system in which the transducer is excited by gated pulses from a constant-amplitude oscillator, the frequency of which is swept through the range 0·3 to 12 MHz. A voltage proportional to the instantaneous value of the frequency is fed to the x-deflection plates of a cathode ray oscilloscope. The transducer is arranged to transmit the pulses into a block of low-loss material, such as aluminium, and to receive the echoes from a reflecting surface. The thickness of the block is made large enough to give a delay which avoids ambiguity between the exciting pulses and the received echoes. The output from the transducer is fed to a wide-band amplifier, the output of which is connected to the y-deflection plates of the oscilloscope. A bright-up pulse is applied to the z-modulation input of the oscilloscope for the duration of each received pulse. Thus, a display appears on the oscilloscope in which the x-deflection is proportional to the frequency, and the y-deflection, to the overall voltage transfer function.

It is important to understand the distinction between the frequency spectrum of an ultrasonic pulse, and the frequency response of a transducer. The frequency response describes the continuous-wave bandwidth of the transducer system, whereas the frequency spectrum depends not only upon the frequency response of the transducer, but also upon the form of the electrical excitation.

The satisfactory generation and detection of very short pulses of ultrasound by a resonant transducer can only be achieved by the use of a non-reflective backing medium. The best backing material currently available seems to be Araldite loaded to a high density with tungsten powder, but even if a mixture with the highest practical characteristic impedance of 16×10^5 c.g.s. Rayl is used, the reflection at the transducer (lead titanate zirconate) to backing interface is only about 20 dB below that from an air backing. The internal reflection at a water loaded face is only about 0·5 dB down, and so the voltage transfer function is small with very short pulses. The Q-factor corresponding to the overall frequency response of the transducer has a value of about 2·5 with most heavily damped probes. It is hard to imagine how the situation could be improved unless transducer materials of characteristic impedance much closer to that of water than that of those which are available today were to be discovered.

2.9 ELECTRICAL IMPEDANCE MATCHING

Maximum electrical efficiency is obtained when the transducer is matched to the electrical impedance of the transmitting and receiving equipment, and the electrical and mechanical resonances are tuned together.

The reactance X_t of the transducer is given by—

$$X_t = \frac{1}{2\pi f C_t} \tag{2.12}$$

where $C_t =$ capacitance of the transducer.

Now $\qquad C_t = \dfrac{\epsilon A_t}{l_t}$ $\qquad\qquad\qquad\qquad$ (2.13)

where $\qquad \epsilon =$ dielectric constant of the transducer,

$\qquad\qquad\quad A_t =$ transducer area,

and $\qquad\qquad l_t =$ transducer thickness.

The design of suitable electrical matching transformers has been described by Walker and Lumb (1964), by means of a specific example. They calculate that the reactance of a 6 MHz lead titanate zirconate transducer of 1 cm diameter is 5·75 Ω. This can be tuned by a transformer of ratio about 3·5 to 1, so that it is matched to 75 Ω, which is a commonly used impedance for electrical transmission. The reflected impedance through the transformer is proportional to the square of the turns ratio.

The resonant frequency f_0 of the electrical circuit is given by

$$f_0 = \frac{1}{2\pi\sqrt{LC}} \qquad\qquad (2.14)$$

where $\qquad C =$ total capacitance of transducer and cable,

and $\qquad L =$ total inductance of the circuit.

In the example of Walker and Lumb (1964), the inductance of the cable is small compared with the transformer inductance, and, to a first approximation,

$$L = \frac{n^2 \mu A_x}{l_x} \qquad\qquad (2.15)$$

where $\qquad n =$ total number of transformer turns,

$\qquad\qquad \mu =$ permeability of transformer

$\qquad\qquad A_x =$ area of transformer core,

and $\qquad\qquad l_x =$ length of transformer core.

Hence, it is possible to arrange for the electrical resonance to be made equal in frequency to that of the mechanical resonance by means of a transformer of suitable size, winding and core material. By using a transformer tuned to 6 MHz, situated within the backing block of the transducer, Walker and Lumb (1964) obtained a substantial increase in probe sensitivity, compared with the sensitivity of a similar probe without a transformer. The actual increase in loop gain was 20 dB, when the probe was used as a combined transmitter and receiver in a pulse-echo system. In spite of the high sensitivity, the pulse length in response to shock excitation was not excessive, the echoes received from a fine wire target being substantially decayed after five vibrations.

The length of the cable has only a small effect on the tuning characteristics of the system. This is because the cable capacitance is relatively small compared with that of the transducer.

It is important for the impedance matching transformer to be mounted close to the transducer, otherwise the loss in the interconnecting cable may become significant. This is because the impedances of the cable and the transducer form a potential divider. Another difficulty with a long cable between the transducer and the transformer is that the signal waveform may become degraded: this effect is particularly troublesome in the case of transmitting transducers.

At low megahertz frequencies, the electrical mismatch of a typical transducer in a 75Ω circuit may be less serious. For example, the reactance of a 1·5 MHz lead titanate zirconate transducer of 2 cm. diameter is about 65Ω, which represents a negligible mismatch. In pulse-echo applications, no significant improvement in system performance is obtained by the electrical tuning of transducers with this degree of mismatch, because the effect is primarily to narrow the effective bandwidth. However, in continuous-wave applications, some improvement in sensitivity may be obtained by electrical tuning.

2.10 DYNAMIC RANGE

The dynamic range of a pulse transducer may be defined as the ratio of the amplitude of the main pulse to the amplitude of the ripple following this pulse, measured with the transducer receiving the echo from a flat reflector normal to the axis of the ultrasonic beam. A large dynamic range is desirable in certain diagnostic applications.

The dynamic range is controlled by a number of factors. The principal limitation arises in the mounting of the transducer. If energy is coupled into the probe casing (which is frequently constructed from metal: see Section 2.6), the casing may ring for some time after the main pulse has been generated. This ringing may be coupled back into the transducer, causing a reduction in dynamic range. The effect may be minimized by the presence of an acoustic insulator between the transducer and the case, as shown in Fig. 2.4. Any tendency of the casing to ring may be reduced by breaking up its profile, and including bands of a damping material such as a plastic.

Another factor which limits the dynamic range is the coupling of energy into resonant radial modes within the transducer. Kossoff et al. (1965) have shown that this effect can be reduced by making the transducer radially asymmetrical. The method they used was to attach a 4 mm cube of rubber to the edge of the transducer, within the backing block. The portion of the transducer covered by the rubber was not excited, thus destroying the radial symmetry. The addition of the rubber increased the dynamic range of a typical probe by 6 dB.

3. THE ULTRASONIC FIELD

3.1 STEADY STATE CONDITIONS

The surface of a transducer of any shape and size may be considered to be represented by small areas, each of which acts as a simple transducer which either radiates energy uniformly in all directions, or has a uniformly non-directional sensitivity as a receiver. Huygen's principle may be applied to show that the directivity of the whole transducer can be analysed by the addition of the contributions of each of these simple transducing elements, provided that due account is taken of phase and amplitude (see Section 1.14).

The most commonly used transducer in diagnostic techniques is in the form of a disc, which is arranged to radiate or to receive energy at its flat surfaces. For theoretical analysis, such a disc may be considered to behave as a cophasally vibrating piston. The directivity of the beam is determined by diffraction in the same way that a plane beam of light is affected by an aperture. Practical transducers do not behave as perfect, cophasally vibrating pistons. Thus, Dye (1932) used an optical interferometer to investigate the modes of vibration of quartz plates, and found that at resonance some portions of the transducer surface do not vibrate at all, and that there may be a phase non-uniformity of as much as 180° between various parts of the surface. Some beautiful photographs obtained by multiple-beam interferometry which show the non-uniformity of vibration amplitude in quartz transducers appear in a book by Tolanksky (1960). Sharaf (1954) has described a non-contact displacement meter, which consists of a capacitor probe of 0·16 cm diameter arranged to frequency modulate a 25 MHz oscillator, and presumably this could be used to investigate the surface vibration of a pulsed transducer. Deferrari *et al.* (1967) have used a laser interferometer to study the displacement of low-frequency transducers, and it might be possible to develop this method for ultrasonic measurements. However, despite the undoubted complexity of vibration in practical transducers, theory based on the assumption that the transducer is a cophasally vibrating piston yields results which generally agree very well with the distributions found in practice.

The application of Huygen's principle is often rather complicated. In the case of a circular piston vibrating cophasally in simple harmonic motion, the

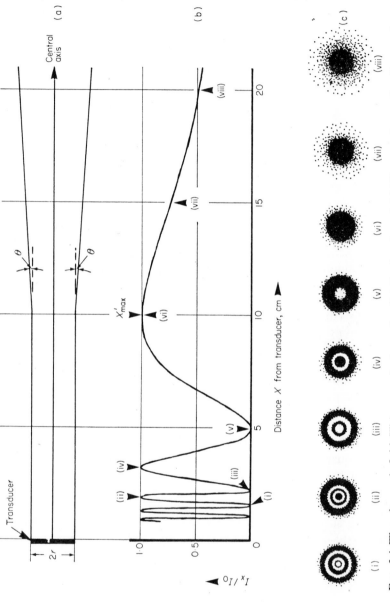

FIG. 3.1 The ultrasonic field. This example shows the distribution for a 1·5 MHz transducer of radius $r = 1$ cm. (a) Almost all the ultrasonic energy lies within the limits shown in this diagram; (b) Relative intensity distribution along the central axis of the beam; (c) Ring diagrams showing the energy distribution of beam sections at positions indicated in (b).

analysis is difficult (Hueter and Bolt (1955), pp. 62–72; Kinsler and Frey (1962), pp. 166–177). However, it can be shown that, for steady state conditions (continuous wave operation with constant drive amplitude) the beam is made up of two distinct regions, as shown in Fig. 3.1. The relationship which applies to the distribution along the central axis of the beam is—

$$\frac{I_x}{I_0} = \sin^2\left[\frac{\pi}{\lambda}(\sqrt{r^2 + x^2} - x)\right] \tag{3.1}$$

where $I_0 =$ maximum intensity,

             $I_x =$ intensity at distance x from the piston,

             $r =$ radius of piston,

and $\lambda =$ wavelength in propagating medium.

Equation 3.1 can be solved to give the position of the axial maxima and minima as follows—

$$x_{max} = \frac{4r^2 - \lambda^2(2m + 1)^2}{4\lambda(2m + 1)} \tag{3.2}$$

where $x_{max} =$ position of maximum amplitude along the x-axis,

and $m = 0, 1, 2, \ldots$

And $$x_{min} = \frac{r^2 - \lambda^2 m^2}{2m\lambda} \tag{3.3}$$

where $x_{min} =$ position of minimum amplitude along the x-axis,

and $m = 1, 2, 3, \ldots$

It can be seen from Equation 3.2 that the last axial maximum occurs at a distance from the transducer given by the expression—

$$x'_{max} = \frac{4r^2 - \lambda^2}{4\lambda} \tag{3.4}$$

If $r^2 \gg \lambda^2$, this expression can be simplified to become—

$$x'_{max} = \frac{r^2}{\lambda} \tag{3.5}$$

The position x'_{max} of the last axial maximum corresponds to the beginning of the transition between the Frésnel and the Fraunhofer zones. For a given radius of transducer, the length of the Frésnel zone increases with decreasing wavelength (or increasing frequency), provided that the wavelength is small compared with the transducer radius.

In the Frésnel zone, the energy is mainly confined within a cylinder of radius r, but the distribution of energy across the beam diameter at any distance x from the transducer ($0 < x < x'_{max}$) is non-uniform, as indicated in Fig. 3.1.c. The number of maxima and minima across the beam diameter depends upon x and $\frac{r}{\lambda}$. In general, the number of peaks increases with decreasing values of x and increasing values of $\frac{r}{\lambda}$. At successive axial maxima and minima, starting at x'_{max} and moving towards the transducer, there are one, two, three, etc., principal maxima across the beam.

It is possible to derive an exact solution for the field distribution in terms of expansions involving known mathematical functions (Carter and Williams, 1951), but calculations employing these exact formulae are exceedingly involved. In the Frésnel zone, even approximate solutions are usually based on the use of rather slowly converging series. However, there is a relatively simple solution due to Dehn (1960) which gives a qualitative indication of the positions of the maxima. The maxima occur at the positions at which the contributions of three rays, one perpendicular to the piston face, and one from each of its extreme edges, are most nearly in phase. Because of symmetry, the figure may be rotated about the beam axis to generate ring patterns such as those shown in Fig. 3.1.c. The situation is so complicated that computations based on the exact solutions do not seem to have been published, and an indication of the shape of the distribution is most easily obtained by direct measurement (see Section 3.3).

The field in the Fraunhofer zone is more amenable to mathematical analysis. The relationship between the intensity and the angle θ defined in Fig. 3.1.a contains a multiplying term, the directivity function D_s, given by

$$D_s = \frac{2J_1(kr \sin \theta)}{kr \sin \theta} \tag{3.6}$$

where $J_1 =$ Bessel's function of the first kind,.

and $k = \dfrac{2\pi}{\lambda}$

Inspection of a table of Bessel's function indicates that $D_s = 0$ when $kr \sin \theta = 3\cdot83$, $7\cdot02$, $10\cdot17$, $13\cdot32$, etc. Therefore, the energy is confined into lobes; the central lobe is reduced to zero at the angles $\pm \theta$ about the axis of the ultrasonic beam, given by—

$$\sin \theta = \frac{3\cdot83}{kr} = \frac{0\cdot61\lambda}{r} \tag{3.7}$$

Equation 3.7 is known as "Fraunhofer's formula". If $kr < 3\cdot83$, D_s is not zero for any real value of θ, and only the main lobe occurs. If kr is very small, D_s has a value of almost unity for all values of θ, and the piston behaves as a simple source which is non-directional.

The energy in the side lobes is usually much smaller than that in the main lobe. For example, calculations based on the values of J_1 show that the maximum intensity of the first side lobe (if it exists) is $17\cdot5$ dB below that of the main lobe, and that the intensities of any subsequent lobes are even smaller.

Along the central axis of the beam, in the region where $x \gg x'_{\max}$, the intensity is governed by the inverse square law, and it is proportional to $\dfrac{1}{x^2}$.

In this discussion, the beam pattern of a transmitting transducer has been considered. The sensitivity of a transducer acting as a receiver has a distribution which is identical to the beam pattern of the same transducer acting as a transmitter. In a system consisting of a separate source and receiver with directivity functions D_s and D_r, the overall directivity is determined by the product $D_s D_r$. If the same transducer acts as a combined transmitter and receiver, the system directivity is determined by the quantity D_s^2.

It has been pointed out by von Haselberg and Krautkramer (1959) that a cophasally vibrating piston is actually a most unfavourable oscillator as far as beam uniformity is concerned. If the edges of the transducer are less strongly excited than the centre, the variations between the maxima and minima in the near field are less pronounced. The ideal solution is represented by an excitation across the diameter in the form of a Gaussian probability curve. The field produced by a transducer the electrodes of which are in the form of a star has a constant axial amplitude in the Frésnel zone, no side lobes and no zero points in the Fraunhofer zone, and a single maximum everywhere normal to the axis.

Bradfield (1960) has shown that the uniformity of the Frésnel zone may also be improved by the use of radially graded excitation. The field is controlled by the number of annuli and the relative amplitudes of their driving voltages. No doubt the same method could be used in a receiver with graded electrical attenuation.

An effect which has attracted a good deal of theoretical attention is due to so-called "geometrical diffraction", for which no satisfactory explanation in physical terms seems to have been yet proposed. Seki et al. (1959) calculated that, in a lossless medium, an attenuation of about 1 dB should occur between the source and $x'_{\max}$, for transducers in which

$$50 < kr < 1000.$$

In addition, McSkimin (1960) found that the velocity in the Frésnel zone is increased by about 0·02% due to geometrical diffraction. Tjaden (1961) concluded that the effect of geometrical diffraction on absorption under pulse-echo conditions is less than would be expected theoretically. Any velocity changes are likewise very small, and the effects of geometrical diffraction can be neglected in medical diagnostic applications. More recent results, which again have no direct bearing on practical applications to diagnosis, have been presented by, for example, Lord (1966) and Papadakis (1966).

3.2 FOCUSSING SYSTEMS

The directivity of an ultrasonic beam may be altered by focussing. There are three different methods by which a beam may be focussed: these are illustrated in Fig. 3.2.

Figure 3.2.a shows how a reflector, in this example a paraboloid, can be arranged to focus an ultrasonic beam at the point F. The distance from the centre of the reflector to F is determined, for a parallel incident beam, by the geometry of the paraboloid. The ultrasonic beam is substantially parallel in the Frésnel zone (see Section 3.1). The increase in intensity at the focus is limited, if losses may be neglected, by the breakdown of simple geometrical theory where the dimensions of the system are not large compared with the wavelength of the ultrasound. The theory of reflecting systems has been discussed by Horton and Naral (1950).

The mechanical construction of a paraboloid of revolution is rather difficult. In practice, it may often be acceptable to use a section of a sphere as the reflecting surface. The theory of such a reflector has been given by Griffing and Fox (1949), and this theory has been tested experimentally by Fox and Griffing (1949).

In addition to simple systems employing a single reflector, it is also possible to construct focussing systems in which two or more reflectors are used. This method has the advantage that it becomes unnecessary to place instruments in the path of the incident beam. For example, Olofsson (1963) has described an arrangement in which the echoes from a transmitting transducer of 2 cm diameter, operating under pulsed conditions at 1 MHz, are detected by a mirror system. The mirror system consists of an ellipsoid of 14·2 cm diameter, and a hyperboloid of 2·8 cm diameter positioned to intercept the energy converging to the near focus of the ellipsoid. The hyperboloid focusses the energy onto a receiving transducer of 0·3 cm diameter placed in the central axis of the system. A small receiver is necessary so that the cone enclosed by the hyperboloid falls within its main lobe. Thus, the arrangement of the mirrors resembles that of the Cassegrainian telescope. The mirrors are constructed from Araldite loaded with fine tungsten powder to give a density of 5·2–5·6 g. cm^{-3}; this mixture has a good reflectivity, and does not give rise to pulse-lengthening such as occurs with a less lossy material. The mirror surface was machined to an accuracy of $\pm 0{\cdot}005$ cm. The resolution of the system, measured using a glass pellet of $0{\cdot}14$ cm diameter as the target, is such that the response is 3 dB down

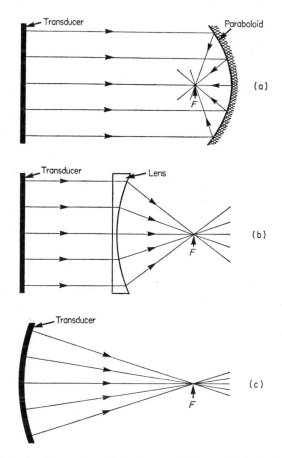

FIG. 3.2 Methods of focussing. (a) Reflector; (b) Lens; (c) Spherical transducer.

from that at the focus, at $\pm 0{\cdot}12$ cm across the beam axis, and at 1.3 cm towards and $1{\cdot}7$ cm away from the focus along the axis. The distance from the focus to the surface of the ellipsoid along the central axis is 20 cm.

A similar system to that of Olofsson (1963) has been described by Hertz and Olofsson (1965). The principle difference seems to be that the frequency is $2{\cdot}5$ MHz, and that the transmitting transducer is focussed at the far focus of the ellipsoid.

Thurstone and McKinney (1966a, 1966b) have described an arrangement in which a parallel beam is made to diverge by the convex surface of a paraboloid: this paraboloid is placed at the focus of the concave section of an ellipsoid, and by this means the beam converges towards the focal point from a large aperture. The lateral resolution at the focus is about 0·05 cm with a dynamic range of 3 dB. The same depth resolution can be obtained by gating the receiver.

A detailed theoretical analysis of double-mirror focussing systems has been given by Belle (1968).

Ultrasonics can also be focussed by means of lenses, as shown, for example, in Fig. 3.2.b. The material from which the lens is constructed should ideally have an absorption coefficient of zero, a characteristic impedance matching that of the loading medium, and a refractive index which is not unity. The refractive index is equal to the ratio of the propagation velocities in the material of the lens and of the adjacent medium. If water is the adjacent medium, there are few materials available from which the lens can be constructed, which in any way satisfy all the ideal conditions. Perspex and polystyrene seem to be the best materials which are readily available. Although the refractive index of polystyrene to water is slightly smaller than that of Perspex to water, its losses due to both mismatch and absorption are lower, and so polystyrene is preferable in high-power applications.

Sette (1949) has investigated the performance of plano-cylindrical and plano-spherical lenses constructed from Perspex. The highest efficiency is obtained when the lens is in contact with the transducer, because its impedance is intermediate between that of the transducer and the water, and so improves the transmission of the system (see Section 1.11). Another advantage of a converging lens is that its greater thickness towards its edge reduces the edge activity of the beam, which results in a reduction in side-lobe intensity.

The laws of geometrical optics can be applied to lens calculations, provided that the aperture of the lens is small, and the diameter of the transducer is large compared with the wavelength. Under these conditions, the focal length f_l is given by—

$$f_l = \frac{A}{1 - \dfrac{c_1}{c_2}} \qquad (3.8)$$

where A = radius of curvature of the spherical or cylindrical surface,

c_1 = propagation velocity in the lens,

and c_2 = propagation velocity in the load.

The sign of f_l given by Equation 3.8 is negative if $c_1 > c_2$, as in the case of a Perspex lens with a water load. This indicates that the lens is concave.

The gain in intensity at the focus of a lens system is limited by diffraction. Thus, the smallest focal diameter which can be obtained in practice is in the order of the wavelength. Sometimes, it is desirable to confine the beam within a narrow section over a chosen range, rather than to focus it into a point. In such cases, the analysis of Kossoff (1963), described later in this section, may be applied. Kossoff *et al.* (1964) have obtained satisfactory results using an Araldite lens. Equation 3.8 may be used to calculate the radius of curvature of the lens, the velocity in Araldite being taken as $2,300 \text{ m.sec}^{-1}$. The lens must be made as thin as possible in order to minimize absorption loss.

Transmission through a lens the characteristic impedance of which differs from that of the loading medium is controlled by interference (see Section 1.11). Maximum transmission occurs in those regions where the lens thickness is an integral number of half wavelengths. Transmission is a minimum where the thickness is an odd integral number of quarter wavelengths. Tarnóczy (1965) quoted data which show that the difference in transmission between interference maxima and minima is about 3 dB in Perspex: these variations are superimposed upon transmission loss due to absorption. In 1953, T. Tarnóczy proposed that efficient lenses could be produced by omitting those concentric rings where interference reduces transmission. It is not necessary for the lens surface to be curved, and excellent results are obtained with a lens constructed in a series of annular zones, spaced in thickness by distances equal to $\frac{\lambda}{2}$.

Focussed ultrasonic beams may also be generated by means of curved transducers, as illustrated in Fig. 3.2.c. Such devices can be constructed from crystals such as quartz, and by careful design the limitations of the fixed piezoelectric axes can be made quite small (Willard, 1949). Large concave transducers can be constructed by arranging a number of small, plane transducers in a mosaic on a suitable curved surface. However, the ferroelectrics (see Section 2.1) can be moulded to shape and then polarized so that the piezoelectric axis always lies along the thickness of the transducer, normal to the transducer surface. This method is often used for the construction of focussing devices with diameters of up to a few centimetres.

An ultrasonic transducer made in the form of a spherical shell radiates spherical waves which converge close to the centre of curvature of the shell. O'Neil (1949) has investigated the theory of devices of this kind, in which the radius of the transducer is large compared both with the wavelength and with the depth of the concave surface. The intensity gain G at the centre of curvature is given by—

$$G = \frac{I_c}{I_i} \simeq \left(\frac{2\pi h}{\lambda}\right)^2 \tag{3.9}$$

where $\qquad I_c =$ intensity at centre of curvature,

$\qquad\qquad\qquad I_i =$ intensity at transducer surface,

and $\qquad\qquad h =$ depth of concave surface.

The point of greatest intensity is not exactly at the centre of curvature, but it approaches this position as the value of $\dfrac{2\pi h}{\lambda}$ becomes greater. In the central part of the focal plane, the directivity function is approximately the same as that given in Equation 3.6, in which r is the radius of the spherical transducer, and θ is the angle from the central axis.

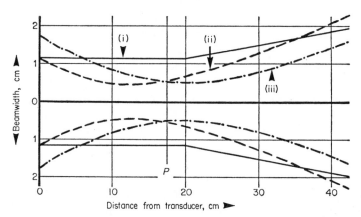

FIG. 3.3 Beamwidths of focussed transducers. (i) $r = 1\cdot15$ cm, $A = \infty$; (ii) $r = 1\cdot15$ cm, $A = 17\cdot5$ cm; (iii) $r = 1\cdot75$ cm, $A = 25$ cm. (Adapted from Fig. 8 of Kossoff et al. 1965).

Kossoff (1963) has developed O'Neil's (1949) theory in order to predict the optimum design for a focussing system to generate a narrow beamwidth over a finite distance. This form of beam is desirable in many diagnostic applications (see Section 4.1.b). The optimization procedure is based on the representation of the solid surface of revolution of the off-axis intensity distribution in a lossless medium as a cone which contains constant energy. The base of the cone is equal to the beam area, and the height of the cone represents the maximum intensity. The criterion for optimization is that the focussed transducer should give the same axial intensity as the "optimum" plane transducer of radius $r = \sqrt{\lambda P}$ at a range $2P$, where P is the required penetration into the patient. In his analysis, Kossoff (1963) was particularly concerned with an investigation in which the transducer stands off in a water bath from the patient by a distance equal to P, so that the maximum operating range is equal to $2P$. In the case of the plane transducer, $r = \sqrt{\lambda P}$ corresponds to $P = x'_{max}$ (see Equation 3.5).

Good results are obtained if the focussing transducer is made equal in radius to the "optimum" plane transducer, and the radius of curvature A is made equal to P (Kossoff $et\ al.$ 1964). Optimum resolution is obtained if the values of both r and A for the focussed transducer are increased by 20% from the values indicated by these considerations, but this improvement is small.

The beamwidths (here defined as the width of the beam which contains 84% of the total energy) of the "optimum" plane and focussed transducers for a penetration of 17.5 cm at a frequency of 2 MHz are compared in Fig. 3.3. However, if a focussed transducer of greater diameter is acceptable, a considerable improvement in beamwidth can be obtained within the range P to $2P$. The intensity distribution of the focussed transducer which, according to Kossoff $et\ al.$ has the best performance, is also shown in Fig. 3.3. This transducer has a diameter of 3·5 cm and a radius of curvature of 25 cm.

3.3 TRANSIENT CONDITIONS

The situation which occurs in a steady state ultrasonic field has been described in Section 3.1. In the steady state, the directivity is determined by interference between contributions from the entire surface of the transducer, and an analysis is possible based upon the application of Huygen's principle to the case of a cophasally vibrating circular piston with uniform amplitude. However, when transient conditions apply, it may not be sufficient to take account only of the phase of each elementary contribution of the transducer surface because the surface vibration is not continuous. For this reason, all the contributions which combine together to form the field in the steady state may not be present at any particular point in space during a transient, particularly at the beginning and the end of the pulse.

The difficulty of analysing the transient conditions depends partly upon the form of the propagated stress transient. Filipczynski (1956) has applied a geometrical analysis to the build-up of the field in the Fraunhofer zone resulting from the sudden commencement of constant-amplitude sinusoidal oscillation of the transducer. By summing the vector contributions of waves derived from elementary strips on the surface of the transducer, he showed that the initial directivity has the shape of an elongated cylinder, and that this alters continuously towards the steady state situation. The speed of this change is very rapid, and is substantially complete within about half a cycle.

Kaspar'yants (1960) analysed the establishment of the stationary régime in response to a suddenly initiated sinusoidal oscillation of constant amplitude at the transducer. At any point in the medium in which the wave is propagated, the field is zero until the arrival of the disturbance which originates from the surface of the transducer closest to the point under consideration. The field changes until the arrival of the disturbance from the most distant surface of the transducer; but, from this instant onwards, steady-state conditions prevail, because contributions then arrive continuously from the entire surface of the transducer. The reverse process occurs when the oscillation of the transducer suddenly ceases. Kaspar'yants' (1960) solution to the problem can be applied to predict the built up and decay in the region which corresponds in the steady state to the Frésnel zone, where the situation is more complicated, and the transition less rapid, than in the Fraunhofer region considered by Filipćzynski (1956).

Both Christie (1962) and Kossoff (1963) have described the transient response in terms of geometrical analyses. However, in their calculations, they assumed that the amplitudes of successive cycles propagated from the source are equal. This implies an infinite transducer bandwidth, and it is a condition which is not satisfied by many forms of short ultrasonic pulse (see Section 2.8). Under these circumstances, the theoretical predictions of the relative magnitudes of the maxima and minima are incorrect, although their positions are defined with reasonable accuracy. Christie (1962) has shown, both by calculation and by direct measurement, that, for most practical purposes, the directivity of the beam becomes close to the steady state condition within about three to six half-cycles. Kossoff (1963) has pointed out that the transient time is zero at the focus of a focussing system, because all the waves arrive simultaneously at this point: this rapid response is a further advantage of the focussed transducer (see Section 3.2).

Oberhettinger (1961) has made a theoretical analysis, using various integral formulae, of the build-up of the field resulting from a generalized form of excitation of the transducer. The same result has been obtained more recently by Farn and Huang (1968), by consideration of the source density. The solution is naturally rather complicated, but should be used if a prediction of the field is required for excitation other than by a suddenly initiated sinusoid of constant amplitude. However, this situation is usually more easily investigated by experimental observation.

There does not seem to be any description in the literature of the directivity of a transient propagated in a medium which possesses dispersive absorption. Biological tissues have absorption coefficients which are frequency-dependent (see Section 1.16), and the short pulses used in many diagnostic applications have amplitude distributions which extend over a wide frequency spectrum (see Section 2.7). Thus, there is a theoretical possibility that the directivity of the beam is degraded with increasing range, in much the same way that the centre of the frequency spectrum is shifted downwards. This problem remains to be investigated.

3.4 METHODS OF OBSERVATION

3.4.a Schlieren Method

Just over a century ago, Töpler (1867) developed a system capable of making very small changes in refractive index visible in a transparent medium. Töpler's work was based on the earlier discovery of Foucault (1859) of a technique for investigating the surface configuration of a concave mirror. Nowadays, there are many variations of the Töpler schlieren (shadow) method for investigating the enormous range of phenomena with which changes in refractive index are associated. The method depends upon the deflection of a ray of light from its undisturbed path when it passes through a medium in which there is a component of refractive index gradient normal to the ray. The technique is exceedingly sensitive, for a change in refractive index of about 1 part in 10^6 can be observed (Barnes and Bellinger, 1945).

The propagation of an ultrasonic wave is associated with changes in the density of the medium through which it travels. Working independently Debye and Sears (1932) in the U.S.A. and Lucas and Biquard (1932) in France, demonstrated that a transparent medium supporting an ultrasonic wave diffracts light. This diffraction occurs because the density of the medium varies in sympathy with the ultrasonic wave, and the refractive index of the medium depends upon its density.

Several schlieren systems have been described in the literature for the visualization of ultrasonic waves. They all share the same basic principles. A beam of light is arranged to pass through a transparent medium, usually water, in which is established the ultrasonic field to be investigated. The light is then focussed on an obstruction, so that none reaches the observer when the field is zero; alternatively, the focus is arranged to fall in an aperture, so that all the light reaches the observer with zero field. However, when ultrasound changes the refractive index of the medium, the light which passes through the disturbed areas no longer falls at the original focus, but it is deviated so that the proportion of light which reaches the observer is changed. In more precise terms, when there is no ultrasonic disturbance, all the light is undiffracted and so falls in the zero order. In the case of a system where the zero order is occult, the light transmission is approximately proportional to the ultrasonic amplitude within the range 10 to 80% transmission for white light (Willard, 1947). However, if the ultrasonic intensity is increased still further, light reappears in the zero order.

Willard (1947) constructed a schlieren system using a slit source of light which was brought into a parallel beam by means of a lens. This beam was arranged to travel through a water tank in which an ultrasonic disturbance was occurring, and was then focussed by means of a second lens on a bar obstruction. A third lens, placed beyond the obstruction, formed an image of the disturbance, either on a screen, or on a photographic plate. A similar system was devised by Barnes and Burton (1949), save that the necessity for the third lens was avoided by a judicious choice of the focal length and the position of the second lens.

The lenses used in schlieren systems need to be free from spherical and other aberrations, and of at least the same diameter as the part of the ultrasonic field to be investigated. It is very difficult, if not practically impossible, to obtain well-corrected lenses of large diameter. Therefore, it is often best to use concave mirrors in place of lenses. Mirrors can be made paraboloid in section, which eliminates spherical aberration, and they are free from chromatic aberration. Such mirrors, with diameters of some 15 cm and focal lengths of around 100 cm are manufactured to high precision for sale quite cheaply, for instance to amateur astronomers. Sjöberg et al. (1963) have described a single-mirror system. Barnes and Bellinger (1945) pointed out that such systems are twice as sensitive as systems in which the light passes only once through the disturbance; but if the disturbance is intense, the image formed is very difficult to interpret.

James et al. (1961) have described a two-mirror system for the visualization of small ultrasonic fields, of up to about 15 cm diameter. A diagram of the arrangement is shown in Fig. 3.4. The light source, mirror axes and occultation assembly are all in the same plane. In setting up such a system, it is important to ensure that the angles formed between the incident and reflected light beams along the optical axis are equal and as small as possible, in order to avoid coma and to minimize astigmatism. James et al. (1961) used cylindrical lenses close to the light source and to the occultation surface, in order to correct for the astigmatism due to using the mirrors off their axes.

The choice of the kind of occultation assembly may be important. A spot of indian ink on a glass slide is suitable if symmetrical observation is required. However, it frequently happens that a large proportion of the field acts along a main axis, and in this case satisfactory results can often be obtained using a knife-edge normal to the direction of the ultrasonic disturbance.

The schlieren image may be observed directly, thrown upon a suitable screen, or photographed. For example, Fig. 3.5 is a schlieren photograph, obtained using the apparatus of James et al. (1961), of the beam from a 1·8 MHz transducer of 2·0 cm diameter. Standing waves are visible because the beam was not completely absorbed at the base of the tank.

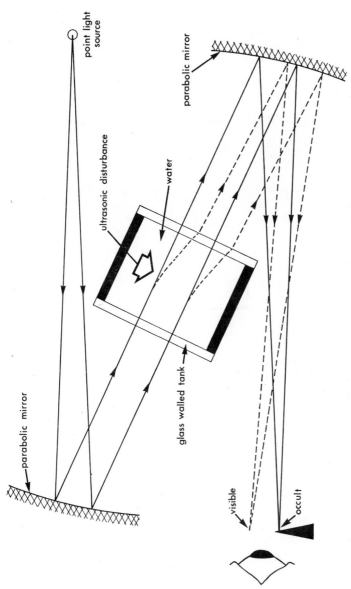

Fig. 3.4 Schlieren optical system using parabolic reflectors. (Adapted from Fig. 4 of James *et al.* 1961.)

The calculated axial intensity distribution is shown beside the schlieren photograph (see Section 3.1).

Qualitative interpretation of the schlieren image is quite simple: the brighter that the image appears, the more intense is the corresponding part of the ultrasonic field. Unfortunately, quantitative analysis may be much more difficult. The intensity of the deviated light depends not only upon the intensity of the ultrasonic disturbance, but also upon its physical extension. The analysis would be quite simple if each ray of light remained in a region of constant density gradient during its passage through the ultrasonic

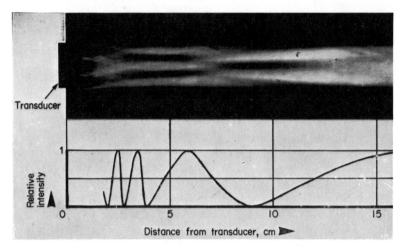

FIG. 3.5 Schlieren photograph of the ultrasonic beam from a 1.8 MHz transducer of 2·0 cm diameter. The graph shows the calculated axial intensity distribution.

disturbance. However, since each ray is continuously refracted this condition may not be satisfied even in a two-dimensional system if the disturbance contains large density gradients. The problem is further complicated in three-dimensional systems by the variation in density across the disturbance.

Ordinary schlieren systems are unsuitable for visualizing very low intensity ultrasonic fields because the light "noise" swamps the schlieren image. This applies not only to continuous wave fields, but also to pulsed beams in which the average intensity is small. However, the ultrasonic power in a single pulse may be quite substantial, and so it may be possible to visualize pulsed fields, which have a low average intensity, by synchronous pulsing of the light source. The time averaged light intensity diffracted by a pulse is equal to that for a continuous wave, reduced by the pulse duty-factor (Lester and Hiedemann, 1962). A pulsed-light technique has been developed by Hunter *et al.* (1964), who used a strobe tube with a flash duration of 0·34 μsec between the ⅓ peak intensity times. Their equipment operated with a pulse repetition frequency of between 100 and 500 Hz, and it was found to be possible to visualize the pulse from a 2·25 MHz transducer. More recently, Aldridge (1967) used a flash tube light source to observe the establishment of standing waves in the ultrasonic field generated by a transducer operating at a frequency of about 2 MHz.

3.4.b Microphones

An ultrasonic field may be plotted by measuring its intensity distribution by means of a non-directional microphone. In addition to being non-directional, a microphone used for investigating pulsed beams must possess non-selective frequency characteristics; in the case of a continuous-wave beam, the microphone must be small in size to avoid the establishment of standing waves. It is not possible to satisfy this last condition at frequencies above about 1 MHz. A probe with cross-sectional dimensions in the order of 0·1 cm has been developed by H. Schilling, and described by Hueter and Bolt (1955), pp. 150–151. The device is satisfactory for continuous-wave operation at frequencies of up to about 150 kHz, where its lateral dimensions are about 0·1 wavelength. However, its frequency response may be substantially flat up to about 1 MHz (Mellen, 1956) and this controls the upper frequency for pulse investigations. Romanenko (1957) has described the construction of a probe consisting of a platinum sphere with a diameter of about 0·01 cm coated with a layer of barium titanate about 0·005 cm thick. This detector element is mounted at the end of a glass rod of about 0·02 cm diameter, and the outside surface is silver plated. The barium titanate layer forms a spherical detector, with the platinum sphere and the silver plating serving as electrodes. For continuous wave investigations, this device is satisfactory at frequencies of up to about 750 kHz, where its lateral dimensions are about 0·1 wavelength; but for plotting pulsed fields, where the establishment of standing waves is not important, the frequency response is satisfactory up to a frequency of about 10 MHz, and the directivity pattern is circular in the plane normal to the axis of the detector mounting.

Schmitt (1961) has described how ceramic capacitors may be used as microphones for plotting ultrasonic field distributions. Such capacitors are inexpensive, and quite small sizes can be obtained.

Koppelmann (1952) has described the construction of microphones in which the ultrasound is conducted along a waveguide, in the form of a slim metal rod, from the liquid supporting the field to the transducer. This form of detector is capable of operating at frequencies of up to at least 500 kHz. Saneyoshi et al. (1966) have constructed microphones similar to those of Koppelmann (1952), apparently without knowledge of his earlier work: their microphones are suitable for operation at frequencies of up to about 1 MHz.

A convenient microphone for plotting pulsed ultrasonic fields may be constructed by collimating a large transducer to a small aperture. A cork annulus forms a suitable collimator. The transducer may either be of wide frequency bandwidth (Aveyard, 1962; Hodgkinson, 1966) or it may have a resonant frequency far removed from the centre frequency of the pulse under investigation (Christie, 1962).

Several systems for beam plotting using this kind of detector have been described in the literature. For example, Christie (1962) constructed a water tank in which the detector could be moved by a manually operated system to any point in the ultrasonic field. Measurements were made from an oscilloscope on which the detected pulse was displayed: the time-base of the oscilloscope was triggered by a pulse appropriately delayed in time from the instant of excitation of the source transducer. In this way, it was possible to deduce the field distribution at various stages during the pulse (see Section 3.3).

Aveyard (1962) developed an automatic beam plotting equipment, with a write-out system employing the Mufax facsimile recorder manufactured by Muirhead and Co. Ltd. The Mufax recorder uses a moist chemically treated paper which is passed between two electrodes. The system was arranged to produce a representation of the intensity distribution of the ultrasonic beam in which the degree of blackening is proportional to the ultrasonic intensity. Hodgkinson (1966) devised a technique by which the write-out of Aveyard's (1962) system was quantized into six discrete grey-tones. The quantizing circuit was designed to accept a continuously varying signal, which was separated into bands of 6 dB intensity range for presentation on the recorder. The lines of transition between adjacent areas of different grey tone correspond to lines of constant intensity separated by 6 dB. For this reason, the recordings are called "isosonographs".

In systems in which a microphone is used to plot the ultrasonic field, the amplitude of the pulse displayed on the write-out generally corresponds to the amplitude of the largest half-cycle in the ultrasonic pulse, if full-wave demodulation is employed (see Section 4.4.e). This half-cycle is normally at least the second, and frequently the third or some subsequent half-cycle, and so the beam pattern corresponds fairly closely to the distribution predicted by continuous wave theory (see Section 3.3).

3.4.c Pulse–echo Methods

A method which is quite widely used for plotting the effective distribution of a pulsed ultrasonic beam is to measure the echo amplitudes from a small target situated in turn at many points in the field propagated in a water bath. The technique has been described, for example, by Panian and van Valkenburg (1961), Gordon (1964), and Wells (1966a, 1966b). The essentials of the pulse–echo system are explained in Section 4.1.a; for echo amplitude measurement, it is usually best to employ a null method, using a calibrated attenuator in the connection between the transducer and the receiver amplifier. The amplitude on the display is kept constant as the target is moved in the field, by making appropriate alterations to the attenuation. Relative echo amplitudes can then be expressed directly in decibels, read from the settings of the attenuator. Because the display amplitude is kept constant, any non-linearities in the receiver amplifier introduce only second-order errors due to alterations in the shape of the echo signal. Alternatively, the attenuator may be inserted in the connection to the transducer so that both the transmitted and received pulses are equally attenuated. In this arrangement, relative echo amplitudes are equal to one half of the difference in the corresponding attenuator settings, provided that the pulse shape is not intensity dependent within the range investigated (see Section 1.17).

A small ball-bearing makes an excellent target for this investigation. Such a target is self aligning, because it is spherical in shape and so non-directional, presenting a similar surface to the beam independent of its position. The target may be attached to a wire soldered to its rear surface, and so be fixed to a support attached to a suitable co-ordinate measuring system. If this wire is made sufficiently long behind the target, no confusion arises between echoes from the target and those from the support. In general, the sphere should be chosen to be as small as possible consistent with an adequate echo amplitude and rigid mounting, and a diameter of about 0·3 cm is usually satisfactory. However, for sensitivity calibration, Gordon (1964) suggested the use of a steel sphere of 1 cm diameter, which could be considered to possess an "echo coefficient" of zero decibels.

The technique produces a representation of the beam which is actually used in the pulse-echo application. The amplitude measured corresponds to the largest half-cycle in the received pulse, if full wave demodulation is employed (see Section 4.4.e). The displayed signal has been generated by the system transmitter, transduced twice, and processed by the amplifier which is actually used for diagnostic observations, and so in many respects this technique for beam plotting is to be commended. Double transduction not only changes the bandwidth of the system, but also modifies the effective directivity of the beam to that corresponding to D_s^2 (see Section 3.1).

An example of an ultrasonic beam plotted by this technique is shown in Fig. 3.6. The transducer diameter was 2.0 cm and the frequency corresponding to the pulse was 1·7 MHz: these conditions resemble the continuous-wave situation illustrated in Fig. 3.5. The results can be presented in several forms. For example, in Fig. 3.6.a, the data are plotted as lines of equal echo amplitude (iso-echo amplitude curves), whereas in Fig. 3.6.b, the same data are shown in the form of the echo amplitude distributions across the beam diameter at various distances from the transducer. It is not possible to measure the distribution very close to the transducer, partly because the pattern is rather complicated, and partly because the paralysis of the receiver amplifier which results from the application of the transmitting pulse continues for a time which corresponds to a centimetre or two of

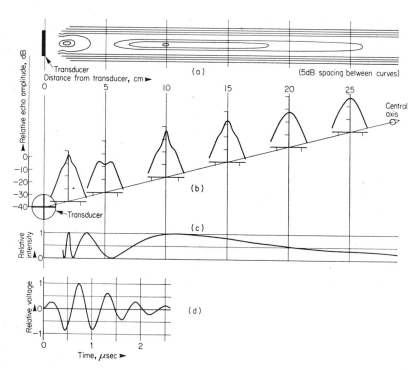

FIG. 3.6 Methods of plotting the ultrasonic field. These examples are for a 1·7 MHz transducer of 2·0 cm diameter. (a) Iso-echo amplitude curves; (b) Diametrical distributions; (c) Theoretical axial intensity distribution; (d) Echo from a flat target, using the transducer with which (a) and (b) were obtained. Diagrams (a) and (b) were plotted experimentally using a 0·32 cm diameter steel ball as a target.

range in front of the transducer (see Section 4.4.a). For comparison, the theoretical axial distribution for a piston of diameter equal to that of the experimental transducer, vibrating cophasally with constant amplitude, at a frequency equal to that of the pulse, is shown in Fig. 3.6.c. The echo detected from a flat reflector situated at a distance equal to less than one half the experimentally determined position of the last axial maximum is shown in Fig. 3.6.d.

3.4.d Other Methods

There are a number of optical methods for investigating ultrasonic fields in addition to the schlieren method described in Section 3.4.a. For example, Barnes and Bellinger (1945) mention the shadowgraph technique, and Nomoto (1954a, 1954b) and Gessert and Hiedemann (1956) describe the theory and application of ultrasonic stroboscopes. However, these methods seem to be only of limited use in the evaluation of diagnostic ultrasonic fields.

Ultrasonic fields can be investigated by means of the image systems described in Section 6.4. Pulsed fields are generally easier to study by this technique than continuous wave fields because the large detector may lead to the establishment of standing waves.

Fry and Fry (1954a, 1954b) devised a method by which the absolute intensity distribution of an ultrasonic field may be investigated. The basis of the technique is the measurement of the time rate of change of temperature of a thermocouple embedded in an absorbing medium, which occurs as a result of irradiation with a pulse of ultrasound with a duration of about one second. Whilst this system is remarkably accurate at medium intensities in the megahertz frequency range, it has the disadvantage that it is not very sensitive, and so it is rather unsuitable for investigating the low intensity fields used in most diagnostic applications.

Various other methods exist for ultrasonoscopy and ultrasonography. These include the use of temperature-sensitive chromotrophic compounds, dyes, and phosphors. These techniques have been reviewed by Ernst and Hoffman (1952). However, their sensitivities are generally too low for the effective study of diagnostic fields.

It is interesting that most attention has been paid in the literature to the study of the field generated by the ultrasonic source: only the technique described in Section 3.4.c takes into account the directivity of the receiver. A natural extension of the use of a microphone to plot the field of the source (see Section 3.4.b) would seem to be to replace the microphone by a small omnidirectional transmitter, and to use this to investigate the sensitivity of the receiver. This method remains to be investigated.

3.5 POWER MEASUREMENT

There are a number of methods by which the power of an ultrasonic beam may be measured. At megahertz frequencies, both calorimetric and radiation pressure methods are satisfactory (Wells et al. 1963). The calorimetric method is based on the complete absorption of the ultrasonic energy which is to be measured: the energy then appears in the form of heat. These techniques can be used to measure powers above about 100 mW, without the need for elaborate apparatus, although difficulties may occur due to confusion between heat due to ultrasonic absorption and heat due to the inefficiency of the transducer.

Radiation pressure measurements are based on the phenomenon described in Section 1.13. The design of the most appropriate detector depends upon the total power and size of the ultrasonic beam cross-section. For example, Newell (1963) has described a radiation pressure balance in which four horizontal torsion wires are used as the suspension: this eliminates friction. The detecting surface is arranged so that measurements are independent of the position and uniformity of the ultrasonic field. This balance has a maximum sensitivity of 0·1 cm deflection for 60 mW of ultrasonic power.

Very sensitive detectors are necessary for the measurement of the radiation pressures produced by the low ultrasonic powers used in most diagnostic applications. The force corresponding to the complete absorption of a beam with a total power of 1 W, travelling in water at 20°C, is about 0·069 g. Twice this force is produced by the same power if the beam is completely reflected, but the potential improvement in sensitivity is largely offset by the probability of the occurrence of errors due to multiple reflections. In diagnostic techniques, total average ultrasonic powers of around 1 mW are quite common: this power corresponds to a force of 69 μg. when completely absorbed.

Two systems capable of measuring such small forces have been described in the literature. Wells et al. (1964) have developed a radiometer, the essential principles of which are shown in Fig. 3.7. The reflecting vane consists of an air-filled box constructed from aluminium, suspended from two fine wires, each about one metre long. The vane itself is buoyant in water, but it is arranged to sink at an angle of 45° to the horizontal by means of two aluminium bars, attached to the vane at each end of its horizontal diameter. The effective net weight of the vane is about 300 mg. Measurements are made by observation of the deflection of the vane when it is struck by the horizontally directed ultrasonic beam. The vane behaves as if it were a perfect absorber, because the reflected ultrasound acts vertically, and so produces no horizontal force component. Multiple reflections are avoided by the use of a static absorbing system. In a typical experiment, the errors in the measuring system were all smaller than the scatter of the separate observations. This scatter was probably due to the effect of dust particles on the surface of the water. Nevertheless, the instrument is accurate to ±3% in measuring a 2 mW beam, and it is sensitive enough to detect powers as small as 0·01 mW.

Kossoff (1965) has described the construction of a radiation pressure detector using a modified analytical balance to measure the force. The sensitivity of this instrument is about 0·01 mg corresponding to an accuracy of about ±7% in the measurement of a power of 2 mW.

Radiation pressure is directional, and so measurement of the associated force yields the value of the total ultrasonic power travelling normal to the detector. Thus the device measures the vector component of the ultrasonic power, and geometrical corrections may be necessary to obtain the value of the total beam power. In the case of a pulsed beam, the detector measures the time average of the ultrasonic power (if its time-constant is long

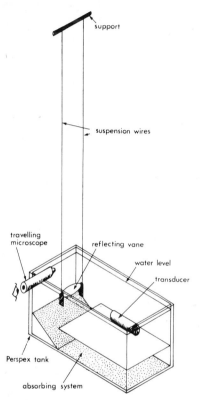

FIG. 3.7 Radiometer of Wells *et al.* (1964), for the measurement of low ultrasonic powers.

compared with the pulse repetition period), and so it is a simple matter to calculate the energy per pulse, if the pulse repetition frequency is known. Similarly, if the shape of the ultrasonic pulse is known, it is possible to calculate the peak power in the pulse.

The absolute intensity of an ultrasonic pulse may also be measured by means of a suitable electrodynamic transducer. Filipczynski and Groniowski (1967) have described two forms of transducer for this purpose, one of which is an electromagnetic device, and the other, electrostatic. The electromagnetic transducer, explained in greater detail by Filipczynski

(1967), consists of a rectangular block of Perspex on which a conductor, in the form of 10 windings of aluminium, 2μ thick, are evaporated. The block is arranged so that one of the flat surfaces on which the conductor is deposited is situated between the poles of a powerful magnet. If this surface is set into vibration by the passage of an ultrasonic pulse, a voltage is induced in the conductor which is proportional to the velocity of the surface. The corresponding ultrasonic power may be calculated by consideration of the characteristic impedances of the media on each side of the conductor, and the strength of the magnetic field. For a typical diagnostic pulse travelling in water, the voltage generated by an electromagnetic transducer might be in the order of a few hundred microvolts.

The electrostatic transducer described by Filipćzynski and Groniowski (1967) is similar to those of Kolsky (1956), Filipćzynski (1966) and Gauster and Breazeale (1966). These instruments were developed independently. The device consists of a parallel plate capacitor, one plate of which is displaced by the reflection of the ultrasonic pulse. The spacing between the two plates is made very small, so that the variation in capacitance due to the reflection of an ultrasonic pulse is large enough to produce a measurable alternating voltage in the presence of a polarizing voltage derived from a high-impedance source. The sensitivity depends upon the spacing, the polarizing voltage, and the effective electrical load impedance. With a spacing of about 30 μ, and a polarizing potential of 212 volts, Filipćzynski's (1966) transducer gave an output in the order of 1 mV when excited by a typical diagnostic pulse travelling in a solid. The sensitivity of the device is substantially reduced if it is used immersed in water, because of the reflection at the water to solid interface. The transducer of Gauster and Breazeale (1966) has a spacing of around 10 μ, and the polarizing voltage (250 volts in series with a 1 MΩ resistor) corresponds to a potential gradient of 250 kV.cm^{-1}. Using special constructional techniques, Arnold et $al.$ (1967) have been able to reduce the spacing to about 3 μ, and to increase the potential gradient to 750 kV.cm^{-1}. These improvements give a useful increase in sensitivity.

Blitz and Warren (1968) have described a capacitor microphone designed specifically for the measurement of ultrasonic transducers used in pulse-echo diagnostic applications. The gap spacing is 70 μ, and the polarizing supply is 300 V in series with a 1 MΩ resistor. The output voltage corresponding to a typical ultrasonic pulse is in the order of 500 μV.

4. PULSE-ECHO TECHNIQUES

4.1 INTRODUCTION

4.1.a Basic Principles

The history of the development of the ultrasonic pulse-echo flaw detector is somewhat uncertain. P. Langevin had already devised his ultrasonic depth sounder before 1920, and some fifteen years later the possibility of using a similar method for detecting defects in metals was proposed by S. Ya. Sokolov. However, the method could not be exploited at that time because electronic pulse techniques were not sufficiently advanced. Suitable pulse circuits were developed in the early 1940's, primarily for use in Radar, and these were soon applied to ultrasonics. Prominent amongst the early pioneers were F. A. Firestone in the U.S.A., and D. O. Sproule in Great Britain. Unfortunately, it is not possible to trace the course of these developments exactly, because of the wartime secrecy by which they were concealed. The earliest publication seems to be that of Firestone (1945). The likely importance of the new technique in medical diagnosis was realized soon after the war: something of the history of the applications to medicine is given in Section 4.7.

The basic principles of the pulse-echo system are illustrated in Fig. 4.1. The diagrams show how an ultrasonic pulse may be used to measure the depth of an echo-producing interface. The ultrasonic probe is arranged to emit a short-duration stress wave into medium (i), in response to an electrical excitation. At the same instant, the luminescent spot on the screen of a cathode ray tube display begins to move at constant velocity from left to right. The vertical deflection plates of the cathode ray tube are connected to the output from an amplifier, the input of which is derived from the ultrasonic probe. Therefore, the luminescent spot is deflected vertically at the instant that the stress wave is transmitted, because the exciting voltage is also applied to the amplifier (Fig. 4.1.a). The stress wave travels at constant velocity through medium (i), and the luminescent spot traces a horizontal line on the display (Fig. 4.1.b). After some time (Fig. 4.1.c), the stress wave encounters the interface between media (i) and (ii). Some of the energy is reflected back into medium (i) at the interface, and some travels on into medium (ii) (Fig. 4.1.d); the reflectivity of the interface is determined by the characteristic impedance ratio, and the configuration of the surface (see Sections 1.8 and 1.9). After some time, the reflected stress wave returns to the transducer, where it generates a voltage which is amplified to deflect the trace on the display (Fig. 4.1.e). The transmitted stress wave travels on into medium (ii), some of the reflected wave is absorbed by the transducer, and the trace on the display has two vertical deflections the distance between which is proportional to the thickness of medium (i)

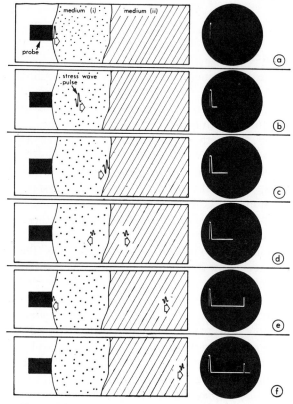

FIG. 4.1 Basic principles of the pulse-echo system.

(Fig. 4.1.f). If the process is repeated sufficiently rapidly (at a frequency of more than about 20 Hz), a steady trace is observed on the display. The method can be extended to the examination of many interfaces lying along the ultrasonic path.

Figure 4.2.a is a block diagram showing the relationships between the various components of an ultrasonic pulse-echo system, such as that which might be used to obtain the display illustrated in Figs. 4.1. This particular kind of display is called an "A-scan" (see Section 4.7.a). The rate generator (Section 4.2) provides a trigger pulse for the transmitter, the swept gain

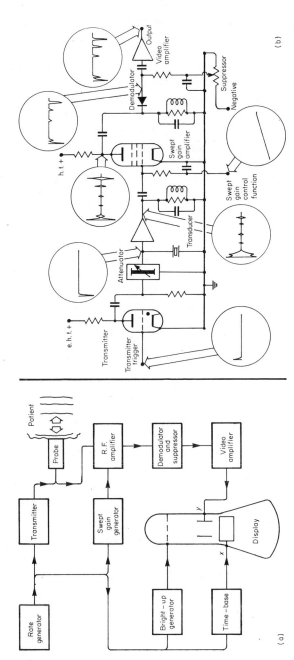

Fig. 4.2 Typical pulse-echo system. (a) Block diagram. The arrangement illustrated employs an ultrasonic probe in direct contact with the patient, and an A-scope display. (b) Typical signal processing circuitry of the pulse-echo system illustrated in (a).

generator, the bright-up pulse generator and the time-base. The minimum repetition rate is that which is required to produce a satisfactory display, in terms of brightness, freedom from flicker, time resolution and scanning rate; the maximum rate is limited by the required penetration, the reverberation decay time, the maximum speed of any associated recording system, and the increasing risk of biological damage.

Figure 4.2.b is a diagram showing typical signal processing circuitry. The transmitter (Section 4.3) generates an electrical pulse which excites the transducer to emit a stress wave. The signal output from the transducer is fed to the radio-frequency amplifier (Section 4.4). The gain of this amplifier may be increased with time by the swept gain generator, to compensate to some extent for the increasing attenuation by absorption of the echoes from deeper structures. In the example illustrated in Fig. 4.2, the swept gain circuits are triggered at the instant that the ultrasonic pulse is transmitted; but in the case of a variable-delay water bath scanner, it is necessary to arrange for the swept gain circuits to be triggered at the instant that the first echo returns from the patient, because of the relatively very low absorption in water (see Section 4.5.d). Sometimes, the receiver is designed to have a logarithmic response. The bright-up pulse generator (Section 4.6.a) provides a rectangular pulse which switches on the display only during the time that echo information is being received; thus, the flyback of the time-base does not appear. The time-base (Section 4.2) generates a voltage ramp which deflects the trace at a constant velocity appropriate to the penetration. The output from the r.f. amplifier is demodulated, and the dynamic range may be restricted by suppression of the smaller echo signals (Section 4.4.e) before being fed to the video amplifier. The output from this amplifier (Section 4.5) is connected to the y-deflection plates of the cathode ray tube to produce an A-scan (Section 4.7.a), or to the cathode of the cathode ray tube to produce a B-scan (Sections 4.7.b and 4.7.c).

Pulse echo systems are suitable for many applications in medical diagnosis. Numerous variations of the circuit arrangement are possible: some of these are described in the following Sections, in relation to the physical and technical aspects of the differences between the systems.

4.1.b Dynamic Range, Swept Gain and Resolution

Within the limitations imposed by noise and maximum transmitted power (see Section 4.4.a), the useful dynamic range of the echoes received in diagnostic pulse systems is in the order of 100 dB. Typically, some 50 dB of this range is due to the attenuation of the echoes from deeper interfaces by absorption, and compensation for this can be partially provided by the use of swept gain. This matter is considered in more detail later in this section. Swept gain is a method by which the gain of the receiver is increased with time so that the echoes from deeper structures are amplified more than those which originate nearer to the transducer, and so arrive earlier. Some of the methods by which swept gain compensation is achieved are discussed in Section 4.4.

The maximum useful signal dynamic range which remains after swept gain compensation is in the order of 50 dB, although this may be restricted by the dynamic range of the transducer (see Section 2.10) if the very small echoes are closely preceeded by echoes of large amplitude. A dynamic range of about 40 dB can be displayed directly on an A-scope. Additional dynamic range compression is required for B-scope presentation. This is because the dynamic range of brightness-modulation for a typical cathode ray tube is around 20 dB (see Section 4.7.b), and much less in the case of an electronic storage tube (Section 4.6.b). If the r.f. amplifier has a linear amplitude response, the dynamic range compression must be applied in the video amplifier (Section 4.5.c).

The resolution of a system may be defined in a number of different ways. For example, the resolution may be taken to be equal to the minimum distance between two point targets at which separate registrations can just be distinguished on the display. An alternative definition, which is usually more convenient in practice, is to specify the area or distance which appears on the display to be occupied by a point target in the field. In ultrasonic systems, two different resolutions are of importance: these are the lateral resolution, which describes the resolution along the beam diameter normal to the axis, and the range resolution, which is the resolution along the axis. Both these quantities depend on a number of factors, including the distance from the transducer. The effect of distance is particularly important in the case of the lateral resolution.

The resolution may be limited by the spot size of the display (see Section 4.6.a). The spot diameter is about 0·05 cm with a good quality cathode ray tube used as a B-scope display, although it is possible to estimate the position of the trace on an A-scan with rather better precision. No advantage is gained if the total resolution of all the other elements is made better than that corresponding to the spot size; however, it is only seldom that the spot size is the limiting factor in practice.

The lateral resolution of pulse-echo systems is usually limited by the signal dynamic range which remains after swept gain compensation. At any given distance from the transducer, structures may be expected to be detected as echoes the amplitudes of which may vary over a range of 50 dB, according to the interface characteristics. Doubtless the dynamic range is really very much larger than this: but it is restricted to not more than about 50 dB by the performance of the system, which determines the maximum overall dynamic range, and by the required penetration, which determines what proportion of the total dynamic range is due to absorption.

The relationship between dynamic range and lateral resolution is of such importance that a detailed discussion is necessary. Some aspects of the ultrasonic field and its distribution have already been considered in Chapter 3; in particular, Fig. 3.1 may be found helpful in the following discussion, in addition to the diagrams which directly illustrate the various points. Thus, Fig. 4.3 shows how the amplitude of the echo received from a small spherical target in water was found to change experimentally as the target was moved across the beam diameter at various distances from the plane transducer, for a series of operating frequencies and transducer diameters. The calculated steady-state positions of the last axial maxima for the corresponding transducers driven cophasally are indicated in the diagrams. Certain features of the data are immediately obvious: for example, the length of the Frésnel zone increases with increasing frequency, for a given transducer diameter, and with increasing transducer diameter, for a given frequency.

The ultrasonic absorption coefficient of water is $0 \cdot 0022$ dB.cm^{-1} at 1 MHz, and is proportional to the square of the frequency (see Table 1.7). For a path length of 40 cm (go-and-return penetration of 20 cm) at a frequency of 5 MHz, the corresponding attenuation due to absorption is $2 \cdot 2$ dB. This absorption is small compared with that which would occur in soft tissues (about 200 dB), and the curves illustrated in Fig. 4.3 may be taken as being for a lossless medium, without fear of introducing qualitative errors into the discussion which follows.

Figure 4.4 shows the effective lateral resolutions for each of the transducers illustrated in Fig. 4.3, for various dynamic ranges. The resolutions were calculated by assuming that the gain of the system was first adjusted so that a non-directional point target of a given reflectivity could just be detected when positioned at the most sensitive part of the field; the gain was then increased by a quantity equal to the dynamic range under consideration. The black areas shown in Fig. 4.4 correspond to those parts of the fields in which the same target would then be detected.

Consider the situation where the system being examined contains two types of non-directional target, randomly distributed. Further, assume that one type of target has a reflectivity of 10 dB more than the other. The beam distribution within which targets are detected is determined by the gain and dynamic range of the pulse-echo system. If the gain is adjusted so that the weaker targets are just not detected, and if the dynamic range is made equal to 10 dB (for example, by adjustment of the suppression level: see Section 4.4.e), then only those stronger targets which lie within the black areas in Fig. 4.4.a will be detected. If the gain is increased by 10 dB, and the dynamic range is kept equal to 10 dB, the stronger targets lying within black areas in Fig. 4.4.b will be detected, and so will all the targets lying within the black areas in Fig. 4.4.a. Similarly, if the gain is increased by a further 10 dB, and the dynamic range remains equal to 10 dB, the stronger

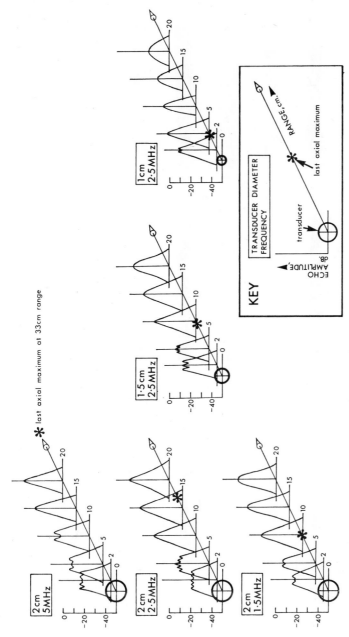

FIG. 4.3 Echo amplitude curves for pulse-echo transducers of various frequencies and diameters, plotted in water. The calculated positions of the last axial maxima for continuous wave conditions are shown. Target: steel sphere, diameter 0·63 cm. (Adapted from Figs 5 and 6 of Wells, 1966b).

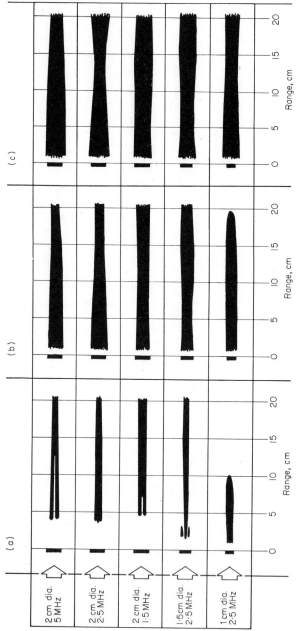

FIG. 4.4 Diagrams showing the lateral resolutions of the ultrasonic beams illustrated in Fig. 4.3. Dynamic range: (a) 10 dB; (b) 20 dB; (c) 30 dB.

targets within the black areas of Fig. 4.4.c, and all the targets in Fig. 4.4.b, will be detected. Under these circumstances, if a third type of target, of 20 dB lower reflectivity than that of the strongest type of target, were to be randomly distributed in the system, only the weakest targets lying within the black areas of Fig. 4.4.a would be detected. This example illustrates how the lateral resolution is determined by the dynamic range of the echoes which are of clinical significance, and also shows how a single weak target might, under some circumstances, appear to be several separate targets lying side by side.

The lateral resolution in the Frésnel zone can be improved if a focussed ultrasonic beam is used. The matter has already been discussed in Section 3.2. The data shown in Fig. 3.3 may be used as the basis for calculations of the resolution improvement which can be obtained under specified conditions.

The preceding discussion applies to targets situated in a relatively lossless medium. In a medium with a constant absorption rate, swept gain can be applied to compensate for absorption. However, correction for dispersive absorption is quite difficult in the case of a pulse observed by electronic systems of finite bandwidth. This is illustrated by Fig. 4.5. The details of this figure are explained in its legend. Figure 4.5.a, curve (iii), is the overall response of the receiving system in this example. Figure 4.5.b shows the various frequency spectra, each spectrum corresponding to a particular target range, which are further modified by the frequency response of the receiver before being fed to the display. The maximum amplitudes corresponding to each particular range are plotted in curve (i) of Fig. 4.5.c. On the same axes, curve (ii) shows the corresponding amplitude for continuous wave reflection (zero bandwidth), and curve (iii) shows the linear relationship which deviates by the minimum amount from curve (i) over a 50 dB dynamic range. The maximum deviation is 6·5 dB, and the slope of curve (iii) is 3·9 dB.cm^{-1}, which is the best rate of exponential swept gain in this example. Extending this result to other frequencies (and assuming similar shapes for the frequency response characteristics), the optimum swept gain rate would be $1·6\alpha N$ dB.cm^{-1}, where α is the absorption coefficient for continuous waves, and N is the frequency of the pulse in megahertz.

The situation is made more complicated if, as is usually the case, varying thicknesses of materials of differing absorption coefficient lie in the ultrasonic path. In practice, the mean value of absorption coefficient seems to be somewhat less than 1 dB.cm^{-1} MHz^{-1} for soft tissues: this is probably due to the presence of blood and other relatively low-loss materials. This is particularly true, for example, in cysts, liver, heart and the pregnant uterus. As a rough guide, a swept gain rate of about 1·3N dB.cm^{-1} is generally satisfactory, but the exact rate needs to be determined for each particular case.

As a consequence of the uncertainty in the effective value of the absorption

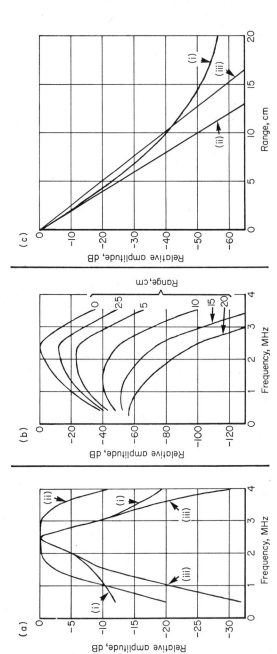

Fig. 4.5 Diagrams to illustrate the effect of system bandwidth on echo amplitude with a dispersive absorber. These diagrams are for a 2·5 MHz transducer and an absorption coefficient of 1 dB cm⁻¹ MHz⁻¹.

(a) Curve (i)   Transducer receiving characteristic; backed by tungsten powder in Araldite. (Adapted from Fig. 6 of Kossoff (1966).)

Curve (ii)   Typical response of r.f. and video amplifier combination.

Curve (iii) Overall response of receiving system.

(b) Pulse frequency spectra after modification by the receiving system, for various target ranges (range = ½ total go-and-return path length).

These spectra were calculated from the data in Fig. 2.8, with the addition of the curve for 15 cm range.

(c) Curve (i)   Relative pulse amplitudes at spectral maxima plotted against range, for a target of constant reflectivity.

Curve (ii)   Corresponding relationship for continuous wave reflection.

Curve (iii) Logarithmic attenuation corresponding to minimum deviation from Curve (i) over 50 dB dynamic range.

coefficient, the accuracy with which swept gain can be applied may not be good, and it becomes necessary to use a wider dynamic range than that which would be required on the basis of variations in target reflectivity alone. Therefore, it is difficult to estimate the lateral resolution of a system at any particular distance from the transducer because of the uncertainty in the value of the effective dynamic range. In addition, it is pointed out in Section 3.3 that there is a theoretical possibility of degradation in the lateral resolution due to beam broadening resulting from the shift to lower frequencies of the pulse energy when propagated in a medium with dispersive absorption.

The range resolution of a pulse-echo system is normally much better than the practical lateral resolution. The range resolution is determined by the precision with which the position in time of the arrival of an echo can be measured. This depends upon the shape of the ultrasonic pulse, and the gain, dynamic range and bandwidth of the receiver. Consider, for example, the received echo pulse shown in Fig. 4.6. Each of the four oscillograms shows the same pulse, transmitted and received by the same transducer, but with the gain of the wideband oscilloscope on which the pulse was displayed set to 0, +10, +20 and +30 dB respectively. However, the set of oscillograms could equally well correspond to the situation where the system sensitivity is kept constant, but the reflectivity of the target is increased in 10 dB steps. The approximate ultrasonic frequency is 1·8 MHz, estimated from the time-positions of the zeroes. Unlike the lateral resolution, the range resolution is only slightly dependent on the diameter of the transducer, and most pulses have a similar shape whatever the frequency. Therefore, the discussion which follows is quite general, and may be extended to the consideration of other situations.

Consider the situation where the threshold of the system is such that only structures which produce echoes whose amplitudes are greater than one major division of the oscilloscope graticule in Fig. 4.6 are registered on the display. If an echo such as that shown in Fig. 4.6 for 0 dB is applied to the system, it will not produce a registration. However, if the gain of the receiver (or reflectivity of the target) is increased by 10 dB, then the range resolution will extend over a distance corresponding to 1·6 μsec (assuming full-wave demodulation is employed: see Section 4.4.e). Similarly, the time-resolution corresponding to increases of 20 and 30 dB can be seen to be 2·7 and 3·5 μsec respectively. These time intervals correspond to distances of about 0·12, 0·20 and 0·26 cm respectively for dynamic ranges of 10, 20 and 30 dB. The dynamic range is equal to the difference between the threshold level and the maximum amplitude of the pulse. For the same transducer, the corresponding lateral resolutions at a distance of 10 cm (see Fig. 4.4) might be about 1·0, 1·6 and 2·5 cm respectively. Thus, in this example, the lateral resolution is around ten times worse than the range resolution.

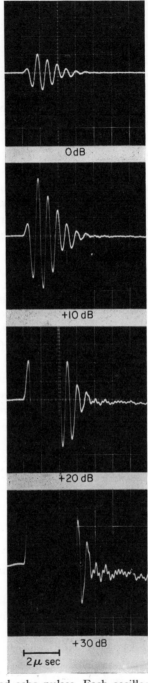

Fig. 4.6 Typical received echo pulses. Each oscillogram shows the same pulse, but for various receiver gains. Frequency 1·8 MHz.

The pulse waveforms illustrated in Fig. 4.6 were obtained directly from the transducer and displayed on a wideband oscilloscope. In a pulse-echo system, the pulses would normally be applied to an amplifier of limited frequency bandwidth. However, if the bandwidths of the r.f. and video amplifiers are each made equal to the centre frequency of the ultrasonic pulse (see Sections 4.4 and 4.5), then the transducer is usually the most important element controlling the frequency response, and the receiver only slightly degrades the range resolution. In general, a typical system will give range resolutions of about 1·5, 2·5 and 3 wavelengths with dynamic ranges of 10, 20 and 30 dB respectively.

The time duration of the displayed pulse is but one aspect of the range resolution of the system. The precision of the system in the estimation of the position of a reflecting surface may sometimes be of equal importance. In Fig. 4.6 the beginning of the echo pulse corresponding to 30 dB dynamic range is quite clearly defined because the pulse amplitude rapidly rises above the threshold when the dynamic range and gain are large. Therefore, only a small error is introduced if the position of the interface is taken to correspond to the beginning of the display registration. All the oscillograms in Fig. 4.6 were photographed with the same time relationship to the oscilloscope graticule. It can be seen that an error of about 0·3 λ occurs if the same criterion is used with a dynamic range of 20 dB; the error increases to about 0·8 λ with a dynamic range of 10 dB. If half-wave demodulation is used, the precision may be degraded by a distance of about 0·5 λ.

It might be expected that half-wave demodulation would be preferable to full wave demodulation, because there is a possibility that, if the pulse is of an appropriate shape, the range resolution may be increased by a distance corresponding to as much as a wavelength. However, the advantage of a range resolution apparently improved by this effect is generally offset by the disadvantage of less efficient demodulation. In addition, any improvement in range resolution which may be achieved by half-wave demodulation is obtained at the expense of a loss in the precision of range resolution, and this may be an important disadvantage.

The estimation of range resolution on the basis of pulse shape and dynamic range becomes more difficult if the pulse is propagated in media which possess dispersive absorption, such as biological soft tissues. Some aspects of the problem have already been discussed in Section 2.7. The fundamental effect is that the stress wave as transmitted contains energy spread over a wide frequency spectrum, and the higher frequency components of the pulse are dissipated with distance more rapidly than those of lower frequencies. The problem is made more complicated, although the magnitude of the overall effect is reduced, by the restricted bandwidth of the receiving system. Thus, if the receiver had a zero bandwidth centred on the transmitted pulse frequency, the effects of dispersion would be eliminated because the system would only respond to energy at this single frequency. However, such a system would be unsuitable for pulse-echo work because it would give rise in the limit to infinite pulse-stretching. On the other hand, a receiver with infinite bandwidth would be best from the point of view of range resolution and precision, but it would be most subject to the effects of dispersion, in addition to possessing a poor signal-to-noise ratio (see Section 4.4.a). Therefore, a compromise is necessary. It has already been explained that the usual arrangement is to make the bandwidth of the electronics sufficiently wide that the transducer is the effective bandwidth limiting component. For example, the overall response of a transducer backed with a mixture of tungsten powder in Araldite and unmatched to the load is typically 6 dB down with a bandwidth of 20% of the centre frequency of the device (see curve (iii), Fig. 2.9).

Pulse stretching due to dispersive absorption and finite system bandwidth certainly degrades the range resolution and the precision. However, in most practical systems, these quantities remain substantially less than the lateral resolution, and so the effects may often be neglected. On the other hand, the effective absorption rate may be significantly modified by the spectral frequency shift which occurs in a dispersive absorber. Such a shift leads to difficulty in swept gain compensation, which in practical terms means that the dynamic range of the system needs to be made larger than would be necessary if the swept gain were accurate. It has already been shown in this section that, as a rough guide, a pulse with a transmitted ultrasonic frequency of N MHz may be taken to be absorbed at a rate of $1{\cdot}3N$ dB.cm^{-1} of penetration (target range) in soft tissues. On this basis, 50 dB of dynamic range due to absorption would correspond to a penetration of about 25 cm at a frequency of $1{\cdot}5$ MHz, and this is about the maximum penetration which would be possible at this frequency.

A constant rate of swept gain, even if it is adjusted to about $1{\cdot}3N$ dB.cm^{-1}, is associated with errors in compensation. This is because the cumulative effects of dispersion become more important as the range is increased. This can be seen by consideration of the data in Fig. 4.5.c. As the dispersive absorption is increased, so the higher-frequency components are lost more rapidly than those of lower frequency. However, if the system has a limited bandwidth, the change in the magnitude of the output from the receiver amplifier for a given change in the range of the reflecting interface decreases as the total range of the interface is increased.

4.1.c Interface Characteristics

The reflectivities of various biological interfaces have already been discussed in Section 1.8, for the rather idealized case of normal incidence on a perfectly flat boundary. The situation becomes much more complicated when the incidence is not normal, or when the interface is very close to the transducer. For example, Fig. 4.7 shows how the echo amplitude depends upon the angle of incidence at various target ranges with a typical pulse-echo system. The amplitudes are expressed in decibels relative to the amplitude at normal incidence. In the particular example illustrated here, the amplitude is reduced by about 22 dB at an angle of incidence of 3° from normal, irrespective of the target range. At greater angulation, the subsequent reduction increases with the range. The maxima and minima which

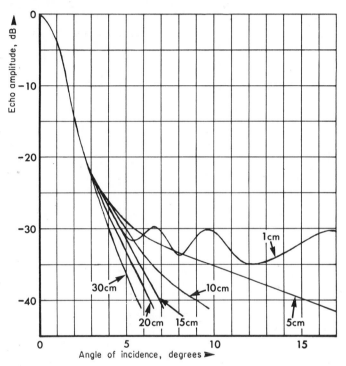

FIG. 4.7 Relationship between echo amplitude and angle of incidence, for a flat target in water at various ranges. Each curve is relative to 0 dB at 0° incidence. Frequency 1·7 MHz, transducer diameter 2·0 cm. (Adapted from Fig. 4 of Wells, 1966a).

occur with increasing angulation when the range is small are due to interference. This is not important in practice, because the transmission pulse (see Section 4.4.a), during which information retrieval is impossible, usually extends beyond this region.

Figure 4.8 shows how the echo amplitude at normal incidence depends upon the target range in water, with a typical pulse-echo system. The levels are relative to 0 dB at a range of 1 cm. Water has an absorption of about 0·0064 dB.cm^{-1} at 1·7 MHz (see Table 1.7). A 2 cm diameter transducer has a Frésnel zone which extends for 11·3 cm at this frequency (see Section 3.1). Therefore, for a target situated at 5·7 cm from the transducer, the echo amplitude is reduced by only 0·07 dB as the result of absorption. The amplitude is actually reduced by 1·2 dB: the excess attenuation is at least partly due to geometrical diffraction. At greater target ranges, the amplitude falls because of the divergence of the beam, which results in an increasing proportion of the reflected energy falling outside the area of the receiving transducer. When the target is very close to the transducer, the echo amplitude

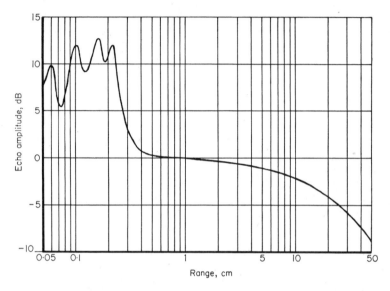

FIG. 4.8 Relationship between echo amplitude and range, for a flat target in water at 0° incidence. Levels relative to 0 dB at 1 cm range. Frequency 1·7 MHz, transducer diameter 2·0 cm.

exhibits a number of maxima and minima with altering range, similar to those produced by changing the angulation of a close-range target. The increase in echo amplitude associated with these fluctuations is due to the pressure amplification which occurs in a standing wave field (see Section 1.10). In clinical diagnosis, this effect is usually unimportant, because it occurs in the region occupied by the transmission pulse.

The examples illustrated in Figs 4.7 and 4.8 are typical of the characteristics of all pulse-echo systems. The relationships between attenuation, angulation and range depend upon the frequency and the diameter of the transducer.

In biological systems, there are usually a number of interfaces spaced in depth along the ultrasonic beam. Each of these interfaces reflects a fraction of the incident energy, and so reduces the quantity of energy which is transmitted. This happens not only as the pulse is travelling away from the transducer, but also as the echo returns, and results in a further reduction in the received echo amplitude which is in addition to the reductions due to absorption, divergence and diffraction.

The situation becomes much more complicated when the reflector is in the form of a rough surface or a small obstacle, and the effective reflectivity in such cases is best estimated experimentally. Some typical values of echo

TABLE 4.1

Typical echo amplitudes for some biological structures, expressed in decibels below the echo amplitude from a perfect reflector at the same range in a lossless medium

Structure	Range, cm	Echo amplitude, dB
Smooth skin surface in water	10	20
Foetal skull, 30 weeks gestation	8	50
Posterior heart surface	10	50
Posterior liver surface	12	50
Brain mid-line	7	60
Cirrhotic liver structures	8	60
Hydatidiform mole structures	8	65
Normal liver structures	8	65
Anterior mitral valve leaflet	7	70
Uterine fibroid structures	8	70

These are mean values, with the alignment of the transducer adjusted for maximum echo amplitude wherever possible. All data obtained using 1·5 MHz, 2 cm diameter transducer. Echo amplitude from perfect reflector in lossless medium: about 5 V peak to peak at 10 cm range.

amplitude, expressed in decibels below the level from a perfect reflector in a lossless medium at the same range, are given in Table 4.1. It is important to realize that these values are only approximate, and that there may be quite wide variations between different individuals and in different clinical conditions.

4.1.d Multiple Reflection Artifacts

The basis of the pulse-echo method is the reflection of ultrasonic energy at acoustic discontinuities. Consider again the simple case illustrated in Fig. 4.1, in which a transducer is directed normally at the flat interface between two homogeneous media of differing characteristic impedance. At the instant that the transmitted ultrasonic pulse leaves the transducer, the time-base circuit associated with the display begins to operate. After a delay which depends on the position of the interface and the velocity of the pulse, an echo returns to the transducer and produces a registration on the display in a position determined by the time-base. This is exactly the same process as that which has already been described in greater detail in Section 4.1.a. However, the process does not end at this stage. There is an acoustic discontinuity at the transducer surface, and although some of the energy in the reflected pulse enters the transducer to produce the registration, quite a large proportion of the pulse is reflected away from the transducer and back towards the target. This pulse behaves as if it were a second transmitted pulse, of smaller amplitude than the first, delayed in time by an interval equal to the delay in the return of the first echo. Consequently, a second echo returns from the interface, and this produces a registration on the display at a position corresponding to twice the range of the interface. Similarly, third and subsequent artifacts appear, until the multiple reflection echoes fall below the threshold level of the display (Wells, 1965).

Multiple reflection artifacts can arise from other sources in addition to those in the simple case of a transducer and single target. For example, multiple reflections can occur between two surfaces lying side by side along the axis of the ultrasonic beam. Again, under some circumstances artifacts can be caused by the reflections of the pulse in directions which do not lie along the axis of the ultrasonic beam: if the pulse strikes a second reflector which returns the echo to the first reflector, an artifact will occur at the corresponding point on the time-base.

In systems in which the transducer stands off from the patient in a water bath, the patient's skin and the surfaces of the water may give rise to quite large-amplitude artifacts. The problem has been discussed, for example, by Robinson et al. (1966). The multiple reflection artifact which occurs between the transducer and the skin is typically some 30 dB below the first skin echo, and its appearance on the scan can be avoided by arranging for the path length in the water bath to be greater than the penetration into the patient which appears on the display. However, multiple reflections between the skin and the surfaces of the water may be more difficult to eliminate, although a substantial improvement is obtained if ultrasonic absorbers are placed at those water surfaces from which artifacts may arise.

The maximum repetition rate in systems employing water bath coupling may be limited by the decay time of the reverberation echoes. The decay time can be quite long because of the relatively low ultrasonic absorption in water.

Contact scanning is less liable to multiple reflection artifacts, but under some circumstances quite large amplitude artifacts which are difficult to recognize may occur. This is because echoes which arise within the patient may cause artifacts due to reflection at the skin-air or skin-transducer interfaces, which have higher reflectivities than the skin-water interface associated with water-bath scanning.

Multiple reflection artifacts which arise from gas-containing structures within the patient are perhaps the most common. Their occurrence is a fundamental limitation of ultrasonic diagnosis. However, such artifacts are usually quite easily recognized, and so they should seldom cause diagnostic errors.

4.1.e Ultrasonic Frequency

The choice of the best ultrasonic frequency for a particular diagnostic application depends upon a number of factors. In general, the potential resolution under ideal conditions is improved as the ultrasonic frequency is increased. However, in practice it is not possible to increase the ultrasonic frequency above a limit which, for a given penetration, target reflectivity and absorption coefficient, is determined mainly by the signal-to-noise ratio (Section 4.4.a), and also partly by the accuracy of swept gain compensation (Section 4.1.b). It is helpful to consider the ultrasonic wavelength as the factor which controls the dimensions of the system: thus, a shorter wavelength gives a higher resolution over a more limited penetration. If a 50 dB dynamic range of swept gain is available, a soft-tissue penetration of around 25 cm can usually be obtained at a frequency of 1·5 MHz. The maximum penetration is inversely proportional to the frequency: thus, at 15 MHz, a penetration of 2·5 cm might be obtained. However, at the present time, few receiving systems are designed so that noise is the limiting factor which determines penetration; restricted gain or the onset of instability are the more common limitations. A dynamic range of swept gain of 30 dB is quite usual, and this allows a penetration of only about 15 cm at 1·5 MHz.

In systems in which the swept gain dynamic range is limited to about 30 dB, it is difficult to do better than to select the maximum frequency which will give the required penetration, and to make the transducer diameter equal to at least about 20 wavelengths. The transducer diameter may be increased slightly above this value with increasing frequency, so that it is for example, 30 wavelengths at 5 MHz. However, if a 50 dB swept gain dynamic range is available, or if the transducer stands off from the patient in a water bath, it may be better to use a rather larger transducer.

The effects of the differing absorption coefficients of different tissues become more pronounced as the frequency is increased. For example, Donald et al. (1958) have shown that a differential diagnosis between fibroids and ovarian cysts is possible, because both are readily transonic at a frequency of 1·5 MHz, whereas, under the same conditions of gain and swept gain, cysts remain transonic at 2·5 MHz, whilst fibroids do not. This method is very convenient if the frequency can be changed readily.

However, in systems designed for optimum performance it is necessary for the frequency to be fixed. Nevertheless, an equivalent diagnosis can be made by testing the effect of changing the swept gain rate.

4.2 TIMING CIRCUITS

The timing circuits in ultrasonic pulse-echo systems fall into three main groups:

(i)   Rate generators;
(ii) Delay generators;
(iii) Time-base generators.

Such circuits are described in many text books on electronics, and no more than a brief discussion of the factors which determine the choice of circuit for each particular application is given here. For complete descriptions of these circuits, see, for example, Millman and Taub (1956).

The rate generator provides a trigger pulse which controls the repetition frequency of the system. This frequency normally lies within the range 25 to 3000 Hz, according to the particular application. The frequency stability of the rate generator is not usually important, because all the other timing circuits are synchronized with the trigger pulse which it generates.

Most systems employ an astable multivibrator as the rate generator. However, it is sometimes necessary to synchronize the rate generator with a particular frequency, such as that of the mains power supply, or the patient's electrocardiogram. Synchronization with the mains frequency can be achieved by applying a voltage derived from the mains to an overdriven amplifier, so that the output from the amplifier consists of a series of pulses at mains frequency. A trigger synchronized with the E.C.G. can be provided by a circuit which is itself triggered by a characteristic part of the E.C.G. signal (usually the R-wave: see for example, Davies and Mitchell, 1960).

Delay generators are required to perform a number of different functions, such as the provision of gating pulses and trigger pulses delayed by time intervals corresponding to fixed ultrasonic path-lengths. The choice of circuitry is governed by the precision with which the delay must be generated. For most gating purposes, the monostable multivibrator is satisfactory. Such circuits can be designed to cover at least a decade of time variation, with a maximum jitter of less than a percent. However, where greater precision and freedom from jitter are required, a circuit such as the phantastron or a voltage comparator fed with an accurate sweep voltage, may be used. This improved performance is usually necessary when the delay is required to equal that introduced by a fixed ultrasonic path length.

Time-base circuits for one-dimensional displays are based on normal oscilloscope practice. The sweep time lies within the range 25 μsec, for examining small organs like the eye, to 500 μsec, for the investigation of the largest abdomen. The special time-base circuits used in some two-dimensional scanned B-scopes are discussed in Section 4.7.c.

4.3 THE TRANSMITTER

The function of the transmitter is to excite the transducer to emit a short-duration pulse of ultrasonic energy. One of the earliest transmitter circuits, which is still in common use today, consists of a capacitor, previously charged to a high voltage, which is suddenly applied to the transducer by means of a thyratron. A typical circuit is shown in Fig. 4.9. The maximum

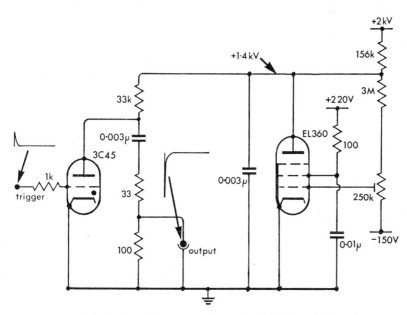

Fig. 4.9 Typical shock-exciting transmitter circuit. (Part of the valve-operated version of the "Diasonograph" type NE 4100. Circuit reproduced by courtesy of Nuclear Enterprises Ltd., who are now the manufacturers.)

voltage applied to the transducer consists of a transient, with an amplitude of about 850 V, a duration of 0·5 μsec, and a rise-time of 0·08 μsec. In response to this form of excitation, the transducer generates a train of stress waves, separated in time by intervals corresponding to its thickness. This mechanism has already been discussed in Section 2.6.a. The electrical energy available from the 0·003 μF capacitor is 4·5 μjoule per pulse, and radiation pressure measurements using the technique of Wells *et al.* (1964) described in Section 3.5 indicate that the ultrasonic power is in the order of

2 μjoule per pulse. The total charge fed to the transducer can be increased by increasing the value of the transmitting capacitor, but this increases the duration of the exciting transient and so limits the operating frequency.

A silicon controlled rectifier can be used as an alternative to the thyratron in shock-excitation circuits. However, there is a delay associated with the triggering of this type of device which may be troublesome in some applications.

When ultrasonic pulses having extremely fast rise-times are required, a mercury wetted relay may be used in place of the thyratron. Mercury wetted relays are limited to repetition frequencies of less than about 1000 Hz, and are

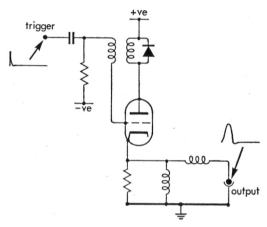

Fig. 4.10 Typical blocking oscillator transmitter circuit. (Adapted from Fig. 2 of Kossoff *et al.* 1965.)

characterized by a rather large jitter. However, this need not be a disadvantage, for the transmitter pulse, as opposed to the transmitter trigger, can be used as the synchronizing signal for the other timing circuits in the system.

Kossoff *et al.* (1965) have described the use of a blocking oscillator as a transmitter. The essential features of their circuit are shown in Fig. 4.10. Designed to operate in a 2 MHz system, it provides a pulse of 0·25 μsec duration. Shunt and series tuning are used to increase the bandwidth. According to the calculations of Kossoff *et al.* (1964), a similar transmitter generates an ultrasonic energy of about 2·5 μjoule per pulse.

At ultrasonic frequencies in the low megahertz range (less than about 3 MHz), the efficiency of a blocking oscillator as a transmitter is greater than that of a thyratron or similar shock exciting system. This is because the electrical energy is supplied mainly at the fundamental ultrasonic frequency by the blocking oscillator, whereas, with shock excitation, much of the ultrasonic energy is generated at high harmonic frequencies. These energy components are rather rapidly attenuated by dispersive absorption, and in any event fall outside the passband of the receiver. The two systems have similar efficiencies at frequencies of around 5 to 10 MHz, where the rise-time of the shock-exciting transient corresponds more closely to that of the fundamental frequency.

A gated sine-wave oscillator is occasionally used as the transmitter in pulse-echo systems. The output from such a transmitter can be arranged to be symmetrical, so that there is no shift of the d.c. level at the transducer. This gives certain advantages in the design of the r.f. amplifier. However, the duration of the transmitter pulse is longer than in the case of shock or half-cycle excitation, and so the use of this type of transmitter is associated with a degradation in range resolution.

4.4 RADIO FREQUENCY AMPLIFIERS

4.4.a General Considerations

The range resolution of a pulse-echo system is determined, other factors being equal, by the total bandwidth and dynamic range. The bandwidth is limited by the performance of the transmitter (Section 4.3), the transducer (Chapter 2), the receiver and the display system. The display system is seldom the limiting factor. However, the performance of the receiver is important. The receiver consists of all the various circuits, some of which may be non-linear, which together process the echo signals fed from the transducer into a form suitable for presentation on the display. In general, the broader the frequency response of the receiver, the smaller will be the range resolution. However, it is explained later in this Section that the signal-to-noise ratio of the system depends upon the bandwidth, and that it is necessary for a compromise to be made between range resolution and sensitivity. A reasonably satisfactory arrangement is to make the r.f. amplifier bandwidth equal to the nominal frequency of the ultrasonic pulse, and to arrange for the passband to be centred on this frequency. The video amplifier frequency response is often chosen to process the signal by restriction of the low-frequency amplification, and this is discussed in Section 4.5.b. The bandwidth of a system is normally taken to be equal to the difference between the frequencies at which the output is reduced by 3 dB from the maximum output, when the input amplitude is kept constant.

The dynamic range of the signal output from a transducer used in a typical pulse-echo diagnostic system is very large. The dynamic range arises partly because of absorption, which reduces the amplitudes of echoes from deeper structures, and partly because of variation in the reflectivities of interfaces between materials of differing characteristics and configurations (see Section 4.1.c). There are so many factors of a controversial nature which control the useful dynamic range that it is not possible to define this quantity with precision. The lower limit is determined by the equivalent input noise of the receiver amplifier: the integrating properties of the system determine the minimum signal-to-noise ratio which can be accepted to give statistically reliable information about the occurrence of an echo. The upper limit is determined, for a given target and transducer sensitivity, by the maximum amplitude of the transmitted pulse. Theoretically, this could be made quite large, simply by increasing the power of the transmitter. However, the risk of biological damage being caused by the ultrasonic energy naturally increases as the energy is increased (see Section 7.4) and so designers should be unwilling to make changes in this direction until the biological processes which are involved are better understood.

The noise of a receiver arises from a variety of different sources. These include thermal-agitation or resistance noise, and noise generated within the amplifying devices. Thermal noise is due to the random nature of electron movements in a conductor. At any instant, there are likely to be more free electrons moving in one direction than another, and this results in the appearance of a voltage across the conductor. The noise energy is uniformly distributed over the whole frequency spectrum; over the range of frequencies f_1 to f_2,

$$E^2 = 4kTR(f_2 - f_1), \tag{4.1}$$

where $E =$ effective value of voltage components in the spectrum lying between the frequencies f_1 and f_2,

$k =$ Boltzman's constant ($1 \cdot 37 \times 10^{-23}$ joule per deg. K),

$T =$ absolute temperature (deg. K),

and $R =$ resistive component of impedance across which the thermal agitation noise is produced.

Thus, a resistor R may be considered as a generator of voltage E and internal resistance R. Similarly, any source of noise voltage uniformly distributed over a frequency spectrum may be considered in terms of the equivalent noise resistance for the spectrum. For example, a resistance of $37 \cdot 5 \ \Omega$ at a temperature of $20°C$ operating in a circuit with a bandwidth of $1 \cdot 5$ MHz generates an equivalent mean-square noise voltage of $0 \cdot 95 \ \mu V$. Under the same conditions, a resistance of $100 \ \Omega$ generates $1 \cdot 55 \ \mu V$, and a noise source of $5 \ \mu V$ is equivalent to a resistance of $1040 \ \Omega$.

Noise is generated in amplifying devices by several different mechanisms. In valve amplifiers, the principal noise sources are:

(i) Shot effect, due to irregular emission from the cathode. This leads to variation in anode current as the number of electrons reaching the anode changes from one instant to another;

(ii) Partition noise, arising from variations in current sharing between the positive electrodes. This noise source does not occur in triodes, which are in principle less noisy than multigrid valves;

(iii) Other noise sources, such as induced grid noise, which is due to random variations in the electron flow adjacent to the grid.

It can be shown (see, for example, Valley and Wallman (1948), p. 625) that, for most valves,

$$R_s = \frac{2 \cdot 5}{g_m}, \tag{4.2}$$

and

$$R_p = \frac{20 I_s}{I_k g_m}, \tag{4.3}$$

where R_s = equivalent resistance for shot noise,

R_p = equivalent resistance for partition noise,

g_m = mutual conductance,

I_s = screen grid current,

and I_k = cathode current.

It can be seen from Equations 4.2 and 4.3 that the noise generated in a valve amplifier is minimized by the use of a valve with a high mutual conductance. In practice, the best performance may not be achieved with a triode valve, but with a pentode, because although the latter has an additional noise contribution due to the partition effect, this may be offset by the difficulty of obtaining high gain from a triode in a high frequency amplifier. In a pentode stage, Equation 4.3 shows that partition noise may be minimized by making I_s small and I_k large.

Two triodes connected in cascade can provide excellent performance as the input circuit of an amplifier (Valley and Wallman (1948), p. 656–666). Such an arrangement has a lower equivalent input noise, and is no more critical in adjustment, than a pentode input stage with the same bandwidth.

Noise in transistor amplifiers arises from the following sources:

(i) Emitter noise, due to fluctuations of diffusion and recombination in the base region;

(ii) Collector noise, due to the same phenomena that are responsible for the emitter noise;

(iii) Base noise, due to the thermal noise of the equivalent base resistance.

The contributions of both the emitter and collector noise sources depend on the junction currents. The best noise performance is obtained with circuits designed to provide the optimum compromise between current and input impedance.

The noise figure F of an amplifier is a quantity which describes its noise performance in a particular system. It is defined as follows:

$$F = \frac{\text{input signal-to-noise ratio}}{\text{output signal-to-noise ratio}} \tag{4.4}$$

An ideal amplifier would make no contribution to the noise content of a signal, and its noise figure as defined by Equation 4.4 would be unity, or 0 dB. Practical amplifiers have noise figures of less than unity. In an amplifier consisting of several stages of amplification in cascade, the noise figure of the whole system is normally determined by the noise of the first stage. This is because the noise contribution of each succeeding stage becomes decreasingly important as the amplitude of the signal fed from the preceeding stage becomes greater.

The noise figure of an amplifier depends upon the operating frequency and bandwidth. The noise power is distributed (usually, but not necessarily, uniformly) throughout the frequency spectrum, and therefore the noise figure is improved as the bandwidth is decreased. In general, for a given bandwidth, the gain of the amplifier falls as the passband frequency is increased: this is because the losses in the system increase with increasing frequency. Consequently, the noise figure deteriorates as the operating frequency is increased, because the noise contribution from an amplifying device may be considered as a constant quantity referred to the input, independent of the stage gain.

In ultrasonic pulse-echo systems, it is rather difficult to estimate the signal-to-noise ratio at the input to the receiver. Most of the noise output from the receiver arises in the input resistance and the first amplifying stage. Therefore, in discussing the performance of a system, the noise figure is not such a useful quantity as the value of the equivalent noise voltage referred to the input. However, the concept of the noise figure is helpful in discussing the performance of a system, particularly in consideration of the effects of alterations in operating frequency and bandwidth.

Another quantity which is often found useful in discussing the performance of an amplifier is the gain-bandwidth product. In any particular amplifier, the product of gain and bandwidth is a constant. In an amplifier consisting of n identical stages, it can be shown (Valley and Wallman, 1948, p. 173) that—

$$\text{overall bandwidth} = \frac{\text{one-stage bandwidth}}{1 \cdot 2\sqrt{n}} \tag{4.5}$$

The receiver in an ultrasonic pulse-echo system is subjected to a grossly overloading signal at the instant that the output from the transmitter is applied to the transducer. This overload is followed by a finite recovery time, during which the receiver is insensitive to small signals such as those which the transducer generates in response to echoes. Some aspects of this paralysis are discussed in Section 4.4.b. A good receiver has a short recovery time: but it is not possible to design a receiver in which the recovery time is zero. The recovery time following the transmission of the ultrasonic pulse is rather loosely known as the transmission "pulse", during which time information retrieval is impossible.

4.4.b Linear r.f. Amplifiers

A radio frequency amplifier for ultrasonic pulse-echo applications needs to satisfy the following requirements:

(i)   Adequate gain-bandwidth product at low noise;
(ii) Provision of swept gain facility;
(iii) Quick recovery from overload;
(iv) Low phase distortion;
(v)   Approximately linear amplitude response;
(vi) Ability to withstand the output from the transmitter.

A wide frequency response can be obtained by using a few (usually two) synchronously tuned stages of low Q-factor, the other stages being untuned, or by staggering the tuning of relatively narrow-band stages in a multistage amplifier (see, for example, Valley and Wallman, 1948, pp. 166–200). The first method is satisfactory for pulse-echo applications at frequencies of less than about 3 MHz; at higher frequencies, the second method is preferable, because it becomes more difficult to obtain high gain with untuned stages. Another possible advantage of the stagger-tuned amplifier is that the pass-band is more sharply defined, but this is not really of great importance with broad-band pulses.

The use of a superheterodyne receiver might at first sight seem to be an attractive possibility. However, this is not the case. Consider, for example, an ultrasonic system operating at 2 MHz, with a bandwidth extending from 1 to 3 MHz. A 2 MHz bandwidth could easily be achieved if the centre frequency was changed to 20 MHz, and this would have the additional advantage that *pin* diodes could be used for swept gain control (see Section 4.4.c). The conversion would require a local oscillator with a frequency of either 18 or 22 MHz. The problem is that the local oscillator frequency is separated by only 1 MHz from either one end or the other of the passband, and it would be very difficult to design filters to prevent the signal from the local oscillator from breaking through to the i.f. amplifier. Systems employing balanced modulators reduce the severity of the filtering requirements, but any advantages of superheterodyne operation are offset by the increased complexity.

At high ultrasonic frequencies (more than 10 MHz), it is possible to use a superheterodyne receiver because the total bandwidth can be rather less than the centre frequency of the pulse. However, it is not usually difficult to obtain adequate bandwidth at such frequencies with a stagger-tuned amplifier. Therefore, the advantages of frequency conversion disappear, unless it is desired to make use of an existing amplifier, such as, for example, an i.f. amplifier designed for Radar applications. This solution was chosen by Reid and Wild (1952), who used a system based on the 15 MHz ultrasonic trainer described by Larsen (1946).

Any tendency of the receiver to paralyze is an undesirable feature, because this results in a long recovery time following an overload. An overloading signal can change the bias conditions of the amplifying stages, as a result of alterations in the charges stored in the coupling and decoupling capacitors. This may be due, for example, to the passage of grid current. The amplifier becomes insensitive to small signals until the biassing conditions have returned to normal. The effects of paralysis can be minimized by making the capacitors which control the biassing so large that overloading signals produce only small changes in the operating conditions, and by arranging for the gain of the system to be low at the times when the largest signals are applied to the input. To some extent, this later protection is afforded by the swept gain of the receiver amplifier, which typically reduces the system gain by up to around 50 dB from the maximum at the time that the transmitter pulse is applied to the receiver. The transmitter pulse is the largest signal which the receiver is required to accept: it is several orders of magnitude greater than the largest echo signal. The paralysis due to the transmitter pulse can be further reduced by some kind of limiting circuit at or near the input to the amplifier.

The requirements for swept gain depend upon many factors. These have already been discussed in Section 4.1.b. For example, in the case of an ultrasonic pulse with a nominal frequency of 2·5 MHz, the swept gain rate needs to be about $3\cdot3$ dB.cm^{-1} in most soft tissues (as opposed to the rate of $3\cdot9$ dB.cm^{-1} when $\alpha = 1$ dB.cm^{-1}MHz^{-1}), which corresponds to about $0\cdot25$ dB.μsec^{-1}. Thus, a 50 dB dynamic range must be covered in about 200 μsec. It is generally best for the gain to be controlled in such a way that it increases by equal fractions for equal increases in time; that is, an exponential swept gain is required. More accurate compensation in which account is taken of variations in the absorption of different materials soon becomes unmanageable.

There are two methods by which swept gain can be obtained. In one method, the gains of suitable stages are controlled by alteration of the biassing conditions. In the other method, the gain of each stage of the r.f. amplifier is kept constant, and electronically controlled attenuation (see Section 4.4.c) is introduced at appropriate points in the circuit. Gain control by bias adjustment is perhaps the simplest method in practice, and so it is considered first in the following discussion. However, the method is not

widely used in transistor amplifiers, because in such amplifiers the input
and output impedances of each stage are essentially dependent on the biassing conditions.

· Consider, for example, the amplifier stage shown in Fig. 4.11.a. The
transconductance characteristic of the type 6CQ6 valve used in this amplifier is shown in Figure 4.11.b. The mutual conductance g_m of the valve is
equal to the slope of the transconductance characteristic, and this decreases
as the control grid is made more negative. This is a feature of variable-mu
valves, of which the 6CQ6 is a typical type. The gain of the stage can be
controlled by variation of the d.c. bias on the control grid. For small-
amplitude signals, the amplifier used to illustrate this example gives a gain
variation of from + 20 to −6 dB with a swept gain controlling bias variation of from 0 to −12 V. The relationship between gain and bias is approximately logarithmic over a limited range; the range of logarithmic operation
depends to some extent upon the value of the cathode resistor. Unfortunately, amongst valves of any given type, there is only a poor correlation
between transconductance and bias voltage, for low values of g_m (Valley and
Wallman, 1948, p. 290). Therefore, in order to obtain a reproducible and
wide dynamic range, it is necessary to apply the bias which controls the
swept gain to several stages connected in cascade. This is done, for example,
in the 2 MHz amplifier of Wells and Evans (1968), in which three stages
identical to that illustrated in Fig. 4.11.a are controlled by the same bias, as
shown in Fig. 4.12. The dynamic range of control of each stage is limited to
about 20 dB (and to much less in practice, as the total swept gain range in
the application to breast scanning for which this amplifier was designed is
only 16 dB), and it is unnecessary to use specially selected valves. In amplifiers for diagnostic applications in which the swept gain requirements are
not critical (for example, in the detection of the mid-line echo of the brain,
and in ultrasonic cardiology), it is usually adequate to apply swept gain to a
single stage; the dynamic range which can be obtained with a single stage
rarely exceeds 40 or 50 dB, but this is seldom an important limitation.

The amplifier of Wells and Evans (1968), of which the complete circuit is
given in Fig. 4.12, is designed so that the application of a linear controlling
voltage ramp results in an exponential increase in gain. The deviation from
this relationship is within 4 dB over a range of 50 dB. This performance is
obtained because the gain of each stage is swept only over a rather restricted
range. If a wide dynamic range is to be obtained from a single stage of swept
gain, it becomes impossible with simple circuits to obtain an exponential
increase in gain with linear controlling voltage. In such cases, it is necessary
to employ a non-linear voltage function for control if an exponential swept
gain is required. The design of suitable function generators is discussed in
Section 4.4.d.

In a multi-stage amplifier, the overall gain is equal to the product of the

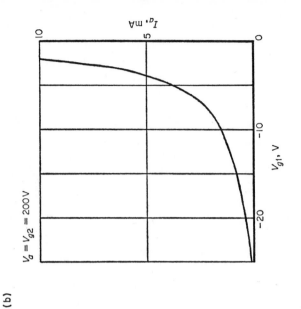

(b)

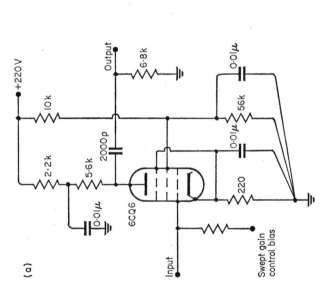

(a)

Fig. 4.11 Amplifier with electronically controlled gain. (a) Circuit diagram; (b) Transconductance characteristic of the type 6CQ6 valve.

gains of each stage. If the gain of any stage is altered, whilst its frequency selectivity characteristic remains unchanged, the overall gain is altered in proportion, whereas the overall frequency response is unaffected. Therefore, the points in the circuit at which gain control is applied to the amplifier are of no consequence to the frequency response, whether the amplifier is syn-chronously-tuned, stagger-tuned or untuned. However, these points are important insofar as they affect the dynamic range and noise figure of the system. The earlier stages of the amplifier are usually designed to operate most satisfactorily with small signals: distortion may be introduced if large signals are applied. Therefore, it is necessary to apply swept gain to the earlier stages, so that they do not become overloaded. It would be both difficult and uneconomic to apply swept gain at a circuit point at which the signal amplitude is already large. A compromise may be necessary when it is desirable to keep the dynamic range of control of each stage as small as possible, so as to maintain a good exponential relationship between gain and controlling voltage. In such cases it may be best to include potentiometric attenuators between the early stages, as shown in Fig. 4.12. Similarly, if swept gain is applied to only one stage, it is generally best if this is also the first stage.

The amplifier of Wells and Evans (1968) (Fig. 4.12) uses a type E810F pentode valve in the input stage. This valve has a maximum g_m of 50 mA.V^{-1}, which gives a good noise performance (see Equations 4.2 and 4.3). The noise referred to the control grid of the first stage is about 5 μV, which is equivalent to a resistance of about 1 kΩ (see Equation 4.1). The additional resistance associated with the input to the two limiting diodes (1 kΩ) raises the overall equivalent input noise to around 7 μV. The first and last stages are tuned to a centre frequency of 2 MHz, and the response is 3 dB down at frequencies of 1·5 and 2·6 MHz. The output from the last stage is fed to a full-wave demodulator (see Section 4.4.e), and the maximum overall gain is about 70 dB.

The design of transistorized gain controlled band-pass amplifiers has been discussed by Wood (1964a, 1964b). Unlike valves, transistors cannot be considered as unilateral devices; for example, in the common emitter configuration, there is internal feedback from the collector to the base. Therefore, changes in load impedance are reflected back as changes in the input impedance, and changes in source impedance alter the output impe-dance. In tuned amplifiers, the input and output impedances of the tran-sistor are in parallel with the tuned circuits. Consequently, the tuning of a stage is coupled to that of its neighbours, and simple cascaded circuits such as are used in valve amplifiers are often unsatisfactory.

One solution to the problem of internal feedback is to arrange for its effects to be cancelled by a process known as unilateralization. This is done by feeding back from the collector to the base a signal which is equal in

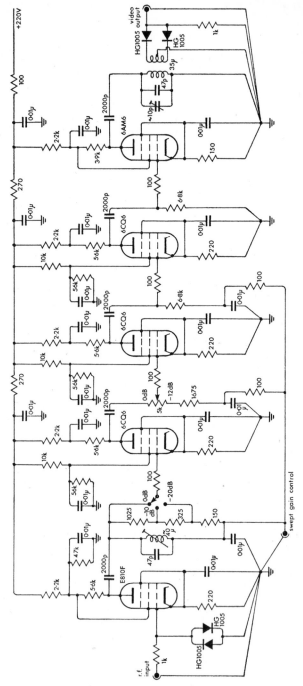

FIG. 4.12 Circuit of typical 2 MHz synchronously-tuned r.f. amplifier and full-wave demodulator. (Adapted from Fig. 6 of Wells and Evans (1968).)

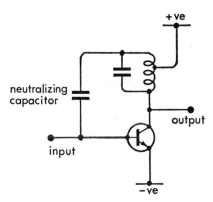

FIG. 4.13 Transistor amplifier with neutralization of internal feedback.

amplitude but opposite in phase to that fed back internally. Exact uni-lateralization is difficult to achieve, but in practice neutralization by capacitive feedback is often adequate. Phase reversal is necessary with this form of feedback, and this can be obtained from an interstage transformer, or a tapped coil. A typical neutralized stage is shown in Fig. 4.13.

As an alternative to neutralization, the cascode circuit illustrated in Fig. 4.14 has certain advantages. T_1 is a common emitter stage, and T_2 is a common base stage. The input impedance of T_2 forms the collector load of

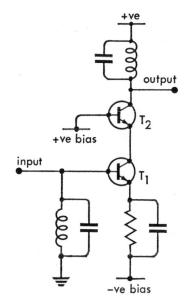

FIG. 4.14 Cascode transistor amplifier providing isolation between input and output circuits.

T_1: this is a gross mismatch because the input impedance of T_2 is very low. This mismatch isolates the effects of changes in the load of T_2 on the input impedance of T_1, and of changes in the source impedance of the input to T_1 on the output impedance of T_2.

Nowadays, the use of integrated circuits as elements in complete systems is gaining in popularity. Some typical circuits for use in r.f. amplifiers have been described, for example, by Gay *et al.* (1967). Single devices can provide maximum gains well in excess of 30 dB over a broad frequency band in the low megahertz range, with controlled gain ranges (see Section 4.4.c) of around 70 dB. Unfortunately, the gain control characteristics of such devices are not usually exponential, and so it is not a simple matter to make use of this feature for accurate swept gain.

4.4.c Electronically Controlled Attenuators

Gain control in transistorized amplifiers by variation of the d.c. bias conditions is associated with alterations in impedances so that considerable difficulties arise with this method, particularly in the case of tuned amplifiers. The best method of gain control in such amplifiers seems to be afforded by the use of a suitable number of variable attenuators connected between appropriate stages. Such attenuators can take the form of networks containing diodes or transistors, the a.c. resistances of which can be controlled by alteration of their d.c. conditions.

The relationship between current and voltage in a semiconductor *pn* junction, according to first order theory (see, for example, Shockley (1950), pp. 309–314), is given by—

$$I = I_s(e^{qV/kT} - 1) \tag{4.6}$$

where $I =$ forward current across the junction corresponding to an applied voltage V,

$I_s =$ reverse saturation current,

$k =$ Boltzman's constant (1.37×10^{-23} joule per deg. K),

$T =$ junction temperature (deg. K),

and $q =$ electronic charge (1.60×10^{-19} coulomb).

From Equation 4.6—

$$V = \frac{kT}{q} \log_e \left[\frac{I}{I_s} + 1 \right]$$

Therefore

$$\frac{dV}{dI} = r_D = \frac{kT}{q} \left[\frac{1}{I + I_s} \right], \tag{4.7}$$

where r_D = dynamic junction resistance corresponding to forward current I,

and $\dfrac{kT}{q}$ = 26 mV at 25 °C (or 29 mV at 60 °C, and so on).

In most diodes, I_s is in the order of 0·01 to 10 μA, and if $I_s \ll I$, Equation 4.7 can be simplified to give—

$$r_D = \frac{kT}{q} \cdot \frac{1}{I},\qquad(4.8)$$

and hence, at constant temperature—

$$r_D \propto \frac{1}{I},\qquad(4.9)$$

and from Equation 4.6 D. U. Follett (1968): personal communication)—

$$r_D \propto \frac{1}{e^{cV}}\qquad(4.10)$$

where c is a constant.

The relationship given in Equation 4.6 is based only on consideration of the diffusion current. More exact theory requires that account is also taken of such factors as the geometry of the junction, the series resistance associated with bulk semiconductor material, and generation and recombination in the space charge region. However, Equations 4.9 and 4.10 are sufficiently accurate to indicate the proportional relationships between the dynamic resistance, and the current and voltage. The resistance of a practical diode may differ from that predicted by simple theory by as many as four or more times (Sah, 1962) and the characteristics of any particular type are best determined experimentally. For example, Fig. 4.15.a shows the forward characteristic of the type 1N916 diffused silicon high-speed switching diode. Figures 4.15.b and 4.15.c show how the dynamic resistance of the same diode varies with current and voltage. It is important to appreciate the distinction between the dynamic resistance r_D, which is given by the slope $\dfrac{dV}{dI}$ of the characteristic, and the static d.c. resistance which is equal to $\dfrac{V}{I}$.

Transistors may be used as controlled resistors in suitable circuit configurations. For example, Morris (1965) has discussed the relationship between the bottomed emitter-collector resistance r_T and the base current I_b of a bipolar transistor, and has shown by making certain simplifying approximations that—

$$r_T = \left(\frac{kT}{q} \cdot \frac{1}{I_b}\right)\left(\frac{1}{\beta_n} + \frac{1}{1 + \beta_i}\right),\qquad(4.11)$$

where β_n = normal common emitter current gain,

and β_i = inverted common emitter current gain.

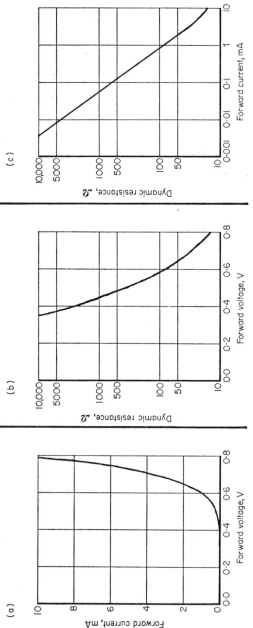

FIG. 4.15 Forward characteristics of type 1N916 diode. (a) Current-voltage characteristic; (b) Variation of dynamic resistance with voltage; (c) Variation of dynamic resistance with current.

It can be seen from Equation 4.11 that r_T depends mainly upon the smaller of the two current gains. In addition, if I_b and β_i are both large, then

$$V_{ce} = \frac{kT}{q} \cdot \frac{1}{(1 + \beta_i)},\qquad(4.12)$$

where V_{ce} = collector-to-emitter voltage.

Of the two possible arrangements, it is better to operate the transistor in the inverted mode, with the base current flowing through the collector. In this situation, $\beta_i = h_{FE}$, and, from Equation 4.12, it can be seen that V_{ce} is quite small (typically less than 1 mV). Also, r_T is determined mainly by $\beta_n = h_{RE}$, which is usually in the order of one percent of h_{FE}. In practice, there is some deviation from the simple theory, and it may be difficult to estimate with accuracy the value of h_{RE}. Therefore, it is generally best to measure r_T experimentally.

Field-effect transistors may also be used as controlled resistors. The effective dynamic drain-to-source resistance r_{DS} can be reduced by forward-biassing the gate with respect to the source. When biassed with drain-to-source voltage below pinch-off, it can be shown (for example, by manipulation of results quoted by Sevin, 1965, pp. 76–77) that—

$$r_{DS} = \frac{V_P^2}{2I_{DSS}(V_{GS} - V_P)},\qquad(4.13)$$

where V_P = gate-to-source voltage cut-off (the "pinch-off" voltage),

I_{DSS} = zero-gate-voltage drain current,

and V_{GS} = gate-to-source voltage.

The value of r_{DS} is a maximum when $V_{GS} = V_P$, and minimum when $V_{GS} = \phi$, where ϕ is the contact potential of the device (around 0·5 V). There is some deviation between the values obtained in practice and from simple theory, but over a limited range r_{DS} is inversely proportional to V_{GS}. It is interesting that the range of linear operation can be increased by arranging for a voltage to be fed back from the drain to the gate, so that this voltage is added to the controlling voltage. A remarkably good improvement can be obtained if half the drain voltage is fed back to the gate (Martin (1962)). The relative values of the feedback resistors can be made quite large compared with the drain-to-source resistance, so that they have little effect apart from providing the desired correction signal.

Similar results to those obtained with the junction field-effect transistor are given with greater inherent stability by the use of the metal-oxide-semiconductor transistor (Bilotti, 1966). An increase in bandwidth of 2·5 times may be obtained by the use of such a device with a distributed drain (Bilotti, 1967).

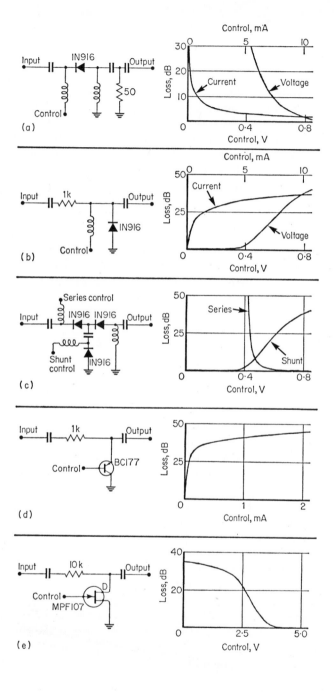

(a)

(b)

(c)

(d)

(e)

Some examples of circuits in which controlled resistors are used as attenuators are given in Fig. 4.16. The control characteristics shown in this figure were obtained experimentally, and some differences may be found due to variations between devices of similar types. In a shunt L-section attenuator, a linear relationship is obtained between the loss in decibels and the controlling function, if the resistance of the controlled element is proportional to the exponent of the controlling function. This relationship exists in the junction diode over a limited range if the device is voltage-controlled (Fig. 4.16.b). However, constant resistance networks, such as the T-section illustrated in Fig. 4.16.c, all require quite complicated control functions to maintain accurate tracking, no matter what devices may be used as the controlled resistors. Similarly, the relationships between controlling function and network loss in decibels is non-linear in every case illustrated in Fig. 4.16, with the sole exception of the voltage-controlled shunt diode attenuator.

All the networks shown in Fig. 4.16 are temperature-sensitive, and some system for temperature correction or control is necessary in precision applications. Because the devices are essentially non-linear, they all introduce signal waveform distortion which increases with increasing signal amplitude across the controlled resistor. The transistor has the steepest slope, and distortion becomes noticeable at peak amplitudes of around 10 mV; the junction diode distorts significantly at 20 mV peak; and the junction field-effect transistor may be operated at up to 150 mV peak before distortion becomes important.

The *pin* diode may be used as a controlled resistor (Heller, 1963). Modern devices behave as linear resistors at frequencies above about 10 MHz. The *pin* diode consists of thin layers of *p*- and *n*-type silicon, between which is placed a relatively wide layer of intrinsic silicon. Such diodes can be designed so that the body resistance is one or two orders of magnitude less than the junction resistance for a given control current. Because the body resistance is not sensitive to high frequency currents, r.f. currents which are much larger than the d.c. control current can be tolerated without serious distortion.

The positions in the r.f. amplifier at which the electronically controlled

---

FIG. 4.16 Examples of electronically controlled attenuators. At r.f., all the coils have high reactances, and all the capacitors have low reactances. Each circuit operates with negative control current or voltage, but the control supplies are shown in the conventional forward directions to simplify the diagrams. For the control characteristics shown (except (c)), the effects of source and load impedances have been made negligible. (a) Series diode attenuator; (b) Shunt diode attenuator; (c) Constant resistance ($600\,\Omega$) T-section attenuator; (d) Transistor shunt attenuator; (e) Junction field-effect transistor shunt attenuator.

attenuators are placed are determined by considerations of signal distortion, dynamic range and noise. The largest echo signals are in the order of a few volts, and it is necessary in the case of a diode attenuator, for example, for a loss of about 40 dB to occur before such signals can be applied to the controlled attenuator if it is operating within its dynamic characteristic. A satisfactory solution is to insert four swept attenuators between the first five stages of the amplifier, and to arrange for these to be controlled in sequence (by suitable biassing), with the attenuator furthest from the input being swept first. In this way, distortion in the early attenuators is minimized because they are saturated when the input signal is greatest. For a swept gain range of 50 dB, the dynamic range of each attenuator is only 12·5 dB, and a linear relationship can be obtained between the controlling voltage and the gain in decibels if shunt diodes are used (see Fig. 4.16.b). Such an arrangement also provides a good noise performance, because the signal-to-noise ratio varies through the range of swept gain to a minimum value when the gain is maximum. However, some improvement in the mid-range noise figure may be obtained if the first attenuator is not swept last (D. H. Follett (1968): personal communication).

4.4.d Swept Gain Function Generators

The swept gain systems described in Sections 4.4.b and 4.4.c require time-varying voltage or current supplies in order to perform the necessary gain control. The simplest controlling function is a linear voltage ramp, which can be generated, for example, by means of a constant current source arranged to charge a capacitor. However, an exponential increase in gain with time is usually required, and it is rather difficult to design circuits in which this is achieved by the use of a linear controlling function. Of the systems described in this Chapter, only the amplifier of Wells and Evans (1968), and the voltage controlled diode shunt attenuator, satisfy this condition. All the other circuits require non-linear controlling functions to provide the gain-time characteristic which corresponds to logarithmic compensation.

There are several methods by which suitable non-linear functions may be generated. The use of the photoelectric waveform generator (Sunstein, 1949) is one of the simplest methods, although the device is rather large and expensive. It consists of a cathode ray tube whose screen is partially obscured by a mask the profile of which is cut to the shape of the required waveform. A time-base is triggered at the appropriate instant to drive the luminescent spot across the display. The other deflection plates are connected to an amplifier which, in the absence of an input signal, allows the spot to fall on the part of the screen not obscured by the mask. Light from the screen is detected by a photomultiplier, which provides an output which is amplified and applied to the deflection plates so that the spot tends

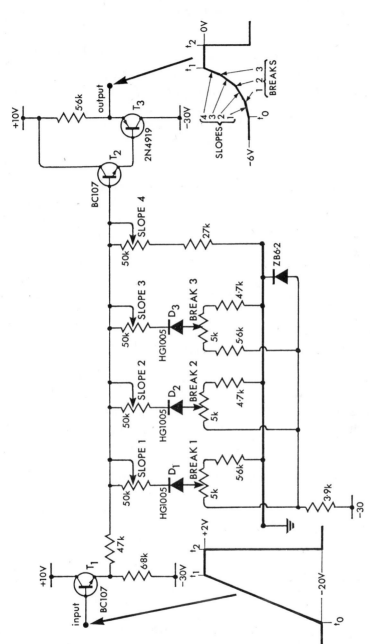

FIG. 4.17 Part of a typical diode function generator for swept gain voltage control.

to be driven behind the mask. Therefore, the spot moves along the edge of the mask, and the output from the amplifier is in the form of the required voltage function.

A satisfactory alternative to the photoformer is provided by the diode function generator (Korn and Korn (1956), pp. 290–299). A diode function generator utilizes the transfer characteristic of a resistive network containing biassed diode switches. The circuit of part of a typical function generator designed for diagnostic ultrasonic use is shown in Fig. 4.17. The input ramp, generated, for example, by a capacitor charged from a constant current source, is fed to the emitter follower T_1. The output from T_1 is connected to R_1, which forms part of a potential divider, the other part of which is the diode-controlled network. In this network, D_1 ceases to conduct when the divided voltage is equal to the first break potential, and this switches out the resistive components adjusted by the first slope potentiometer. Similarly, the diodes D_2 and D_3 switch out in turn as the divided voltage increases. Thus, the output, which is fed through the voltage followers T_2 and T_3, consists of a voltage which increases with time as indicated in the diagram. This form of control voltage gives an exponential swept gain when used, for example, with the Diasonograph, Nuclear Enterprises Ltd. type NE4100.

4.4.e Demodulation and Suppression

The output from the r.f. amplifier consists of signals extending in amplitude over a dynamic range which is typically in the order of 50 dB. It is normally necessary to demodulate these signals so that further amplification and processing may occur in the video amplifier.

Demodulation in ultrasonic systems is usually carried out by means of suitable diode networks, such as that illustrated in Fig. 4.18.a. The characteristic of the ideal diode (Fig. 4.18.b) is such that $r_D = \infty$ when $V < 0$, and $r_D = r_0$ when $V > 0$, where r_D is the equivalent resistance of the diode, V is the voltage across the diode, and r_0 is the forward resistance of the diode (a constant in the ideal case). Thus—

$$\frac{v_{\text{out}}}{v_{\text{in}}} = \frac{R_L}{R_S + R_L + r_0} \quad \text{when} \quad V > 0, \tag{4.14}$$

and $\quad\quad \dfrac{v_{\text{out}}}{v_{\text{in}}} = 0 \quad\quad\quad \text{when} \quad V < 0, \tag{4.15}$

assuming that the input impedance of the video amplifier is either very large, or is included in the value of R_L. Consequently the circuit shown in Fig. 4.18.a provides a half-wave demodulated output signal, the amplitude of which is proportional to the instantaneous forward value of the r.f. input signal.

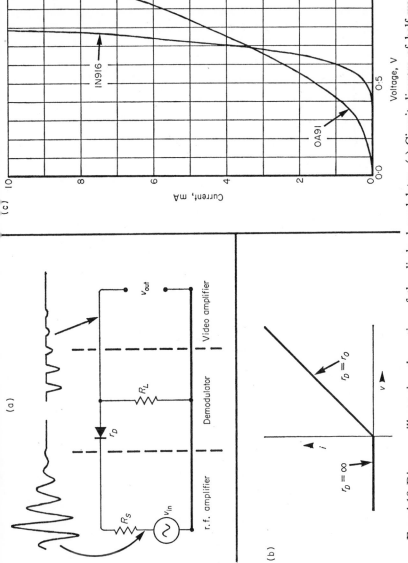

Fig. 4.18 Diagrams illustrating the action of the diode demodulator. (a) Circuit diagram of half-wave demodulator with negative-going video output; (b) Relationship between current i and voltage v in an ideal demodulating diode; (c) Current-voltage characteristics of two typical semiconductor diodes. That of the type 0A91 (point-contact) diode approaches more closely to (b).

Practical diodes do not possess the ideal linear characteristic. For example, Fig. 4.18.c shows the forward characteristics of typical germanium point-contact and silicon junction diodes. The point-contact diode approximates more closely to the ideal diode, but even this device has a much higher resistance at lower forward voltages than at higher voltages. The non-linearity of the forward characteristic of the diode demodulator determines the lower limit of the dynamic range of the signals which the circuit can

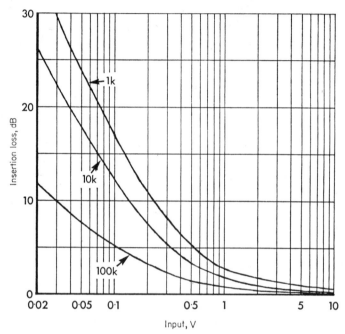

FIG. 4.19 Insertion loss characteristics for a type OA91 half-wave demodulator similar to that illustrated in Fig. 4.18.a. Each curve is for a different total value of resistance ($R_S + R_L$).

accept. The upper limit is controlled by the maximum output voltage available from the r.f. amplifier, provided that this is not so large that the diode carries an excessive current. Consider, for example, a r.f. signal the maximum amplitude of which is 10 V peak, and a type OA91 diode demodulator. Figure 4.19 shows how the insertion loss of such a demodulator varies with the forward input voltage, for various values of $R = R_L$, with $R_S = 0$. Curves of the same shape correspond to situations in which $R_S > 0$, but for which $(R_S + R_L) = R$; R_S and R_L simply form a potential divider to share that part of the input voltage which is not developed across the diode, and the curves are shifted by an additional insertion loss which is independent of the input voltage. The effect of demodulator non-linearity is to expand the dynamic range of the video signal. Thus, if the input to the demodulator has a dynamic range of 50 dB, and a maximum amplitude of 10 V peak, then the minimum input signal is 0·0316 V peak. The dynamic range of the demodulated output (video) signal depends upon the total value of $(R_S + R_L)$; in the example illustrated in Fig. 4.19, the video dynamic range varies from about 60 dB when $(R_L + R_S) = 100$ kΩ, to 78 dB when $(R_L + R_S) = 1$ kΩ.

Although the effect of the non-linearity of the demodulator can be reduced by increasing the total value of $(R_S + R_L)$, there are in practice certain factors which limit this improvement. The input impedance of the video amplifier is generally in the order of 1 kΩ, and this sets an upper limit to the value of R_L. In any event, R_L must be kept quite small so that the effects of the stray capacitances do not become significant. R_S can be increased, for example by means of a series resistor, but R_S and R_L form a potential divider which reduces the amplitude of the signal fed to the video amplifier. In addition, the reverse current of the type OA91 diode, for example, is around 1 μA at 0·5 V, and the efficiency of the device as a rectifier is reduced if it is operated in a high impedance circuit. However, it is usually possible to make the value of $(R_S + R_L)$ as high as 10 kΩ.

It follows from this discussion that, even if the r.f. amplifier is able to supply 10 V peak into a 10 kΩ load, the effect of diode demodulator non-linearity is to expand a 50 dB r.f. dynamic range by about 22 dB. Such an expansion is rather serious if a linear video amplifier is used. The effect of demodulator non-linearity is minimized if a logarithmic video amplifier is used, because such an amplifier performs the reverse function of dynamic range compression. For example, the 2 MHz logarithmic amplifier of Kossoff (1965) (see Section 4.5.c) is designed to accept input signals with the 63 dB range of 0·4 mV to 0·6 V. A 63 dB video range corresponds to a r.f. range before diode demodulation of about 40 dB, if $(R_S + R_L) = 10$ kΩ. However, it seems clear from a limited circulation Report—Report C.A.L. no. 31 (1965): "The C.A.L. abdominal ultrasonic echoscope", by G. Kossoff, D. E. Robinson and W. J. Garrett. (Commonwealth Acoustic Laboratories, Sydney, Australia) that, in the particular system for which it was designed, this video amplifier is actually used as a wide-band r.f. amplifier. The signal is demodulated after logarithmic compression, so that the consequent dynamic range expansion is negligible.

A very small improvement in the performance of the demodulator can be obtained if the diode is biassed in the forward direction. The difficulty with this technique is that the efficiency of the device as a rectifier is reduced, and the output signal contains an increasing proportion of the alternating current signal.

Full-wave demodulators, typical examples of which are shown in Fig. 4.20, are more efficient than half-wave demodulators. Such circuits have the additional advantage that the demodulated output accurately conveys the information contained in the input (apart from degradation due to dynamic range expansion). Thus there is less possibility of ambiguity as to the time-position of the pulse: an error equal to about half the period can occur in the case of half-wave demodulation when the phase of the signal is such that the diode is open-circuit to the first half-cycle.

Although such a circuit is apparently not widely used in ultrasonic pulse-echo systems, a full-wave infinite impedance demodulator gives a small-signal dynamic range expansion of some 20 dB less than the corresponding full-wave diode arrangement (D. H. Follett, 1968: personal communication).

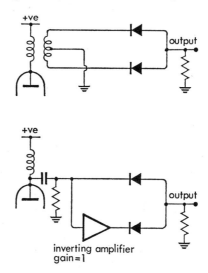

FIG. 4.20 Diagrams illustrating two types of full-wave demodulator.

The dynamic range of the signals fed to the display is usually deliberately restricted. This is the case, for example, when only the signals which exceed some particular amplitude are considered to be of clinical significance. Perhaps equally important, the resolution becomes rather poor when a wide dynamic range is displayed (see Section 4.1.b), and a r.f. dynamic range of as little as 20 dB may represent the best compromise, in which case a diode demodulator is perfectly satisfactory. The process of dynamic range restriction is known as "suppression". It is important to appreciate the distinction between suppression and dynamic range compression. Suppression is equivalent to the action of a non-linear demodulator. This is because such a demodulator expands the signal dynamic range so that the weak signals become relatively even weaker. Variable signal suppression can be introduced by reverse-biassing either the demodulator, or a separate diode which is connected in the forward direction in the video signal path. The use of a separate diode is generally preferable, because the demodulator can be designed to give the minimum dynamic range expansion, and the suppression diode can be forward biassed when zero suppression is required. In most clinical applications, the adjustment of the suppression level is empirical. The degree of suppression may be measured either in volts, or in decibels relative to some fixed reference level.

4.5 VIDEO AMPLIFIERS

4.5.a General Considerations

The demodulated output from the r.f. amplifier consists of video signals with a useful dynamic range in the order of 50 dB and maximum amplitude of around 1 V peak. It is necessary for these signals to be amplified to a level suitable for driving the particular display which is being used. Usually, the display is a cathode ray tube arranged as an A-scope or as a B-scope (see Section 4.7). In most cases, the maximum small-signal gain required in the video amplifier is around 50 dB, although it can often be much less in practice.

The video amplifier must be designed to meet the following requirements:

(i) Adequate gain to drive the display when the input signal is of the smallest value of clinical significance;

(ii) Adequate bandwidth to maintain the pulse characteristics, unless it is deliberately desired to process the signal, for example by differentiation; and

(iii) Dynamic range compression to avoid overdriving the display with large amplitude signals. This may be achieved if necessary by limiting the maximum value of the output of a linear amplifier, or by logarithmic amplification.

The degree of dynamic range compression which is required depends upon the type of display which is being used. An A-scope display normally has a dynamic range of around 40 dB, and in any event overloading signals do not confuse the interpretation, and so it may not be necessary to apply compression. Simple limiting by amplitude clipping in the linear amplifier is usually satisfactory, unless measurements of echo amplitude throughout the whole dynamic range are required, in which case a logarithmic amplifier may be necessary. However, the dynamic range of a B-scope is not greater than around 20 dB, and dynamic range compression by limiting in a linear amplifier is not ideal, unless the dynamic range is deliberately restricted to improve the resolution (see Section 4.1.b). In other cases, a logarithmic video amplifier provides a satisfactory characteristic.

Brinker (1966) and Brinker and Taveras (1966) have mentioned the use of a video amplifier in which the output dynamic range is effectively zero.

The device consists of a video activated monostable multivibrator which generates a 0·4 μsec pulse for every echo which is greater than some fixed amplitude. The monostable cannot be retriggered by another video signal until an additional time has elapsed, so that the B-scan produced by this system consists of a large number of appropriately positioned bright spots, each of an equal size. This method seems to be valuable in brain scanning through the intact skull, where the signal dynamic range is very large.

4.5.b Linear Video Amplifiers

The various aspects of the design of linear video amplifiers have been discussed in many textbooks on electronics: see, for example, Millman and Taub (1956), pp. 58–103. The simplest and most commonly used type of video amplifier is made up of several amplifying stages coupled together by resistance-capacitance networks. At low megahertz frequencies, the upper limit of frequency response (3 dB down from mid-band gain) is conveniently made equal to the centre frequency of the ultrasonic pulse. For operation at higher frequencies, a somewhat narrower bandwidth may be satisfactory: thus, the 15 MHz system of Reid and Wild (1952) has an overall bandwidth of 4 MHz. The design of suitable amplifiers presents no special problems, except that at frequencies in excess of around 3 MHz, it may be necessary to include some kind of frequency compensation, in order to obtain an adequately fast rise-time. Such compensation may be provided by shunt-peaking inductors connected in series with the load resistors of appropriate stages.

The low frequency response may be modified to process the signal fed to the display. For example, in the 2 MHz system of Wells and Evans (1968), provision is made to limit the low frequency gain to 3 dB down from that at mid-band at a frequency of around 300 kHz. The amplifier differentiates the signal applied to the display, and this emphasizes the positional information (Wells, 1967), because the positions of the leading edges of the echoes are recorded, rather than information about the durations of the echoes. Differentiation also introduces some signal suppression, because the output is proportional to the rate of change of signal amplitude: for a given pulse shape, this becomes smaller as the signal amplitude is reduced. Another consideration which applies particularly in differentiating systems is the degree of smoothing which is necessary after demodulation to generate a suitable video envelope shape. There is no doubt that differentiation is employed in many diagnostic systems, particularly those in which the display is a two-dimensional B-scan (see Section 4.7.c), but unfortunately the details of the circuit arrangements are seldom described in the literature. However, Kossoff et al. (1965) consider that differentiation leads to a loss of information, and gives no real improvement in the quality of the scan. This is probably because their system employs a logarithmic video amplifier, which makes good use of the echo information. In systems using linear amplification, the improvement in the clarity of the scan which results from differentiation is generally more important than the loss of information. This information loss seems to arise mainly from the suppression, and partly from the small shift in the system threshold which is associated with the recovery, of the differentiating network.

Difficulties can arise if the video amplifier response cuts off at a frequency within the range 10 kHz to 100 kHz. Such a response results in serious degradation of long pulses, and the recovery time following large signals becomes excessive. Therefore, unless differentiation associated with time-constants of a few microseconds is required, it is necessary for the low frequency response to extend to about 1 kHz.

The amplitude limiting of the video output signal level is usually achieved by driving an appropriate amplifying stage to cutoff. It is best to include the limiter in an early part of the amplifier, so that the following stages are protected from excessively large signals. Alternatively, limiting can be provided by means of a diode clamp, arranged so that it does not degrade the recovery characteristic of the amplifier.

4.5.c Logarithmic Video Amplifiers

Amplifiers in which the output voltage is proportional to the logarithm of the input voltage have been used for at least twenty years in anti-clutter Radar systems. Thus, Alred and Reiss (1948) described a r.f. amplifier with a bandwidth of 2 MHz centred on 13·5 MHz, in which the output of each of five non-linear stages is shunted by a pair of appropriately biassed diodes. Typical diode characteristics are shown in Fig. 4.15. Over a limited range, the characteristic is such that, to a first approximation, the forward voltage is proportional to the logarithm of the input voltage (see Equation 4.10) if the diode is used as part of a potential divider of which a fixed impedance, or constant source impedance, forms the other part. For example, if two diodes are connected in parallel but with opposite polarity, the combination forms a logarithmic element if it is used as the load in a r.f. amplifier. A difficulty with this method is that if the diodes are connected in parallel with a tuned circuit, the bandwidth increases as the gain of the stage is reduced, because the Q-factor is also reduced. In addition, a diode used as a non-linear element generates harmonics because the instantaneous value of the dynamic resistance depends upon the forward voltage.

The five non-linear stages of Alred and Reiss's (1948) amplifier are followed by a linear stage with a gain of 20 dB, so that the effects of demodulator non-linearity are minimized (see Section 4.4.e). The amplitude response is logarithmic over the output range 1 to 12 V (22 dB). The maximum gain is 108 dB with an input of 4 μV, and the minimum gain is 30 dB with an input of 0·4 V.

Amplifiers of this type suffer from a number of practical disadvantages. Very careful selection of components and operating conditions is necessary, and in particular the performance is critically dependent on the biassing voltages of the diodes which form the non-linear elements. If the diodes are included in the anode circuit, as shown in Fig. 4.21.a, the biassing depends on the characteristics of the valve. On the other hand, the biassing conditions do not require stabilization in the arrangement shown in Fig. 4.21.b, but the transient response is degraded and the recovery time is increased by the tendency of charge stored in the coupling capacitor C to alter as a result of the occurrence of large signals.

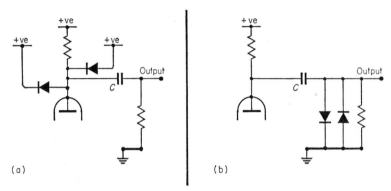

FIG. 4.21 Output limitation by shunt diodes in a single-ended amplifier. (a) Limiting at the anode by appropriately biassed diodes; (b) Limiting after d.c. decoupling by zero biassed diodes.

The nature of the logarithmic characteristic makes it difficult to apply swept gain to a logarithmic amplifier. This presents a serious restriction on the use of logarithmic r.f. amplifiers in ultrasonic pulse-echo systems. It is generally necessary to apply swept gain before the logarithmic amplifier. A suitable r.f. amplifier might have an overall gain swept through a range of from 20 to 70 dB, and might be designed along the lines indicated in Section 4.4.b. The output from the r.f. amplifier may be fed either to a second r.f. amplifier with a logarithmic response, or it may be demodulated and fed to a logarithmic video amplifier. The second alternative is often the more attractive, because the r.f. amplifier output can be made large enough to avoid excessive dynamic range expansion as a result of the demodulator non-linearity, and suppression can be conveniently applied if required (see Section 4.4.e).

The performance of a system employing both linear and logarithmic amplifiers is controlled by the range of input signals to the logarithmic amplifier. The logarithmic characteristic extends only over a limited range, and it may be necessary to shift the output level from the r.f. amplifier to match this range. For example, if the output from the r.f. amplifier has a range of 30 mV to 10 V, and the input range to the logarithmic amplifier needs to be 3 mV to 1 V for correct operation, then a 20 dB attenuator will be required between the two amplifiers. The insertion loss of a suitable demodulator might be in this order. In effect, the input noise level is adjusted by the gain of the r.f. preamplifier, and the system output, by the video amplifier which follows the logarithmic amplifier.

A logarithmic response over a dynamic range of 60 dB can be obtained in a video amplifier by the use of a single Zener diode as the non-linear element (Ophir and Galil, 1961). The diode is biassed so that a Zener current is drawn in the absence of a signal; the signal polarity is arranged so that the Zener current increases with increasing signal amplitude. At input levels corresponding to a diode current of about 100 μA (which would typically

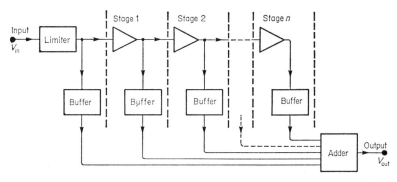

Fig. 4.22 Successive addition logarithmic video amplifier with in-phase stage gain. (Adapted from Fig. 1 of Kossoff, Liu and Robinson (1965).)

correspond to maximum gain for a dynamic range of 60 dB), the rise-time is in the order of 1 μsec because of the high capacitance of the Zener diode. This capacitance falls with increasing current. A satisfactory performance could probably be obtained for dynamic range compression in ultrasonic pulse-echo systems at low megahertz frequencies with an input range of 40 dB and a minimum Zener diode current of 1 mA, although this does not seem to have been tried in practice.

Kossoff *et al.* (1965) have described two logarithmic video amplifiers specially designed for dynamic range compression in ultrasonic pulse-echo systems. Their circuits were developed from the "successive detection and addition" logarithmic r.f. amplifier of Croney (1951). The basic principles of the technique have been discussed by Alcock (1962).

Amplifiers in which successive addition is used to obtain a logarithmic response consist of several stages connected in cascade, as shown in Fig. 4.22. Each stage is linear for very small input signals, and becomes non-linear as the input level is increased until the stages become saturated and no further increase in output level can occur. As the input to the amplifier is increased from a low level, each stage in turn becomes saturated, beginning with the final stage, until there is sufficient signal to saturate all the stages. The output signals from every stage are combined so that the amplifier output is proportional to the sum of the outputs from each stage. The input limiter is required to ensure that the direct input signal contribution to the output has a maximum value equal to that of a saturated stage, even when the input signal exceeds this value.

There are several methods by which the non-linear stage response may be achieved. For example, in Croney's (1951) r.f. amplifier, stage limitation is provided by valve overloading. This method is associated with a rather long recovery time, and diode limitation is generally better in this respect. The difficulty of arranging the appropriate limiting diode biasing is avoided in

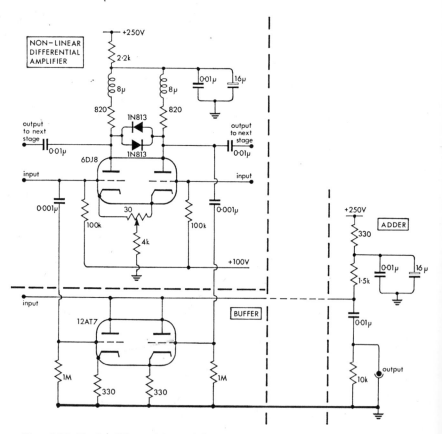

FIG. 4.23 Single differential amplifier stage and associated circuits for 2 MHz logarithmic video amplifier. (Adapted from Fig. 5 of Kossoff *et al.* 1965.)

the design of Kossoff *et al.* (1965), by placing the diodes between the anodes of cathode-coupled differential amplifiers, as illustrated in Fig. 4.23. The d.c. levels of the anodes of each stage are balanced by the potentiometer at the cathodes. The use of low-capacity, high-speed diodes minimizes the recovery time.

In amplifiers employing unbalanced stages, the outputs cannot be added directly owing to the phase inversion in each amplifying stage. Therefore, it is necessary to feed the output from alternate stages through phase inverting amplifiers before the addition takes place. However, in amplifiers employing differential stages, in-phase outputs are available: this is the situation illustrated in Figs 4.22 and 4.23.

Consider an amplifier with n stages, each with a gain of g in the linear range.

Let V_{in} = peak input signal to the amplifier,

V_i = peak input signal to saturate a stage,

V_s = peak output amplitude from a saturated stage,

α = gain of the adding circuit,

and V_{out} = peak output signal from the amplifier.

For input signals which are so small that the last stage is operating within the linear range, the amplifier response is linear. As the input level is increased, successive stages becomes saturated, and the output is the sum of the outputs from each stage. The maximum output occurs when all the stages including the input limiter have become saturated.

The input and output levels can be calculated at the transition points for stage saturation, as shown in Table 4.2. These values are plotted in Fig. 4.24

TABLE 4.2

Signal levels in a logarithmic amplifier with n stages of successive addition. For explanation, see Section 4.5.c.

No. of saturated stages	V_{in}	V_{out}
0	$< \dfrac{V_i}{g^{n-1}}$	$\alpha V_{in}(g^n + g^{n-1} + \ldots + g + 1)$
1	$\dfrac{V_i}{g^{n-1}}$	$\alpha V_S \left(1 + \dfrac{1}{g} + \dfrac{1}{g^2} + \ldots + \dfrac{1}{g^n}\right)$
2	$\dfrac{V_i}{g^{n-2}}$	$\alpha V_S \left(2 + \dfrac{1}{g} + \dfrac{1}{g^2} + \ldots + \dfrac{1}{g^{n-1}}\right)$
n (all stages)	V_i	$\alpha V_S \left(n + \dfrac{1}{g}\right)$
$(n + 1)$ (all stages + input limiter)	gV_i	$\alpha V_S(n + 1)$

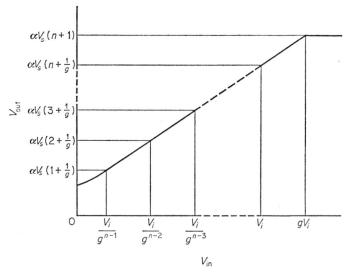

FIG. 4.24 Transfer characteristic of a logarithmic amplifier with n stages of successive addition. The ordinate has a linear scale, and the abscissa has a logarithmic scale. (Adapted from Fig. 3 of Alcock, 1962).

to give the transfer characteristic of the amplifier. The transfer characteristic deviates only by small amounts from the logarithmic relationship between the levels for stage saturation, because each stage has a non-linear response below saturation due to the limiting diodes. In most practical amplifiers, g is sufficiently large to allow $\dfrac{1}{g^2}$ and higher terms to be neglected in the expression for V_{out}, and this is done for simplicity in Fig. 4.24. The amplifier has a logarithmic characteristic over an input range of $\dfrac{V_i}{g^{n-1}}$ to gV_i, and the corresponding output range is $\alpha V_s \left(1 + \dfrac{1}{g}\right)$ to $\alpha V_s (n + 1)$. Expressed as ratios these values correspond to an input dynamic range of g^n, and an output dynamic range of $\left(\dfrac{n + 1}{1 + 1/g}\right)$. Therefore, the input dynamic range is approximately equal to the small-signal gain, and the output dynamic range increases with the number of stages, and is only slightly affected by the stage gain.

Kossoff *et al.* (1965) have given complete circuit diagrams for logarithmic video amplifiers for operation at frequencies of 2 and 8 MHz. Their 2 MHz amplifier has five differential stages, each of which has a maximum gain of 15 dB and a bandwidth of 11 MHz. The recovery time is less than 0·5 μsec. The bandwidth of the video amplifier is 4 MHz for small signals, and that of the adder is 5 MHz. The input coupling time-constant of the final stage is chosen to give a low frequency response cut-off at 500 kHz. It has already been pointed out that such a response differentiates the video signal (see Section 4.5.b); but in the system in which this amplifier is used, the demodulator apparently follows the so-called "video" amplifier, which is really used as a wide-band r.f. amplifier (see Section 4.4.e). The amplifier has a logarithmic characteristic over the input range 0·4 mV to 0·6 V (63 dB), and the corresponding output range is 0·8 to 3·8 V (14 dB). Similarly, their 8 MHz amplifier consists of four differential stages and a single-ended output stage. The single-ended stage reduces the power requirements and improves the stability of the amplifier. Pentodes are used in

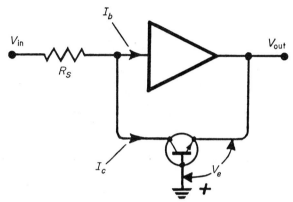

FIG. 4.25 Arrangement of a transistor to apply negative feedback to an amplifier, resulting in a logarithmic amplitude response.

this amplifier to give the required high-frequency response, and the recovery time is less than 0·15 μsec. The bandwidth is 12 MHz. The input dynamic range is 0·4 mV to 1 V (80 dB); the corresponding output range is 0·5 V to 4·6 V (19 dB). An additional stage of linear video amplification is required with both these amplifiers to drive the display.

A satisfactory logarithmic response can also be obtained by the use of a transistor as the negative feedback element in an amplifier, although this approach does not yet seem to have been used in an ultrasonic system. The basic principles are shown in Fig. 4.25. It can be shown (Paterson, 1963) that, provided $V_e > 100$ mV,

$$I_C = \alpha_n I_{ES}\, e^{\frac{qV_e}{kT}}, \qquad (4.16)$$

where $\quad \alpha_n$ = normal common base current gain,

I_{ES} = emitter reverse saturation current,

k = Boltzman's constant ($1·37 \times 10^{-23}$ joules per deg. K),

T = temperature (deg. K),

and $\quad q$ = electronic charge ($1·60 \times 10^{-19}$ coulomb).

An accurate conversion device requires that α_n is independent of the current, so that feedback degeneration increases with the exponent of the output. This condition is almost perfectly satisfied by silicon diffused transistors of the mesa or planar types, and such devices exhibit ideal logarithmic behaviour over extremely wide ranges. For example, Lunsford (1965) has described a pulse amplifier in which a type 2N2219 transistor is used as the feedback element, and in which an input range of from 10 mV to 10 V (60 dB) is compressed, with a logarithmic linearity of about 2·5%, into an output range of from 2 to 10 V (14 dB). The rise-time of this amplifier is less than 0·1 μsec, the droop is negligible with a 1 msec pulse, and high thermal stability is achieved by maintaining the critical transistors at constant temperature.

4.5.d First Echo Swept Gain Trigger Circuits

In systems in which the transducer is in direct contact with the patient, the swept gain circuits are triggered by the same pulse as that which is used to trigger the transmitter. However, this method is not satisfactory in systems in which the transducer is separated from the patient by a variable length water delay path. The attenuation of the ultrasonic pulse when travelling in water may generally be neglected, and swept gain is only required from the instant that the first echo returns from the patient. Because the distance between the transducer and the skin surface is not constant in a scanning system, it is necessary to derive a trigger pulse from the echo information at the instant that the first echo returns from the skin surface, and to arrange for this pulse to trigger the swept gain generator.

Unfortunately, the circuits which have been used to derive a trigger pulse from the first echo are seldom described in the literature. In one method, described only in a limited circulation Report—Report C.A.L. no. 31 (1965): "The C.A.L. abdominal ultrasonic echoscope", by G. Kossoff, D. E. Robinson and W. J. Garrett. (Commonwealth Acoustic Laboratories, Sydney, Australia), the main trigger pulse, which also triggers the transmitter, is fed to a monostable multivibrator. In this particular scanner, the echoes of clinical importance are arranged to return during an interval of 232 μsec, which begins 232 μsec after the transmission pulse. The multivibrator provides a delay of 200 μsec, so that the swept gain generator is not triggered by the transmitter. At the end of this delay, a second multivibrator is triggered to generate a gate of 100 μsec duration. The first echo to return during this interval is arranged to trigger the swept gain generator.

A somewhat similar method has been described by Wells and Evans (1968). A block diagram of their arrangement is shown in Fig. 4.26.a. At time t_0, the transmitter trigger is applied to a monostable multivibrator which generates an output pulse at time t_1, delayed by 100 μsec after t_0. 100 μsec corresponds to a range of 7·5 cm in water, and in the particular scanner for which this circuit was designed the skin surface could not be so close to the transducer. The pulse at t_1 triggers the bistable multivibrator, which opens the signal gate. The circuit remains in this condition until a pulse of sufficient amplitude to trigger the bistable passes along the video channel and through the signal gate. The first echo from the patient's skin, at t_2, normally performs this operation: the triggering of the bistable closes the

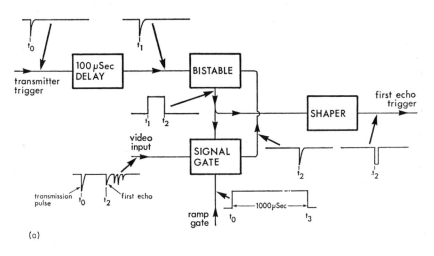

(a)

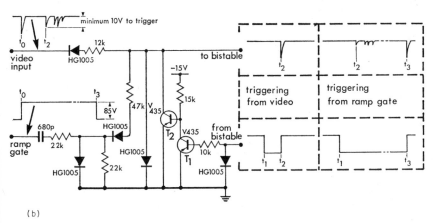

(b)

Fig. 4.26 Diagrams illustrating the derivation of a trigger pulse at the instant that the first echo returns from the patient. (Adapted from Figs. 10 and 11 of Wells and Evans, 1968). (a) Block diagram; (b) Circuit diagram of the signal gate. An additional amplifier (not shown in the diagram) is necessary to invert the output from the bistable to drive this circuit.

signal gate, and the negative-going pulse from the bistable is differentiated and shaped to provide the first echo trigger output.

The circuit of the signal gate is shown in Fig. 4.26.b. When the gate is open, the minimum video signal required to trigger the bistable is 10 V. Under some circumstances, the first echo does not have an amplitude large enough to trigger the bistable. Therefore, a large-amplitude pulse is applied along the video channel, at time t_3, 1000 μsec after t_0: this pulse is derived from the time-base gate (see Section 4.7.c). Consequently, if the bistable has not been previously triggered by the first echo, it is triggered at t_3; this prevents the circuit from coming out of sequence and so being triggered by the arrival of the next transmission pulse.

4.6 CATHODE RAY TUBE DISPLAYS

4.6.a Conventional Cathode Ray Tubes

Cathode ray tubes are extensively employed for the presentation of ultrasonic pulse-echo information. Modern cathode ray tubes are precision instruments possessing a linear deflection sensitivity, and are capable of providing excellent resolution. Their design is a specialized subject (Soller et al. 1948) and no more than a brief account of the most important considerations is given here.

Cathode ray tubes are classified into two broad groups, according to their deflection systems which may be either electrostatic or electromagnetic. The principal features of the two types of tube are illustrated in Fig. 4.27. The electron gun is designed to produce a beam of electrons which is focussed on to the fluorescent screen, either by means of a suitable anode assembly in an electrostatic tube, or by the magnetic field of the focus coil in an electromagnetic tube. In an electrostatic tube, the spot deflection is proportional to the potential difference between the deflection plates. The y-deflection plates are normally further from the screen than the x-deflection plates, and so the y-deflection sensitivity is usually the higher. The design of suitable coils to produce uniform deflection of the beam in an electromagnetic tube presents a number of problems, but electromagnetic deflection is associated with a smaller degree of defocussing. For this reason, electromagnetic tubes are preferable where a large display is required.

The accelerating voltage is made as high as possible in order to develop the maximum energy at the screen for conversion into visible radiation. The most economical technique by which this can be achieved is to accelerate the electron beam after it has been deflected. In this way, the high deflection sensitivity of a low energy beam is maintained. Post deflection acceleration is achieved by means of a conductive coating on the inside of the front part of the tube, which is kept at a high voltage relative to the last anode in the electron gun. The ratio of these two voltages may be as high as 10 : 1, but with high ratios the field from the post deflection acceleration anode tends to penetrate behind the deflectors and to accelerate the beam before deflection. In some tubes, this effect is reduced by forming the post deflection acceleration electrode into a helix, which acts as a potential divider and reduces the accelerating field as the distance from the screen increases.

A disadvantage of post deflection acceleration is that if the beam is deflected off the screen it may strike the post deflection acceleration electrode

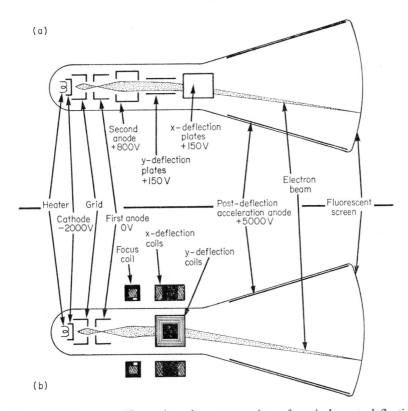

Fig. 4.27 Diagrams illustrating the construction of typical post deflection acceleration cathode ray tubes. (a) Electrostatic deflection and focussing type; (b) Electromagnetic deflection and focussing type. Typical electrode voltages are shown. Arrangements are normally made to prevent the control grid from being driven positive with respect to the cathode. The grid-cathode cut-off voltage is typically around −40 V. In the electrostatic tube, focussing is accomplished by variation of the second anode potential, and the deflection sensitivity is around 100 V for a deflection of one screen radius. The coils of a typical electromagnetic tube designed for use with thermionic valve circuits draw 20 mA for focussing, and 50 mA to produce a one-radius deflection.

and generate secondary electrons: these secondaries produce large areas of fluorescence on the screen, which tend to obscure the trace. The effect can be reduced by careful selection of the operating voltages. However, because of the rather low duty cycle in many ultrasonic diagnostic applications, the advantages of a bright trace combined with high deflection sensitivity outweigh any such disadvantages associated with post deflection acceleration.

The screen is formed by coating the inside surface of the tube with a suitable phosphor, which emits luminous radiation under the impact of the electron beam. The best type of phosphor depends upon the particular application. The characteristics of some of the more common phosphors are given in Table 4.3. Of the two general purpose phosphors included in this

TABLE 4.3

Characteristics of some common phosphors used in cathode ray tubes

Designation	Colour	Decay characteristic	Typical application
P1	Yellow-green	25 m.sec to 10%	General purpose
P11	Blue	35 μsec to 10%	Photography
P31	Green	50 μsec to 10%	General purpose
P33	Orange	60 sec to 1%	Long persistence

Table, the type P31 is more efficient in terms of light intensity than the type P1. Long persistence phosphors, such as the type P33, can be used in displays from which, for example, the operator can gain an impression of a complete scan as a preliminary to photographic recording.

The resolution of a cathode ray tube display is determined by the relationship between the size of the screen and the diameter of the luminescent spot. In practical tubes, imperfections in the electron optics deform the shape of the spot, especially near the edge of the screen. In addition, the brightness of the spot is greatest at the spot centre, and falls off towards its edge: therefore, the spot has no sharp boundary. The edge of the spot is defined as the contour at which the brightness has fallen to some specific fraction of the maximum brightness. This fraction is usually chosen so that if the centres of two spots are one spot diameter apart, the two spots can just be resolved. The spot diameter is conveniently measured by the "shrinking raster" method. A series of, say, 100 lines is drawn on the screen by means of two time-base circuits as in a television raster. Under conditions of optimum focus, the lines are brought closer together by decreasing the amplitude of the slower time-base, until the screen appears to be uniformly illuminated in the raster area. The height of the raster divided by the number of lines then gives the line width, which is equal to the spot diameter.

The measurement of the spot size is further complicated by non-linearity in the luminescent intensity with changing beam current, which causes variation in the spot diameter as previously defined. As a general guide, however, the spot diameter may be taken as being about 0·05 cm for a display tube with a diameter or diagonal size of around 15 cm. When other display sizes are used, it is usual to assume that the ratio of spot sizes is equal to the ratio of screen diameters for similar electron gun assemblies. The spot size not only determines the maximum potential resolution of a diagnostic ultrasonic system, but also to some extent controls criteria, such as the maximum useful scanning speed, upon which the design of the complete system is based.

In ultrasonic scanning, the echo information is often displayed on a brightness-modulated cathode ray tube. There are two characteristics of the tube which are especially important in such applications. Firstly, the dynamic range of the display system, which is determined by the linearity of the phosphor as a luminescent source, limits the signal dynamic range which can be accepted from the video amplifier. This is typically in the order of 20 dB. This is much less than the dynamic range of vision, which is normally at least 50 dB, and considerably more if time is available for adaptation. The video signal may be applied either to the cathode or the grid of the cathode ray tube. Cathode drive has the advantage that the cathode is readily accessible by capacitive coupling. However, capacitive coupling makes it suitable only for low-duty-cycle, short-duration pulses as the time constant of the circuit is typically in the order of 100 μsec. Another difficulty with cathode modulation in electrostatic tubes is that the effective deflection sensitivity and the focussing field are directly dependent on the cathode potential: these effects limit the maximum cathode drive to about 20–30 V. Grid modulation is free from these disadvantages, and direct coupling is normally possible. In brightness-modulated displays, it is often most convenient to apply the echo information in the form of negative-going pulses to the cathode, whilst the grid is controlled by the bright-up pulse.

The second characteristic of the cathode ray tube which is important in ultrasonic scanning is the extent to which it contributes to the integration of the video information. Video integration is dependent upon the signal-to-noise ratio and the scanning parameters (beam width, speed of scanning, pulse repetition frequency and time-base velocity), but it is also affected by the dynamic range of the display system, and the integrating characteristics of the screen of the cathode ray tube and of the observer or the recording process. It is important to realize that the storage which can be accomplished in the eye and mind of an observer is extremely effective, and, at least in high-speed scanners, it may be substantially better to use a directly observed display than to present the image on an electronic storage tube, or even to record it photographically (see Sections 4.6.b and 4.6.c). However, visual integration by the observer is not satisfactory over long periods of time.

4.6.b Electronic Storage Tubes

The need frequently arises in ultrasonic pulse-echo diagnosis for the storage of information presented on a cathode ray tube display, either for subsequent study or as part of an integrating process. This kind of storage can generally be achieved photographically; but the photographic process suffers from certain disadvantages, particularly in time delay and expense (see Section 4.6.c). However, it is possible to record many of such data

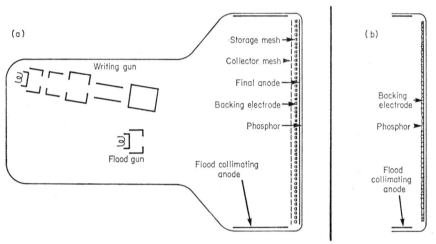

FIG. 4.28 Diagrams illustrating the construction of typical electronic storage tubes. (a) Transmission-control type. Certain electrodes, particularly those associated with the collimation of the flooding electron beam, have been omitted from the diagram in the interest of simplicity; (b) Construction of the target area of the bistable type. The electron gun arrangements are similar to those shown in (a).

quite adequately on an electronic storage tube, and thus avoid the disadvantages of photography. This method of storage is not satisfactory in every situation, but it is quite widely used.

Two types of direct-view storage tube are in common use. They differ in the method of modulating the viewing beam: this may be achieved either by transmission control, or by bistable landing-velocity control. Storage tubes of either type have poorer resolution (larger spot size) than conventional cathode ray tubes of similar screen dimensions. Typically, the spot diameters might be 0·1 cm and 0·05 cm respectively.

Figure 4.28.a is a diagram showing the main features of a transmission-control electronic storage tube. The operation of this type of tube has been described by Knoll and Kazan (1956). The writing gun deposits a charge pattern on the storage surface, which consists of an insulator coating on a metal mesh backing electrode. The quantity of charge deposited depends on the writing beam density and the speed and number of the superimposed scans. Low velocity electrons from the flood gun (which must be operating during the writing process to avoid runaway charging) approach the storage mesh normally at constant current density. These electrons penetrate the mesh in those areas on which a charge pattern has been written, and are accelerated to the viewing screen where they produce an image. The brightness of the image is determined by the stored information, and so this type of tube is capable of displaying several shades of tone; the dynamic range is typically around 10 dB. The image can be completely erased by the application of a small positive pulse (about 1 sec duration) to the backing electrode. Such a pulse produces an instantaneous rise in the storage mesh potential as a result of capacitive coupling, and this allows the flood beam electrons to land on the entire surface of the storage mesh. The potential of the storage mesh is consequently reduced to near flood gun potential, so that the stored potential pattern becomes erased. The flow of flood beam electrons to the screen is cut off at the end of the erasing pulse, and the tube is then ready for the next writing operation. Varying degrees of display persistence can be obtained by the application of a continuous train of short-duration pulses to the backing electrode.

A typical transmission-control storage tube (the type E702C of the English Electric Valve Co. Ltd.) has a screen diameter of just over 10 cm, and gives a viewing time of at least 10 min. Storage times of several days can be obtained by cutting off the flood beam. The maximum writing speed is about 2·5 cm per μsec, which corresponds to a maximum display size in ultrasonic diagnosis of over 30 times the dimensions of the soft-tissue structures being examined.

The bistable category of direct-viewing storage tube is a relatively recent development. Bistable tubes differ from those which employ transmission-control modulation chiefly in the construction and performance of the target area. The target of a modern bistable tube (Anderson, 1967) is shown diagrammatically in Fig. 4.28.b. The writing gun forms a charge image on the dielectric storage layer which controls the transmission of flood current to the storage screen. Where the target background is unwritten the screen is at low potential, and the flooding electrons bombard the target at low velocity: this results in only a low secondary emission ratio. Consequently, these areas become negative. However, the areas of the target which have been written are at increased potential: the flooding electrons cause a high secondary emission ratio, and the target becomes positive. Thus, the target has bistable properties, and may be charged in opposite directions by flood gun bombardment from a single source. The image can be erased by reducing the voltage applied to the backing electrode.

The performance of a bistable storage tube is largely dependent on the design of the target area. The phosphor is deposited in the form of a porous layer with a semi-continuous surface. The storage time is limited by the migration of charge across the dielectric layer; useful storage times of up to about one hour are obtainable under optimum conditions. Writing speeds of over 0·025 cm per μsec are quite common, and some specially selected tubes (for example, the type T5640-201 of Tektronix, Inc.) are capable of writing at speeds of over 0·1 cm per μsec. However, the fastest writing speed corresponds to a maximum display size in ultrasonic diagnosis of only just slightly more than the dimensions of the soft-tissue structures being examined; and the maximum writing speed of this type of tube becomes substantially less as the tube ages.

The dynamic range of a bistable storage tube is effectively zero, as the image is either stored or not stored. This severely restricts the usefulness of this type of tube as the display in B-scope systems.

4.6.c Photographic Recording

Although the diagnostic information available from an ultrasonic investigation may often be studied directly on the cathode ray tube display, the need frequently arises for a photographic recording to be made. This may be required either as a step in the process of video integration, or for subsequent reference or publication. Single events or transients which occur in a very short time interval can only be studied in the form of recordings, and photography is frequently the best method.

The most convenient cameras for oscilloscope photography generally employ either 35 mm film, or Polaroid-Land material ("Polaroid" is a registered trade-mark of the Polaroid Corporation). The Polaroid-Land process in invaluable where a positive print is required very rapidly: with type 47 or type 107 films, both of which are available with a speed of 3000 A.S.A., the print is ready only 10 sec after the exposure has been completed. No darkroom facilities are required. Modern Polaroid-Land materials have been developed from the original techniques described by Land (1947).

In ultrasonic diagnostic applications employing brightness modulation of the display, the dynamic range of the photographic recording process may be a limiting factor controlling the system resolution. The effect is similar to the non-linearity of the brightness-modulation of the cathode ray tube (see Section 4.6.a). In general, higher speed emulsions produce images of higher contrast, or smaller dynamic range. For example, a film with a speed of 500 A.S.A. might have a dynamic range of 10 dB, whilst a speed of 2 A.S.A. might correspond to 40 dB.

Photographic recording depends upon a change being produced by light in the photographic emulsion to form a latent image which can be developed by suitable chemicals. The action of light on the emulsion may be considered in terms of the statistical probability that it will produce such a change. For a given light intensity, the probability that a latent image will be formed increases with the exposure time. This property of photographic recording gives rise to a theoretical possibility of resolution enhancement in certain ultrasonic scanning systems. Thus, due to the finite width of the scanning beam, the registration of a small target may appear on a two-dimensional compound sector B-scan (see Section 4.7.c) as a series of lines. These lines intersect at the point corresponding to the true position of the target on the display. If the conditions of exposure are carefully chosen, a latent image is only formed on the photographic emulsion at the centre of the image of the crossed lines, because it is only there that there has been sufficient light to produce a chemical change. However, practical realization of this theoretical improvement can seldom be achieved, because the wide dynamic range of the echo information usually makes it impossible to adjust the exposure conditions with enough precision and at the same time to record all the echoes of clinical significance.

It is not possible to state the exposure times required for every diagnostic application, as they depend on so many different factors. However, as a rough guide, and using 3000 A.S.A. material, an A-scan of normal brightness can be photographed using an exposure of $\frac{1}{25}$ sec at $f8$; an abdominal B-scan made up of about 1000 lines requires an aperture of $f4$ for satisfactory recording. Other conditions of brightness and film speed require exposures calculated on a proportional basis.

4.7 DATA PRESENTATION SYSTEMS AND CLINICAL APPLICATIONS

4.7.a The A-Scope

The basic principles of the A-scope are described in Section 4.1.a. Wild (1950), using a 15 MHz ultrasonic system developed by the U.S. Navy, demonstrated that the method can be used to measure tissue thickness, and for the detection of changes of tissue density. More precisely, the method indicates the presence of discontinuities in characteristic impedance. French, Wild and Neal (1950) confirmed that cerebral tumours can be detected, using brain removed from the skull immediately after death. Ludwig and Struthers (1950) were able to detect isolated gall-stones using an echo method at frequencies between 1–5 MHz, and considered that the method might be used for searching at operation, but that external application was unlikely to be possible.

Although D. Gordon and others had previously and independently used the A-scope technique on the intact living human skull, the first publication describing the method is that of Leksell (1956). Leksell's results were based on work apparently begun in 1953. Echoencephalography has become a subject of continuous development, and all the individual improvements which have taken place are too numerous to mention here. Similarly, it is outside the scope of this book to describe the separate contributions of the many investigators who have developed the applications of the method in other clinical fields. However, information on some of the more important clinical applications is included in Table 4.4. This Table is not comprehensive: but it may be useful as a guide to representative articles which contain references to the work of other investigators.

The application of the A-scope to the diagnosis of certain clinical conditions has been advanced by the development of special techniques of instrumentation and measurement. Some of these are described in the following Subsections: the numbering of these Subsections corresponds to the Notes of Table 4.4. In most medical applications of the A-scope, the ultrasonic probe is held in direct contact with the patient's skin. It is important to ensure that the ultrasonic transmission is not interrupted by the presence of air, and so some form of liquid coupling medium is used. Water is not very satisfactory, because it tends to dry up rather quickly, and so constant replenishment is necessary. For this reason, liquid paraffin or olive oil are preferable. A water-soluble couplant such as a mixture of polyethylene glycols (de Vlieger, 1967) is sometimes used. In investigations in which maximum transmission uniformity is required, washing with a detergent removes the microscopic bubbles which otherwise adhere to the skin (Pätzold *et al.* 1951).

(i) *Differential diagnosis of malignant and benign tumours*

Wild and Reid (1952b) analyzed the 15 MHz A-scans obtained from 21 patients with various abnormalities of the breast, in order to determine whether or not a quantitative measurement could be found to indicate the degree of malignancy of the corresponding lesions. The diagnosis was confirmed in each case by histological examination. The A-scans were analysed in terms of the ratios of tumour to control, for the number of echoes, the area under the A-scan tracing, and the length of the time-base along which the echoes extended. Very small echoes were neglected. It was shown that the area estimate provides a statistically significant difference between malignant and benign tumours of the breast. The area estimate is a measure of the total energy reflected by the tissue. With malignant tissue, the ratio of the area under the A-scan to that corresponding to the control (normal tissue) is greater than unity; the same ratio is less than unity with benign tissue. Subjective analysis of the A-scan is possible, although less accurate, because malignant lesions give rise to areas of increased echo density, whereas benign tumours have a decreased reflectivity.

TABLE 4.4

Some clinical applications of the A-scope

Site	Application	Reference	Note
Breast	Differential diagnosis of malignant and benign tumours	Wild and Reid (1952b)	i
	Localization of tumours	Wagai *et al.* (1965)	
Cardiovascular	Aortic aneurism	Segal *et al.* (1966)	
	Pericardial effusion	Feigenbaum *et al.* (1967)	ii
	Pulmonary embolism	Miller *et al.* (1967)	
	Septal defects (using intra-cardiac probe)	Kimoto *et al.* (1964)	
Dentistry	Examination of pulp cavity	Kossoff and Sharpe (1966)	
Gastro-enterology	Liver A–P dimensions	Holmes (1966a)	
	Liver abscess	Wang *et al.* (1964)	ii
	Liver disease	An *et al.* (1962)	iii
		Schentke and Renger (1966)	
	Operative use in cholelithiasis	Knight and Newell (1963)	
Genito-urinary	Bladder dimensions	Holmes (1967a)	
	Localization of renal calculi at operation	Schlegal *et al.* (1961)	
Miscellaneous	Disease at various sites	An *et al.* (1962)	
		Pell (1964)	
		Wagai *et al.* (1965)	
	Differentiation of cystic and solid masses	Ostrum *et al.* (1967)	ii
	Pleural effusion	Pell (1964)	ii
	Soft tissue thickness	Ramsden *et al.* (1967)	
Neurology	Amplitude-averaging technique	White and Blanchard (1966)	iv
	Brain mid-line localization: basis of method	Jeppsson (1961)	iv
	Comparator technique: basic principle electronic switching duplicate systems	Gordon (1959) Robinson and Kossoff (1966) Brinker (1967) White and Blanchard (1966)	iv
	Control technique by transmission time	Lithander (1960)	iv
	Clinical results	Ford and Ambrose (1963) Brinker *et al.* (1965) White (1966, 1967)	v
	Intracranial pressure	Jeppsson (1964)	vi
Obstetrics and Gynaecology	Foetal cephalometry	Willocks *et al.* (1964)	vii
	Hydatidiform mole	An *et al.* (1962)	viii
	Placental localization	Bang and Holm (1968)	viii
Ophthalmology	Axial length measurement of eye	Jansson (1963) Coleman and Carlin (1967)	ix
	Diagnosis of disease	Oksala (1967)	
	Foreign body localization and extraction	Bronson (1965)	
	Special probes	Buschmann (1965) Leary (1967)	x

The Notes detailed in this Table appear as Subsections in Section 4.7.a.

It is important to realize that the distinction between malignant and benign tumours made possible by this method is not necessarily satisfactory at other ultrasonic frequencies. Thus, at frequencies in the low megahertz range, solid abnormalities often appear as areas of increased echo density, no matter what their histological nature may be (see, for example, Subsection (iii) of this Section). This is probably because it is not possible to compensate by swept gain for the differing absorptions of normal, benign and malignant tissues at 15 MHz. At lower frequencies the absorption differentials are reduced, and the swept gain is consequently more accurate.

(ii) Differential diagnosis of cystic and solid masses

When an ultrasonic pulse travels through an apparently homogeneous mass of tissue, it suffers multiple small reflections at the interfaces between the various constituent parts of the mass which differ in characteristic impedance. This results in the appearance on the A-scan of many small echoes on those parts of the time-base corresponding to tissue masses, in addition to the large echoes which mark the interfaces between the various organs. However, propagation of a pulse through a cavity containing water, or a uniform liquid, is relatively free from such small echoes. Therefore, it is possible to differentiate between cystic and solid masses by the absence or presence of small echoes on the corresponding part of the A-scan when observed with high system sensitivity. Such echo-free areas are said to be "transonic". It is important for the test to be made at high sensitivity, because otherwise the small echoes which originate in a solid mass may not appear on the display. The method is illustrated in Fig. 4.29.

The presence of a cyst or similar structure can complicate the interpretation of the A-scan. This is because the absorption coefficient of watery liquids is much less than that of soft tissues, and so echoes which originate from beyond the cyst are of larger amplitude than would be the case if the mass were solid. The swept gain of the receiver (see Section 4.1.b) is normally adjusted to a rate which gives good visualization of soft tissues, and, in the case of transmission through a cyst, the echoes from distant structures are displayed with disproportionately large amplitudes.

(iii) Diagnosis of liver disease

The diagnosis of liver disease by A-scan ultrasonography is based on two kinds of observation. Firstly, the positions of echoes on the time-base give an indication of the size of the liver. Secondly, the amplitudes of echoes from within the liver are related to the configurations and magnitudes of the corresponding characteristic impedance discontinuities. The analysis of the information available from echo amplitude measurements is rather difficult. This is partly because there is quite a wide variation in this respect between so-called "normal" livers, partly because of the difficulty in recognizing

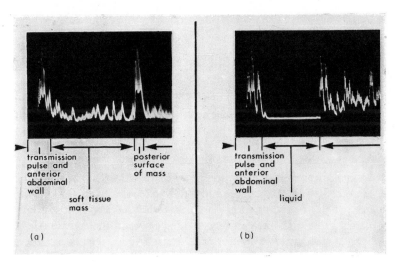

Fig. 4.29 A-scans illustrating the differentiation of solid and cystic masses. Scans obtained using 1·5 MHz transducer of 2·0 cm diameter. Swept gain 1·8 dB cm^{-1}. System sensitivity and timebase velocity equal in both scans. (a) Soft tissue mass (hydatidiform mole); (b) Liquid mass (ovarian cyst).

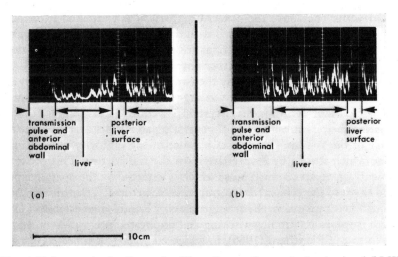

Fig. 4.30 A-scans in the diagnosis of liver disease. Scans obtained using 1·5 MHz transducer of 2·0 cm diameter. Swept gain 1·8 dB cm^{-1}. System sensitivity and timebase velocity equal in both scans. (a) Normal liver; (b) Liver cirrhosis.

artifacts, and partly because the thickness and transmission characteristics of the body wall differ from one individual to another. These problems are discussed further in Section 4.7.d. Despite these difficulties, the method seems to be quite reliable; for example, An *et al.* (1962) achieved an overall accuracy of 94% in 3554 patients (including 1541 with normal livers) examined by this method. Examples of A-scans obtained from patients with normal and diseased livers are shown in Fig. 4.30.

(iv) Localization of brain mid-line

This is perhaps the most widely-used application of diagnostic ultrasound. The basis of the method is that, in the normal, the mid-line structures of the brain lie in a plane at the geometrical centre of the skull. This is at the time-centre of the corresponding A-scan produced by holding the ultrasonic probe in contact with the temporoparietal region just above the tip of the ear. The mid-line echo can be identified on the A-scan because it normally has the largest amplitude of the intracranial echoes. Adequate swept gain compensation is normally provided, at frequencies below 2 MHz, by arranging for the gain to increase to maximum over a range of about 5 cm (67 μsec). 1·5 MHz is the most commonly used frequency for brain scanning, because the skull-bone attenuation is inconveniently large at higher frequencies. If a substantially higher frequency is used, a two-stage swept gain is necessary to compensate at the appropriate rates for the different absorptions in bone and brain.

Measurements made from a single A-scan are not very reliable. It is much better to examine the skull from each side in turn, and to display the two A-scans one above the other. Comparison is simplified if one of the A-scans (usually the one obtained with the probe on the left side) is electrically inverted, so that the deflections are in opposite directions from the two time-bases, which lie close together near the centre of the display. A rather attractive possibility is to display the two A-scans simultaneously, by using two probes operating alternately, as suggested by Gordon (1959). However, this comparator technique has certain practical disadvantages, the most important being the possibility of generating an artifact exactly at the time-centre of the A-scan. This arises because of the difficulty of isolating the probe which should be inoperative from the transmitter. This probe consequently generates a small pulse which is detected by the operative probe, in addition to the echoes from intracranial structures. Transmission breakthrough is eliminated in the arrangements of Robinson and Kossoff (1966), which employs electronic switching and duplicated preamplifiers, and that of White and Blanchard (1966), in which completely duplicated ultrasonic systems are used.

Lithander (1960) developed the method, nowadays widely used, in which the time-centre of the skull is determined by transmission, and compared with the position of the mid-line structures as determined by reflection. This technique is illustrated in Fig. 4.31. A displacement of 0·2–0·3 cm is generally considered to be within normal limits: to some extent, this reflects the inherent errors in the ultrasonic measurement, because it is unlikely that so large a shift would actually be found in a normal patient.

A serious criticism of the pulse-echo method for brain mid-line localization is that it seems to be a rather subjective examination. The problem is that a clinician who knows something of the history of the patient is likely to obtain a more accurate A-scan than that obtained by an operator who is ignorant of the clinical condition. In pointing this out, White and Blanchard (1966) suggested that the objectivity of the test can be improved if the A-scan display is photographed with a time-exposure whilst small changes

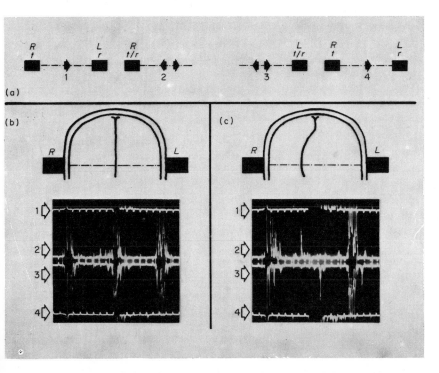

FIG. 4.31 A-scan localization of brain mid-line structures. (a) Diagrams indicating positions of probes in standardized examination. Transmitting probe: t; receiving probe: r. Each of the positions 1 to 4 correspond to the appropriate scans in the composite displays (b) and (c); (b) Scans of a patient with central brain mid-line structures; (c) Scans of a patient with brain mid-line structures displaced by 1·4 cm towards the right side by an intracerebral haemorrhage on the left side. The time markers on the scan correspond to 1 cm distances in soft tissues. Scans obtained using 1·5 MHz transducer of 2·0 cm diameter.

are made in the position and direction of the probe. This technique seems to reduce the ambiguity in determining the position of the mid-line echo.

(v) *Clinical results in neurological examinations*

The most reliable index of intracranial abnormality afforded by ultrasonic pulse-echo diagnosis is the measurement of the extent of shift of the mid-line echo from the central position. Other examinations, based on the identification of abnormal echoes from within the brain, require considerable skill in interpretation, although it is possible, for example, to measure the widths of the third and lateral ventricles (Ford and McRae, 1966).

There is quite a wide divergence between various authors in estimating the accuracy with which the mid-line can be localized. This is partly due to differing definitions of accuracy, but it is also due to the surprisingly subjective nature of the test. Whether or not this is a valid criticism is a matter for personal opinion. There is no doubt that a skilled clinician can obtain a very high diagnostic accuracy with pulse-echo ultrasonics: for example, Brinker *et al.* (1965) achieved an overall accuracy of 97% in a series of 469 patients. However, White (1966) examined the results obtained in a series of 310 patients investigated by the technique of amplitude-averaged A-scanning, and concluded that the echograms of nearly half of the patients with radiologically confirmed shifts could not be satisfactorily analysed, as compared with 10% of the whole group. This was presumed to be due to a distortion of the mid-line structures which alters the characteristics of the mid-line echo so that it is no longer the echo of the largest amplitude. As a screening method, the technique seems to be reliable: there were no errors when satisfactory echograms were obtained and no shift of the mid-line structures was diagnosed. In a further analysis, White (1967) reported no false-negative errors in 2500 examinations.

(vi) *Estimation of intracranial pressure*

The amplitude of the echo from the mid-line structure of the brain oscillates in sympathy with the cardiac cycle. Jeppsson (1964) demonstrated that the rise-time of the maximum excursion of the mid-line echo amplitude, normalized to the heart rate, is significantly decreased in patients with raised intracranial pressure. The ultrasonic information may be presented in the form of a time-amplitude recording of the signals fed from an electronic integrator. ter Braak and de Vlieger (1965) suggested that the change in echo amplitude may be due to alterations in the curvature of the surface from which the mid-line echo originates, and that the extent of these alterations depends upon the pulsating intracranial pressure. This theory is supported by the apparent existence of horizontal echo pulsations along the time-base, associated with the variations in echo amplitude (see Section 4.7.e).

The character of intracerebral echo amplitude pulsations seems to be related to other clinical conditions in addition to the pressure of the cerebro-spinal fluid: see, for example, de Vlieger (1967).

(vii) Foetal cephalometry

The distance between the parietal bones of the foetal skull can be measured with quite high precision by means of a suitably calibrated A-scope. The basis of the method is that the amplitudes of the echoes from both parietal bones are most nearly equal when the ultrasonic beam encounters both bones at normal incidence. Good agreement has been demonstrated between ultrasonic measurements and measurements made using calipers immediately after birth (Willocks et al. 1964). The accuracy of the method is improved if a two-dimensional B-scan (see Section 4.7.c) is made as a preliminary to cephalometry, to ensure that the A-scope probe is properly orientated (Campbell, 1968). The measurement is most easily made by means of a calibrated variable time delay generator, which provides some form of marker on the display.

Unfortunately, there is only a poor correlation between the foetal biparietal diameter and the weight of the foetus (Thompson et al. 1965, and Thompson, 1966). However, the technique is useful in the diagnosis of placental insufficiency, which reduces the rate of foetal growth, and in the assessment of foetal maturity (Donald, 1968).

There is some reason to doubt, on purely physical grounds, that an accuracy of measurement of much better than 0·1 cm could be possible with present techniques of ultrasonic foetal cephalometry. Ultrasonic frequencies of 2·5 MHz and less seem to be used. At 2·5 MHz, a distance of 0·1 cm corresponds to 1·7 wavelengths. The measurement is based on the estimation of the time-position of two echoes: for an overall accuracy of 0·1 cm at 2·5 MHz, the position of each echo needs to be estimated to better than about 0·9 wavelengths. It is explained in Section 4.1.b that such a resolution would require quite stringent conditions of dynamic range. The situation is proportionately worse at lower frequencies.

(viii) Diagnosis of hydatidiform mole and localization of placenta

The A-scan echo complex from a hydatidiform mole is distinguished from that of a normal pregnancy by the relatively larger number of echoes of more uniform amplitude which arise from within the uterus. In a series of 200 patients, An et al. (1962) correctly diagnosed the presence of hydatidiform moles in 100 out of 112 patients, and the absence of moles in 74 out of 88 patients.

Bang and Holm (1968) have described how the placenta may be identified on an A-scan. The placenta appears as a homogeneous area from which uniformly distributed echoes can be detected with high sensitivity. The width of the placenta does not alter as a result of changing pressure on the probe, whereas a variation in width does occur in fluid-filled spaces.

(ix) Measurement of the axial length of the eye
The axial length of the eye can be measured with good precision using an A-scope. Quite high ultrasonic frequencies (up to about 15 MHz) are commonly used. The accuracy and convenience of the method compare favourably with other techniques. The physical considerations have been reviewed by Freeman (1963), who also gave an extensive bibliography. The method is more convenient and rapid than phacometry (Sorsby *et al.* 1963). Jansson (1963) compared X-radiological and (4 MHz) ultrasonic measurements of the axial lengths of 36 normal eyes, and found that the ultrasonic method has the smaller error. Coleman and Carlin (1967) have developed an improved technique for axial length measurement, in which the axis of the eye is optically aligned with that of the ultrasonic beam; they claim a precision of 0·01 cm, using a 50 MHz clock as the timing reference.

(x) Special probes for ophthalmology
The difficulties of examining the eye ultrasonically have led to the development of several probes of ingenious design. Perhaps the most widely used is the water delay probe described by, for example, Leary (1967). This

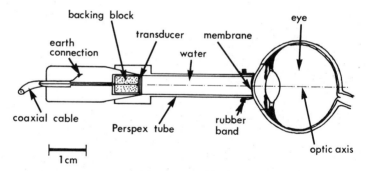

Fig. 4.32 Ultrasonic probe for measurement of the axial length of the eye, shown in relation to an adult human eye.

probe is shown diagrammatically in Fig. 4.32. Its use enables the anterior components of the eye to be examined without interference from the transmission pulse. The transducer is spaced from the cornea by a distance which is at least equal to the required penetration: this prevents the formation of multiple reflection artifacts within the eye (see Section 4.1.d). Silicone-coated rubber seems to be a satisfactory material for the membrane which closes the end of the extension tube.

Buschmann (1965) has developed miniature probes, some of which are provided with focussing lenses, for examinations other than the measurement of the axial length. For example, a probe consisting of a flat blade 0·25 cm wide, with two transducers set side-by-side in the flat surface, can be used for investigations in the equatorial region of the globe. The construction of such small probes is possible because adequate performance can be obtained at frequencies in the range 8–12 MHz.

4.7.b The B-scope

The information obtained by a pulse-echo system is a combination of range and amplitude data. This information may be presented in the form of an amplitude-modulated time-base (on an A-scope; see Section 4.7.a). However, the information may, in principle, be displayed equally well on a brightness-modulated time-base, in such a way that the brightness is proportional to the echo amplitude. This kind of display, called a B-scope, is compared with the A-scope in Fig. 4.33.b.

Practical B-scope displays have certain limitations when compared with their corresponding A-scans. The dynamic range of brightness-modulation of a conventional cathode-ray tube is about 20 dB (see Section 4.6.a), and it may be between 0 and 10 dB in an electronic storage tube (see Section 4.6.b). A typical A-scope is capable of displaying around 40 dB. Dynamic range compression is often necessary to obtain satisfactory results with a B-scope in ultrasonic diagnosis, and it is difficult to make quantitative measurements of echo amplitude. Brightness-modulation is associated with some degree of spot defocussing, and so the display resolution is rather worse in the B-scope than the A-scope.

Despite its limitations, the B-scope is used as the basis of several important diagnostic systems, some of which are described in the following sections.

4.7.c The Two-dimensional Scanned B-scope

The B-scan illustrated in diagram (ii) of Fig. 4.33.b corresponds to the pulse-echo information obtained along a typical scan line. Its interpretation requires a knowledge of the anatomical situation which it represents, so that at least some of the echoes may be identified as arising from particular structures. Thus, it is a one-dimensional display which can only be recognized and used by an experienced observer.

It is a simple matter in principle to link the direction of the time-base across the display to the direction of the ultrasonic beam across the patient, as shown in Fig. 4.33.c. The B-scan then represents the space-position of each echo-producing interface, and not simply its range from the transducer. If the probe is moved around the patient, and all the separate B-scans (each one similar to that shown in Fig. 4.33.c, but corresponding to a different transducer position and beam direction) are integrated, for example on a photographic plate, then a picture such as that shown in Fig. 4.33.d is produced. This is a compound B-scan, and it represents a two-dimensional section through the patient in the plane of the scan.

Several two-dimensional ultrasonic scanning systems are possible. As a matter of convenience, such scanners are often considered to be divided

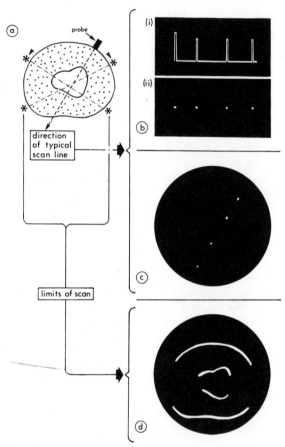

FIG. 4.33 A-scope and B-scope methods for display ultrasonic pulse-echo information. (a) Schematic representation of a section through a patient; (b) (i) A-scope presentation of a typical scan line; (ii) B-scope presentation of the same scan line; (c) B-scan as in (b) (ii), but with the direction of the timebase linked to the direction of the ultrasonic beam; (d) Compound B-scan, integrated from many individual scans, each one similar to (c).

into two main groups, according to whether the transducer scans the patient through an intervening water bath or by direct contact with the patient's skin. This division is somewhat arbitrary, and the pattern of the scan is really just as important as the coupling system.

The various scanning systems which have been described in the literature are illustrated diagrammatically in Fig. 4.34. The diagrams in this figure are arranged in chronological order of the first descriptions of the various systems. Methods a, b, c, j and k are simple scanning systems in which each reflecting interface is examined from only one direction. This severely restricts the capability of the technique on account of the specular nature of ultrasonic reflection (see Section 4.1.c). The likelihood of detecting the presence of any given interface is increased if the ultrasonic beam is arranged to scan from many different directions, as in methods d, e, f, g, h and i. However, even the most complete two-dimensional scanning system cannot detect the maximum echoes from interfaces which are curved out of the plane of the scan.

Water bath scanners can be arranged so that the part of the patient which is being examined is either actually immersed in the water, or is in acoustic contact with the water by transmission through a thin membrane and some kind of coupling medium. Coupling problems are eliminated by immersion, but the method is not always acceptable to the patient. The useful life of the water can be extended, both in immersion and non-immersion scanners, by the addition of a sterilizing chemical such as ICI "Savlon" concentrate (chlorhexidine gluconate 1·5% w/v, cetrimide B.P. 15% w/v) diluted 1 part in 5000 (Wells and Evans, 1968).

A major difficulty with water-bath scanners is due to the occurrence of artifacts which arise by multiple reflections between the transducer and the patient's skin (see Section 4.1.d). It is necessary to make the water path length at least equal to the required penetration into the patient. The difficulty can be minimized by gating the bright-up pulse (Section 4.6.a) so that the time-base only appears when useful echoes are being displayed. Multiple reflections within the water bath may take a substantial time to decay. This is particularly so if the echoes arise from primary reflections at the walls of the tank, and so have large amplitudes. The maximum repetition rate may be limited by the decay time of these reverberations.

Most two-dimensional scanners employ quite conventional transducer arrangements, similar to that described in Section 2.6.a. Focussing devices (Section 3.2) are often used to improve the lateral resolution. Howry (1955) proposed that it might be possible to obtain up to a 20 dB improvement in lateral resolution by comparing the amplitude of the echo pulse with the amplitudes of the two previous corresponding echoes as the beam is swept across the target. A simple computer could select the peak or inflection point of the beam, and modify the registration accordingly.

Probes designed to be introduced into the patient's body, as in method c of Fig. 4.34, need to be quite small and special constructional techniques are necessary. Such a probe may consist either of an unbacked transducer element (Kimoto *et al.* 1964), or be a miniature version of a full-sized conventional probe (Wells, 1966c). It has been pointed out by Kossoff (1966) that the performance of an unbacked transducer can be improved by matching its characteristic impedance to that of the loading medium (see Section 2.8). However, the lateral resolution of a miniature probe is rather poor on account of the wide divergence of the beam (see Equation 3.7), which also results in low sensitivity.

The mirror system illustrated in Fig. 4.34.j has been described in Section 3.2. This system gives two advantages in scanning the heart. Firstly, the lateral resolution is improved in the focal region; and secondly, the effective aperture of the system is relatively large, so that the amplitude variations (due to the presence of costal cartilage, sternum and lung) are minimized.

A high-speed system giving a linear scan is illustrated in Fig. 4.34.k. The transducer oscillates at the focus of a parabolic reflector. A radial scan can be obtained by using an elliptical reflector.

The direction and position of the time-base on the display can be coupled to that of the ultrasonic beam across the patient by either an electrical or a mechanical system. Electronic scanning is a third possibility. The three methods are discussed in the following Subsections.

In all three methods of coupling, the requirements are the same. It is necessary for the display to be related by some fixed scale factor to the scanned anatomy. The x and y scale factors are usually (but not necessarily always) equal. For example, the display might be $\frac{1}{5}$ actual size in the case of an abdominal scan presented on a cathode ray tube with a 10×8 cm screen: a movement of the transducer by a distance of 5 cm in any direction would produce a deflection of 1 cm in the same direction on the display. The angular direction is not altered by the scale factor. In order to maintain the correct spatial relationships, it is necessary to choose the time-base velocity (in the direction of the scan line) so that the scale factor remains constant. Thus, in the example of the $\frac{1}{5}$ actual size display, the time-base velocity would need to be about $\frac{1500}{2} \times \frac{1}{5} = 150$ m.sec^{-1} (0·015 cm per μsec). The exact time-base velocity must be adjusted with considerable precision to match both the actual propagation velocity and the scale factor, so as to obtain satisfactory registration (except in the case of simple scanning systems such as those illustrated in Fig. 4.34.a, b, c and k, in which an error in the time-base velocity simply distorts the scan without spoiling the registration).

Two factors which may limit the registration in water-bath scanners are due to the differences in velocity in water and in tissue. Such differences may be typically as much as 4% (Kossoff *et al.* 1964). At an angle of incidence of $30°$, a 4% velocity variation refracts the ray by $1·5°$ from its original direction (see Section 1.8). This corresponds to an error of $0·25$ cm for a target at a range of 10 cm beyond the skin surface. Similarly, if the scanner is adjusted for accurate registration in water, a 4% velocity variation corresponds to an error of $0·4$ cm for a target at a range of 10 cm beyond the skin surface. Similar velocity variations occur at the interfaces between soft tissues of different kinds (see Table 1.2), and in practice such variations constitute a fundamental limitation in the registration. The mean value of velocity in soft tissue is 1540 m.sec^{-1}, and this is equal to the velocity in water at $50°C$ (see Fig. 1.2). Such a temperature is rather too high to be comfortable for the patient, and the temperature of most water-bath scanners is maintained at $37°C$ (body temperature): this corresponds to a velocity of 1520 m.sec^{-1}.

Water-bath scanners are generally motor-driven. This ensures a uniform scan pattern. Best results are obtained if the transducer moves at constant velocity, and in the case of reciprocating angular motion special mechanical systems are necessary to satisfy this condition. The motors need to be chosen so that they do not generate electrical interference which would confuse the echo information.

Contact scanners may be either motor or manually driven. Manual drive has the disadvantage that the uniformity of the scan depends to a large extent on the skill of the operator. In some scanners, only one of the available motions is motor driven: this allows the operator to concentrate on obtaining better uniformity in the movements which he is controlling.

(i) Electrical coupling

The co-ordinates of the transducer (either its position or its direction, or both, according to the scanning system) are measured by means of resolvers. Potentiometers are widely used for this purpose: linear potentiometers can be coupled mechanically to the probe to give information about linear movements in rectangular co-ordinates, and sine/cosine potentiometers can be used to give angular information in polar co-ordinates. Some typical systems are illustrated in Fig. 4.35.

High-precision linear potentiometers, which in the arrangements shown in Fig. 4.35 are only required to handle d.c. signals, can be obtained in both wirewound and conducting-film types. The film type can be designed to give better resolution combined with longer life than the wirewound type.

Sine/cosine potentiometers are likewise available in both wirewound and film types. A large wirewound potentiometer, such as the type CLR96 of Colvern Ltd., may have a conformity of as good as $0·05\%$, but its life may be only about 300,000 revolutions, and the maximum speed of rotation is in the order of a few revolutions per second. Film potentiometers may be obtained with conformities of at least as good as $0·25\%$, and have a much longer life

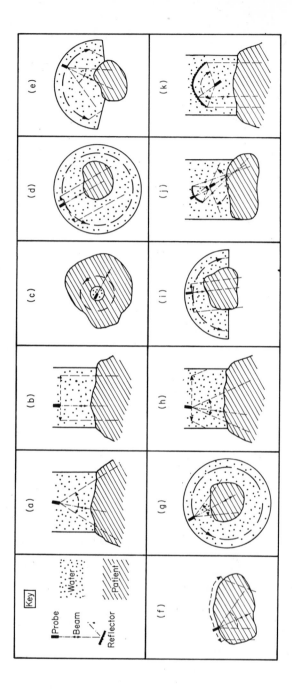

Diagram	Principal diagnostic site	Reference
a	Breast	Wild and Reid (1952a, 1952b)
	Miscellaneous	Howry and Bliss (1952)
b	Breast	Wild and Reid (1954)
	Breast and abdomen	Kikuchi et al. (1957)
c	Rectum	Wild and Reid (1957)
	Liver and heart	Kimoto et al. (1964)
d	Miscellaneous	Howry (1957)
e	Eye	Baum and Greenwood (1958)
	Uterus	Kossoff et al. (1965)
	Eye	Filipézynski et al. (1967)
	Breast	Wells and Evans (1968)
f	Abdomen	Brown (1960)
	Brain	Greatorex and Ireland (1964)
		de Vlieger et al. (1963)
	Abdomen	Holmes et al. (1965)
		Wells (1966c)
		Filipézynski and Gronioski (1967)
		Holm and Northeved (1968)
g	Miscellaneous	Gordon (1962)
	Brain	Makow and Real (1966)
h	Brain	de Vlieger et al. (1963)
	Abdomen	Evans et al. (1966)
i	Miscellaneous	Howry (1965)
j	Heart	Hertz and Olofsson (1965)
k	Miscellaneous	Krause and Soldner (1967)

FIG. 4.34 Two-dimensional compound B-scanning systems. The Table gives references to articles in which the systems are described.

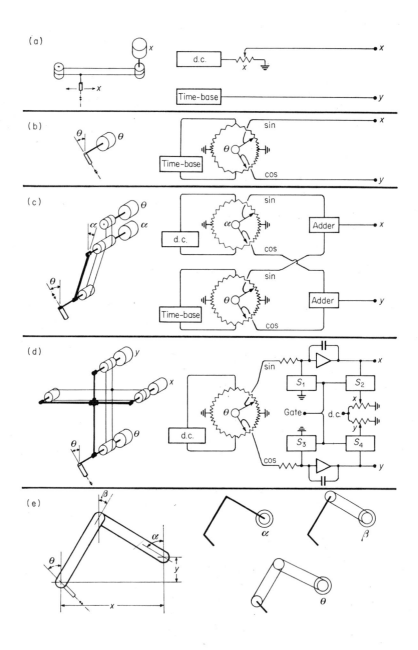

(typically 30 million revolutions) than corresponding wirewound units. Their maximum speed of rotation is a few tens of revolutions per second.

In the arrangements shown in Figs 4.35.b and c, the time-base voltages are applied directly to the sine/cosine potentiometers. This may not be entirely satisfactory if the sweep time is very fast, on account of the capacitive loading of the potentiometer and, in the case of wirewound devices, its inductance. The effects of capacitive loading can be minimized by using a low resistance potentiometer, and taking the outputs to high input-impedance amplifiers situated close to the potentiometer.

A sine/cosine potentiometer is designed to maintain accurate conformity only when it is driving a specified load impedance. This impedance is usually chosen to be as large as possible, so as to minimize the current drawn through the brushes of the potentiometer. A typical potentiometer might have a resistance of 20 kΩ per quadrant, and so its outputs are liable to interference from external fields (such as mains-induced hum voltages). For this reason, it is often necessary to change the impedance to a low level, for example by means of cathode followers placed close to the potentiometer, if the electronic system is physically an appreciable distance from the scanner. This

---

FIG. 4.35 Systems for electrical coupling of the probe co-ordinates to the display. (a) Simple linear scan. The voltage developed by the potentiometer is proportional to the x-co-ordinate of the probe. The timebase velocity is chosen to match the scale factor; (b) Simple radial scan. Balanced, antiphase timebase ramps are applied to the sine/cosine potentiometer; (c) Compound sector scan (water bath scanner). Balanced, antiphase timebase ramps are applied to the θ sine/cosine potentiometer. The d.c. supply to the α sine/cosine potentiometer is adjusted to match the scale factor; (d) Compound sector scan (contact scanner). The potentiometers are supplied with d.c. The x and y timebase ramps are generated by feedback integrators. The electronic switches S_1, S_2, S_3 and S_4 are normally closed, and are opened by an appropriately timed gating pulse. When the switches are closed, S_1 and S_3 short-circuit the inputs of the two amplifiers to earth; S_2 and S_4 set the output levels of the integrators to V_x and V_y respectively. Consequently, the beam of the cathode ray tube is stationary at the position corresponding to the position of the probe. When the switches are opened by the gating pulse, the two integrators generate voltage ramps, the signs and amplitudes of which depend on sin θ and cos θ respectively. Consequently, the movement of the spot on the display is a linear sweep at constant velocity in a direction θ from the y-axis. (Block diagram adapted from Fig. 2 of Brown (1960); (e) Compound sector scan (contact scanner). Conversion of x and y co-ordinates from polar to rectangular form is carried out by the sine/cosine potentiometers measuring the angles α and β. The appropriate outputs from these potentiometers are added together as follows:

$$x \propto \sin \alpha + \sin \beta$$
$$y \propto \cos \beta - \cos \alpha$$

(Adapted from Fig. 8 of Wells, 1966c).

precaution is unnecessary if the repetition rate is synchronized with the mains supply, as in the scanner of Brown (1960).

The electronic system illustrated in Fig. 4.35.d, which is also used with the mechanical system in Fig. 4.35.e, avoids the necessity for the time-base voltage to be applied directly to the potentiometers. The potentiometers operate at d.c., and the x and y time-bases are generated from the d.c. information by means of feedback integrators, as explained in the legend of Fig. 4.35.d. The circuit diagram of the time-base generator and switching arrangements for a single axis (either x or y) is given in Fig. 4.36. This circuit was developed by T. G. Brown and J. E. E. Fleming. Variations of this type of circuit, in which ramps proportional to sin θ and cos θ are first generated, and subsequently shifted in d.c. level by the additions of x and y voltages, have been described by Holmes et al. (1965) and by Kossoff et al. (1965).

The x, y, θ co-ordinate information is processed in the systems described here in such a way that the x, y position defined on the display is the centre about which θ rotates. No further difficulty arises if the ultrasonic probe is placed so that this centre of rotation passes along a diameter of the front face of the transducer. Unfortunately, this cannot always be so arranged in practice; for example, it would not be possible to maintain proper contact with the patient when using a compound scanner similar to those illustrated in Figs 4.35.d and e. The problem can be solved by arranging for the front face of the transducer to be at some fixed radius (usually 5–10 cm) from the centre of rotation corresponding to the x, y co-ordinates. The correct spatial relationships of the display are maintained by delaying the triggering of the transmitter until the time-base generators have been functioning for a period equal to the time corresponding to the radial distance. It is necessary for this delay to be generated quite accurately (see Section 4.2) to avoid distortion of the spatial information.

Fleming and Hall (1968) have discussed the various factors which control the display registration in electrically coupled scanners. They define the registration as the accuracy with which a point reflector is represented as a single point on the display when viewed ultrasonically from a number of different positions, assuming a system with zero beamwidth and perfect range resolution. Within the terms of this definition, the registration is limited by the precision of the mechanical and electrical parts of the scanning system. Although concerned primarily with a scanner similar to that of Donald and Brown (1961) (the principles of which are illustrated in Fig. 4.35.d), much of the discussion in their article is relevant to other forms of two-dimensional scanner. They considered the effects of imperfections in the sine/cosine and linear potentiometers, and of errors in the mechanical alignment of the measuring axes, in the time-base generators and deflection amplifiers, and in the adjustment of the transmitter delay and the time-base

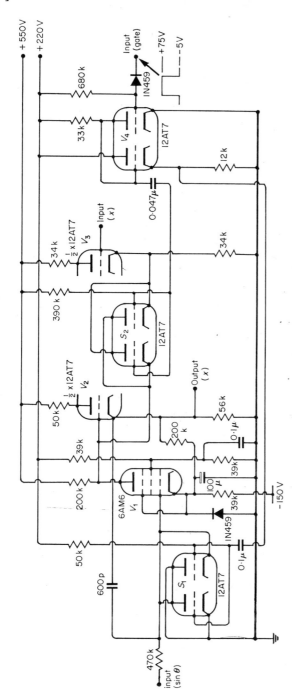

Fig. 4.36 Circuit diagram of the x-time-base generator which forms part of the block diagram in Fig. 4.35.d. V_1 is the integrating amplifier, S_1 and S_2 are the clamps. The x-input voltage is fed through the cathode follower V_3, and is arranged to vary around a mean potential of about $+150$ V. The output from the integrator is fed through the cathode follower V_2. V_4 provides the gating pulses for both the x- and y-time-base generators. The x- and y-time-base generators are identical. (Part of the valve-operated version of the "Diasonograph" type NE 4100. Circuit reproduced by courtesy of Nuclear Enterprises Ltd, who are now the manufacturers.)

velocity. They concluded that, in the system which they analysed, there is more than a 90% probability that the spot will fall within three spot diameters (0·15 cm) of the true position at a range of 20 cm on a $\frac{1}{5}$ actual size display. This is an acceptable performance in relation to the lateral and range resolutions which can be achieved in practice.

(ii) Mechanical coupling

It is possible to couple by means of a mechanical linkage a movable cathode ray tube to the ultrasonic probe in such a way that a B-scan in a fixed position on the screen of the tube is related by a suitable scale factor to the position and direction of the ultrasonic beam in space. This method of generating a compound B-scan display was proposed by Gordon (1962), who described the construction of a water-bath scanner based on the principle. Figure 4.37.a shows the main features of his instrument. A similar arrangement was used by Filipczynski and Gronioski (1967) in an abdominal contact scanner; their machine employed a pantograph constructed from articulated arms, as illustrated in Fig. 4.37.b. Again, Filipczynski et al. (1967) used a system of articulated linkages in a water-bath scanner for examining the eye.

Mechanical coupling avoids some of the complications of electrical systems, and essentially operates without distortion. The principle disadvantage of the method is its lack of versatility. Although Gordon's (1962) scanner has provision for adjustment of the scale factor of the scan, this is necessarily a much more elaborate procedure than the simple alteration of deflection amplifier sensitivity which is all that is required in an electrically coupled system. Again, it may be difficult to arrange for alteration of the plane of the scan on account of the large size of the combined electro-mechanical system, and it is often easier to move the patient than the machine. The electronic and scanning systems must be constructed as an integrated unit if mechanical coupling is employed, whereas they can be physically separated with electrical coupling. Therefore, the electronics of an electrically coupled system can be used with several different scanners, each designed for a particular diagnostic area, thus affecting a substantial economy.

Although mechanically coupled scanners are simple in principle, in practice their registration performance depends to a large extent upon the precision of their mechanical construction, and the accuracy of the timebase and the positioning of the trace on the screen of the cathode-ray tube are also very important. The registration of the best electrically coupled scanners is at least as good as that of the best mechanically coupled systems. Mechanical systems are generally rather less expensive than the corresponding electrical systems (chiefly because of the high cost of precision sine/ cosine potentiometers). However, electrically coupled scanners are almost always preferable on every other consideration except that of cost.

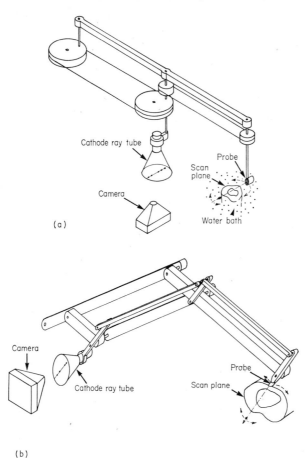

Fig. 4.37 Systems for mechanical coupling of the probe co-ordinates to the display. (a) Water bath scanner for compound sector scanning. (Adapted from Figs. 1 and 6 of Gordon, 1962); (b) Contact scanner for compound sector scanning. (Adapted from Fig. 1 of Filipczynski and Groniowski, 1967).

(*iii*) *Electronic scanning*

Electrical and mechanical systems for generating a two-dimensional B-scan are both complicated in construction and slow in operation. The limitation of speed at least would be greatly reduced if it were possible for the ultrasonic beam to be electronically steered to any desired angle from a stationary array of small transducers. The theory of such a technique is based on an extension of Huygen's principle, which is mentioned in Sections 1.14 and 3.1.

Somer (1968) has reviewed the problems of electronic beam steering, and has described the construction of a 1·3 MHz, 21 element array with dimensions of 1·1 × 1·0 cm. Each element of the array is energized by a separate transmitter; but each transmitter is triggered by the same pulse applied through separate voltage-controlled delay circuits. Thus, the phase across the array can be adjusted by altering the main control voltage, a different proportion of which is applied to each delay circuit according to the position in the array of the corresponding transducer. Alteration of the phase distribution causes the ultrasonic beam to swing through a sector: the instantaneous value of the main control voltage is related to the beam direction, and may be used to control the time-base direction on the display oscilloscope.

Unfortunately, electronically scanned beams have rather large side-lobe amplitudes, which would restrict the dynamic range in a practical diagnostic system. Again, the design of suitable circuitry to steer the receiving beam in synchronism with the transmitting beam presents formidable problems. Somer (1968) avoided this difficulty by using the central element alone of his array as a non-directional receiver. However, it is doubtful if such a solution would be practicable in clinical applications, because of its low sensitivity.

It is unlikely that the resolution of an electronically scanned arrangement could be as good as that of a mechanically scanned system employing a transducer of similar size and frequency to the array. Consequently, the main advantage of electronic scanning is its high speed capability. However, it should be understood that the ultimate limit to scanning speed is fixed (provided that adequate ultrasonic information is available despite the high scanning speed) by the deviation between the actual position of the echo-producing interface and the position at which it is recorded on the display. This deviation, which is due to the rotation of the beam which occurs during the propagation of the pulse, is equivalent to a degradation in lateral resolution. For a given speed of rotation, the angular deviation is proportional to the target range.

4.7.d Clinical Application of the Two-dimensional Scanned B-scope

The first two dimensional ultrasonic scans were obtained by Howry and Bliss (1952) and Wild and Reid (1952a, 1952b). They used rather crude water-bath scanners, operating respectively at frequencies of 2 MHz and 15 MHz. D. H. Howry and his colleagues set out from the start to produce tissue maps, or accurate cross-sectional representations of the scanned anatomy; J. J. Wild and J. M. Reid, on the other hand, were more concerned with measuring the quantity of reflected ultrasound, and trying to use this as an indication of histology. Since the time of these early investigations, most research has been concentrated on the development of the method for cross-sectional representation.

It is remarkable that D. H. Howry had already proposed in various articles published during the first few years of his work (Howry, 1955, 1957) many of the ultrasonic techniques which are nowadays sometimes thought to be quite novel. Although he was unable to test all his ideas in practice, he was able to develop equipment of outstandingly good performance. The results presented in a review article (Howry, 1965) are so excellent that it is only recently that scans of a similar quality have been obtained by other investigators. The improved systems which have been constructed are capable of making scans which contain enough information about echo amplitude for certain inferences to be made about the histology of the structures being examined.

A most important development was the invention of the contact scanner (Brown, 1960). The ability to scan patients without the use of a bulky water tank enabled I. Donald and his colleagues to demonstrate the great value of ultrasonic diagnosis in obstetrics and gynaecology. There is no doubt that it is as a result of their work that the method is now receiving increasing attention, particularly in Great Britain.

It is outside the scope of this book to describe all the clinical applications of the two-dimensional scanned B-scope. However, information on some of the more important applications is given in Table 4.5. This table, which is not comprehensive, is arranged for each diagnostic site in chronological order of recent articles, one from each particular group of investigators. Each of these articles contains a bibliography which gives references to earlier relevant publications.

The appearances of some typical scans, obtained with both water-bath and contact scanners, are discussed in the following Subsections. The numbering of these Subsections corresponds to the Notes of Table 4.5.

(i) Diagnosis of abnormalities of the breast

Typical two-dimensional ultrasonic scans of the breast are shown in Fig. 4.38. The breast is most conveniently examined by a water immersion technique. It seems to be possible to identify quite small abnormalities. The useful resolution of these scans is somewhat spoilt by the rather small number of lines from which they are composed. This is because the pulse repetition frequency of the scanner with which they were obtained is only 50 Hz, and the scanning time was about 15 sec. The result is that the scans seem to be rather speckly. No doubt the quality of the scans would be improved if the number of lines were to be increased.

The swept gain rate ($1 \cdot 4$ dB.cm^{-1}) is less than might be expected to give the optimum visualization. There is some evidence in the scans that the swept gain is undercompensating, and that echoes from deeper structures are not displayed with adequate amplitude. This is particularly noticeable in Fig. 4.38.c. A rate of about $2 \cdot 6$ dB.cm^{-1} would probably give rather better results (see Section 4.1.b).

TABLE 4.5

Some clinical applications of the two-dimensional scanned B-scope

Site	Comments	Reference	Note
Brain	Water bath and contact scanners. Encouraging results in hydrocephalic children. Many problems due to effects of skull and hair.	de Vlieger et al. (1963) Grossman (1965) Brinker and Taveras (1966) Makow and McRae (1967)	
Breast	Water bath scanners. Differentiation of cystic and solid masses. Diagnosis of carcinoma. Detection of small lesions.	Wild and Reid (1957) Hayashi et al. (1962) Howry (1965) Wagai et al. (1965) Wells and Evans (1968)	i
Heart	Demonstration of a.s.d. by intracardiac probe. High-speed cinématography (7 frames per sec.)	Kimoto et al. (1964) Åsberg (1967)	
Liver	Intravenous, water bath and contact scanners. Differentiation of cystic and solid masses. Diagnosis of various abnormalities, particularly cirrhosis and metastases.	Kimoto et al. (1964) Wang et al. (1964) Howry (1965) Holmes (1966a) McCarthy et al. (1967)	ii
Miscellaneous	Genito-urinary investigations	Holmes (1966b) Damascelli et al. (1968)	
	High-speed linear scanning Spleen Thyroid	Krause and Soldner (1967) Lehman et al. (1966) Fujimoto et al. (1967)	
Obstetrics and Gynaecology	Water bath and contact scanners. Diagnosis of multiple pregnancy, complications of pregnancy, placental localization, foetal position. Diagnosis of hydatiform mole cysts, fibroids and carcinomatosis.	Sundén (1964) Gottesfeld (1966) Kossoff et al. (1966) von Micsky (1966) Bang and Holm (1968) Donald (1968)	iii
Ophthalmology	Differential diagnosis of intraocular tumours, retinal detachment and vitreous haemorrhage. Location of foreign bodies.	Baum and Greenwood (1965)	

The Notes detailed in this Table appear as subsections in Section 4.7.d.

The sensitivity used to demonstrate the presence of most solid abnormalities is chosen so that the normal breast tissue appears on the scan as a uniform fine background. At this sensitivity, it may be rather difficult to detect cystic masses. However, cysts are quite easily seen as transonic areas if the sensitivity is increased so that echoes from the surrounding tissues are

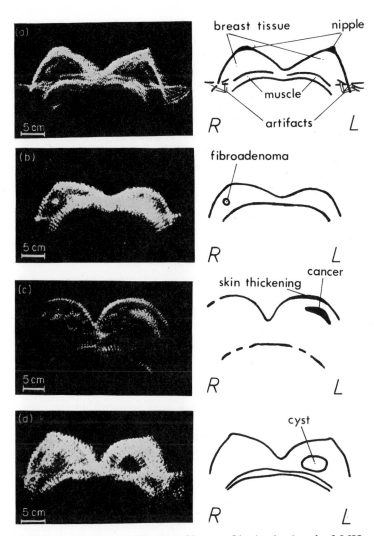

FIG. 4.38 Compound sector B-scans of breast. Obtained using the 2 MHz water bath scanner of Wells and Evans (1968). Swept gain 1·4 dB cm^{-1}. Differentiated display. Approximately 800 lines per scan. (a) Scan of normal breasts; (b) Scan showing fibroadenoma (diameter 0·8 cm) in right breast. Left breast normal; (c) Scan showing carcinoma in left breast, with associated skin thickening. Right breast normal; (d) Scan showing solitary cyst (diameter 5 cm) in left breast. Right breast normal. Scans (a), (b) and (c) were obtained using the same system sensitivity; scan (d) was obtained using increased sensitivity.

registered on the display at high amplitudes. The identification of an abnormality is made easier in breast scanning if both breasts are shown on the same scan, so that any asymmetry is obvious.

(*ii*) *Diagnosis of abnormalities of the liver*

Diagnosis of liver abnormalities by two-dimensional ultrasonic scanning is based either on the visualization of abnormal structures within the liver, or on the recognition of differential reflection. There is no difference in principle between these two criteria: but in the case of diffuse abnormalities, the structure dimensions may be too small to be resolved.

Either water-bath or contact scanners can be used for examining the liver. The most usual method is to scan in a transverse plane through the patient, if necessary through the ribs. Unfortunately, this approach is liable to error because of uncertainty in the transmission loss. More consistent results are obtained if the scan is made in an oblique plane from just below the costal margin. This is conveniently done using a contact scanner (McCarthy, *et al.* 1967). Some typical scans obtained by this method are shown in Fig. 4.39. Certain artifacts and the appearance of normal scans are soon learned from experience. For example, if the angle of the scan is not sufficiently acute relative to the skin, a group of echoes may appear in the centre of the liver area corresponding to the concave inferior liver surface. Again, echoes grouped into arrangements which resemble sections through tubes are often seen in normal livers.

The accurate diagnosis of diffuse liver abnormality depends on the maintenance of a good degree of system stability (better than about 2 dB at 1·5 MHz), and the use of an exponential swept gain applied at the correct rate. This is because the interpretation of the scan is based on the estimation of the quantity of the reflections which arise from within the liver, rather than on the actual distribution of the echoes.

It has been suggested that it is reasonable for the clinician who interprets the scan to be told the clinical history of the patient (as is certainly the case in most routine interpretations of X-radiographs). In a series of 220 scans

---

FIG. 4.39 Compound sector B-scans of liver. Scans made from the subcostal area, using the "Diasonograph" type NE 4100 of Nuclear Enterprises Ltd. Frequency 1·5 MHz. Swept gain 1·8 dB cm^{-1}, controlled by a function generator similar to that illustrated in Fig. 4·17. Differentiated display. Approximately 500 lines per scan. (a) Scan of normal liver; with explanatory diagram; (b) Scan showing cirrhosis of liver; (c) Scan showing fatty liver; (d) Scan showing secondary carcinoma of liver; (e) Scan showing liver with solitary cyst in posterior right lobe. All these scans were obtained using the same system sensitivity, except (e), for which the sensitivity was increased by 5 dB.

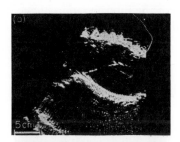

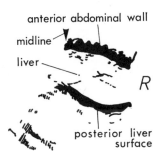

anterior abdominal wall

midline

liver

R

posterior liver surface

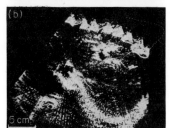

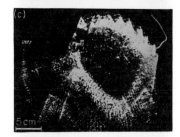

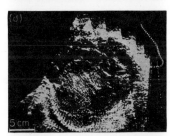

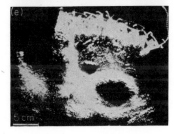

analysed in this way, the correlation of the interpretation of the ultrasonic pattern with the confirmed clinical diagnosis in many different liver conditions was around 90% (Holmes, 1966a). However, it might be considered that a better assessment of diagnostic accuracy is afforded by an analysis in which no clinical information is available for guidance. Thus, in a series of 47 patients with cirrhosis, McCarthy *et al.* (1967) obtained a diagnostic accuracy of about 87%.

It seems clear that, under appropriate conditions, two-dimensional ultrasonic scanning can be used to detect liver abnormality due to, for example, cirrhosis, metastases, obstructive jaundice and hepatic cysts. Cysts and abscesses can be clearly distinguished from other abnormalities, particularly if the sensitivity of the system is increased so that the cysts appear as transonic areas surrounded by echoes from the liver tissue. In any event, the absorption which occurs within a fluid-filled cyst is much less than that in normal liver, and so echoes from structures beyond the cyst are of larger amplitude than in the normal at the same range.

The diagnostic accuracy seems to be rather poor in obese patients (except for the detection of fluid-filled cavities). This is probably because the intrahepatic echoes are received with larger amplitude than in the normal at the same range, because of the relatively low absorption which occurs in fat (see Table 1.8). These echoes are displayed at inappropriately large amplitudes because no allowance is made for the fat thickness in the swept gain calibration.

At the present time (1968), the accuracy of ultrasonic diagnosis in liver abnormalities is highest in the case of cysts and abscesses. Accurately calibrated equipment is necessary to obtain results of significant value in other disorders, except possibly when an isolated mass can be demonstrated beyond doubt.

(iii) Application in obstetrics and gynaecology

Two-dimensional ultrasonic scanning is of established value as a diagnostic method in obstetrics and gynaecology. The various applications have been described by, for example, Donald and Abdulla (1967), and may be summarized as follows:

(a) *Early diagnosis of pregnancy.* During the first few weeks of pregnancy, the uterus is normally situated within the pelvis and so it is inaccessible to ultrasonic examination. However, Donald (1963) demonstrated that it is possible to scan the uterus in very early pregnancy through the bladder, if the bladder is first allowed to become filled with urine. Pregnancy can thus be diagnosed within the first six weeks after the last menstrual period in a normal cycle, and occasionally even before the urine tests are positive. Figure 4.40.a shows a scan obtained by this technique.

(b) *Diagnosis of multiple pregnancy.* Multiple pregnancy can be reliably diagnosed by the demonstration of more than one foetal head. Caution is necessary because it sometimes happens that a section through the foetal trunk is mistaken for a head. In order to avoid such an error, it is necessary either to demonstrate the mid-line structures of each foetal brain, or to make serial scans so that the foetal heads can be identified with certainty. Figure 4.40.b shows a scan in which the two heads of twins appear together.

(c) *Localization of placenta.* The placenta gives rise to a characteristic echo pattern (Gottesfeld *et al.* 1966). Figure 4.40.c shows the appearance. When scanned at reduced sensitivity, the echoes from within the placenta disappear. The technique can be used reliably from the 26th week onwards (Donald, 1968).

(d) *Diagnosis of hydatidiform mole.* A hydatidiform mole can be identified as it appears on the scan as a mass of uniformly distributed echoes filling the uterus (Donald and Brown, 1961); MacVicar and Donald, 1963). The echoes almost all disappear when the sensitivity of the system is reduced, although the mass remains transonic so that the posterior uterine wall can still be seen. The appearance of the scan of a mole made at high sensitivity is shown in Fig. 4.40.d.

(e) *Diagnosis of ovarian cyst.* A cystic mass appears on the scan as a transonic area, even when the system sensitivity is high. The deeper surface of the cyst gives rise to strong echoes because of the relatively low loss of the liquid of which the mass is composed. Malignant cysts can be identified by the occurrence of bizarre groups of echoes from within the mass. Figure 4.40.e is an example of a scan of a simple ovarian cyst.

(f) *Diagnosis of fibroids.* Fibroids absorb ultrasound more rapidly than cysts, but give rise to fewer echoes than occur with hydatidiform moles. Therefore, differential diagnosis is possible.

(g) *Diagnosis of other conditions.* Two-dimensional ultrasonic scanning is useful as an aid in the diagnosis of ectopic gestation, abortion, blighted ovum, hydramnios, malpresentation, ascites and carcinomatosis.

4.7.e Time-Position Recording

Pulse-echo information is a combination of time and amplitude data. The instantaneous position of a moving reflector can be determined from the time data. This can be presented in the form of a recording, in which a waveform represents the variation with time in the position of the reflector.

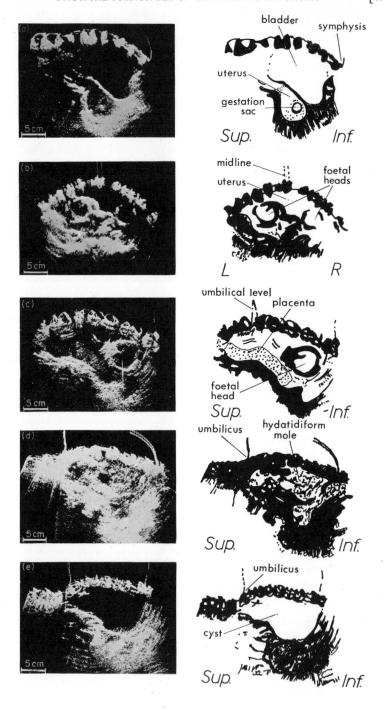

It is explained later in this Section that such a recording may frequently be useful as an aid to diagnosis.

The two most commonly used methods by which time-position recordings can be obtained are illustrated in Fig. 4.41. In Fig. 4.41.a, the ultrasonic probe is arranged to measure the position of a reflector moving regularly between positions (1) and (2), situated respectively at distances d_1 and d_2 from the transducer. The corresponding B-scans are shown in Fig. 4.41.b, with the start of the vertical time-base at the top of the display. If this display is photographed by a camera in which the film moves at constant velocity in a direction normal to the ultrasonic time-base, then the result is a waveform showing how the instantaneous position of the reflector varies with time. This recording may be seen to be made up of separate B-scans lying side-by-side if the time-resolution of the system is sufficiently good; but for simplicity the recording is shown as a continuous line in Fig. 4.41.b. As an alternative to the use of a moving film camera, a fixed film camera may be used if the B-scan is moved across the display by a second, relatively slow-speed time-base connected to the other pair of deflection plates. The photographic method of recording enables the movements of several reflectors to be studied simultaneously. Kossoff and Wilcken (1967) have developed this method so that several related time-dependent functions can be displayed together with the B-scan on a single-beam storage oscilloscope, each function being processed by a separate voltage-to-time converter.

As an alternative to photographic recording, it is possible to design apparatus which provides a representation of the motion of a selected reflector on a strip-chart recorder. This method avoids the delay and some of the difficulties associated with photographic recording, and is capable of providing a time-resolution which is at least as good as that obtained with photographic recordings.

Most soft-tissue structures can be examined at a range of not more than about 20 cm when the ultrasonic probe is placed on the skin. This corresponds to a time delay of about 270 μsec. Such a short interval is beyond

---

Fig. 4.40 Compound sector B-scans in obstetrics and gynaecology. Obtained using the "Diasonograph" type NE 4100 of Nuclear Enterprises Ltd. Frequency 1·5 MHz. Swept gain 1·8 dB cm^{-1}, controlled by a function generator similar to that illustrated in Fig. 4.17. Differentiated display. Approximately 1000 lines per scan. (a) 10 week pregnancy scanned through full bladder. Longitudinal section, 2 cm left mid-line; (b) Twins at 19 weeks gestation. Both heads visible. Transverse section, 4 cm below umbilicus; (c) Placenta demonstrated in 28 week pregnancy; Longitudinal section, 2 cm left mid-line. High sensitivity; (d) Hydatidiform mole: 14 weeks amenorrhoea. Longitudinal mid-line section. High sensitivity; (e) Ovarian cyst. Longitudinal mid-line section.

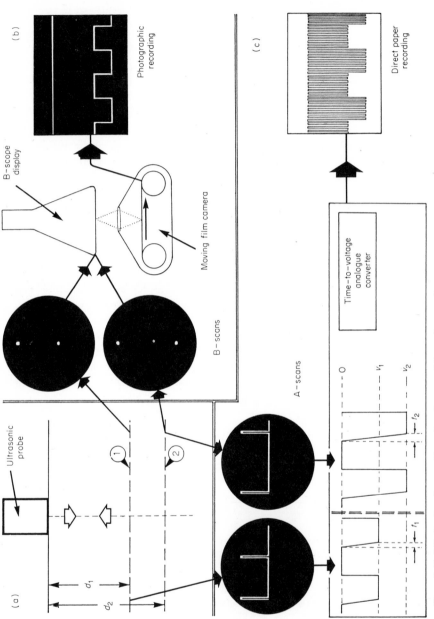

FIG. 4.41 Methods of recording the time-position of a moving structure.

the response of a conventional strip-chart recorder. However, the pulse repetition frequency of diagnostic pulse-echo systems is typically a few hundred per second, and square-wave signals at such a frequency can be recorded by high-speed instruments. Figure 4.41.c shows how the ultrasonic information can be converted into a series of square-wave pulses with periods corresponding to that of the pulse repetition frequency, in such a way that the amplitude of each square-wave pulse is proportional to the corresponding time delay. The basic principles of a suitable analogue converter have been described by Effert *et al.* (1959). A linear voltage ramp starts from a fixed voltage at the instant that the ultrasonic pulse is transmitted; the ramp is stopped at the instant that the echo returns from the reflector. The voltage at which the ramp is stopped is proportional to the distance from the transducer to the reflector, and the voltage can be maintained at this level for an interval which may extend until just before the transmission of the next ultrasonic pulse. In Fig. 4.41.c, the voltage is maintained at the measuring level for nearly half the interval between ultrasonic pulses, and so the recording consists of a series of square waves, fluctuating in amplitude between v_1 and v_2, which correspond to d_1 and d_2 respectively. This method of recording allows the movement of only one reflector to be studied at a time, and the system will operate only under certain conditions of echo amplitude.

Wells and Ross (1969) have described a time-to-voltage analogue converter for direct recording of reflector movement, which has some advantages in comparison with systems which have previously been described. Details of the circuit, and the waveforms corresponding to certain circuit points, are shown in Fig. 4.42. For proper operation, it is necessary for the echo from the reflector under investigation to be always of such an amplitude that no larger echo precedes it on that part of the time-base along which it moves. An electronic gate is arranged to be closed to ultrasonic signals during the interval between the transmitter pulse and the beginning of that part of the time-base on which the echo from the moving reflector is always first. The first echo (of sufficient amplitude to operate the following circuits) to pass through the open gate is then the echo from the moving reflector. The input to the analogue converter is the interval between the instant that the signal gate opens, and the time of arrival of this echo. The converter generates a voltage which is proportional to this time interval. In the apparatus of Wells and Ross (1969), the pulse repetition frequency is about 150 Hz, so that the interval between pulses is about 6·6 msec. The output from the analogue converter is returned to zero at 3·3 msec after the signal gate has opened, so that a 150 Hz square wave is generated: the amplitude of each cycle of the square wave corresponds to a single pulse-echo measurement of the position of the moving reflector. The circuit is designed to operate with signals readily available from a typical A-scope. In

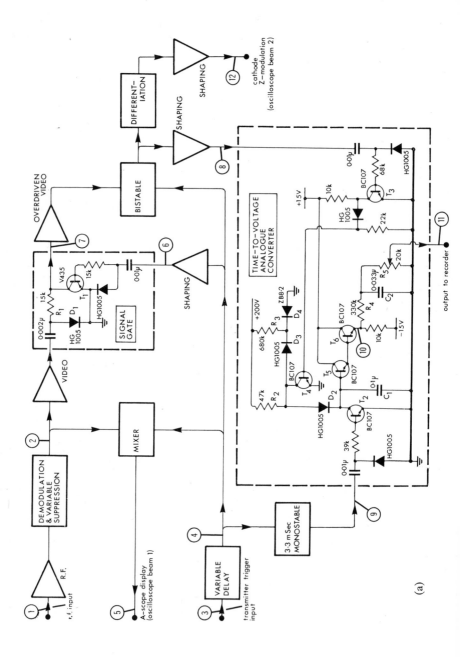

(a)

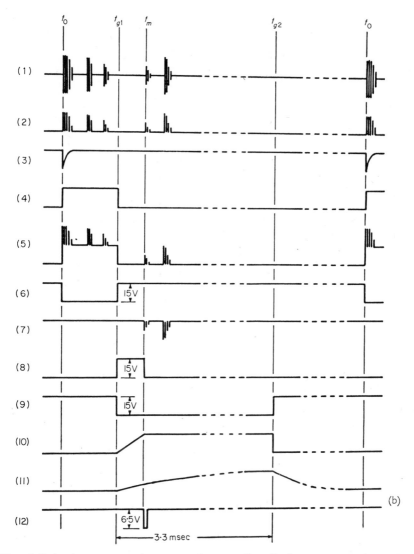

Fig. 4.42 Analogue conversion system for recording displacement waveform of a moving reflector. (a) Block diagram, showing circuits of signal gate and time-to-voltage analogue converter; (b) Waveforms at points corresponding to those shown in (a). (After Fig. 2 of Wells and Ross, 1969.)

the following description, the numbers in brackets refer to the corresponding circuit points and waveforms indicated in Fig. 4.42.

The radio-frequency signals (1) are amplified and demodulated. Variable suppression is used to control the system sensitivity because this method restricts the useful dynamic range (see Section 4.4.e), and so minimizes the possibility of spurious triggering of the converter before the arrival of the echo from the moving reflector. The transmitter trigger (3) is fed to a monostable, the delay of which is set to slightly less than that corresponding to the minimum range of the moving reflector from the transducer. The output of this monostable (4) is mixed with the output from the suppressor (2), to generate an A-scan signal with a step corresponding to the end of the delay. The output from the suppressor (2) is also fed to a video amplifier, the negative-going output of which is applied to the signal gate and clamped by D_1. T_1 is controlled by a current pulse (6) derived from the output (4) of the delay circuit. T_1 is saturated during the interval t_0 to t_{g1}, and so the gate is closed, the input voltage appearing across R_1. t_0 corresponds to the transmission of the ultrasonic pulse. The gate is open except during this period, and the first echo to pass through the gate (7) after t_{g1} is normally the echo from the moving reflector, which occurs at t_m. This signal (7) is fed to the overdriven video amplifier. The output (4) of the delay circuit is arranged to trigger the bistable at t_{g1}; the bistable is again triggered at t_m by the output from the overdriven amplifier. Therefore, the output from the bistable consists of a pulse which starts at t_{g1} and ends at t_m; this pulse is squared in an amplifier to provide one of the controlling gates (8) for the time-to-voltage analogue converter. The other gate (9) for the converter is a pulse of 3·3 msec duration, starting at t_{g1} and ending at t_{g2}, which is generated by a monostable triggered by the output (4) from the variable delay.

The analogue converter operates by clamping the voltage across C_1. Until t_{g1}, C_1 is short-circuited by T_2. T_2 and T_4 are unsaturated at t_{g1} by the gating pulse (9) from the 3·3 msec monostable. C_1 begins to charge up a voltage ramp as current flows through R_2, until T_4 is again saturated at t_m by the gating pulse (8) fed through T_3. After t_m, the voltage across C_1 remains constant because the discharge path is blocked by D_2, until it is clamped back to zero volts by T_2 at t_{g2}. The maximum voltage across C_1 is limited to 8·2 V (developed across D_4) by D_3. This corresponds to a range of about 14·5 cm beyond t_{g1}, and the converter output is limited to this value if no suitable triggering echo occurs. The voltage across C_1 is sampled by two emitter followers T_5 and T_6 in cascade.

The output (10) from the converter has fast rise times. If such a signal is fed directly to a recorder (even to a high-speed instrument such as an Elema-Schönander "Mingograf"), the recording is spoilt by transient overshoots. This is avoided by the network R_4, R_5 and C_2, which causes the deflections to approach their maximum values along exponentials (11).

The output of the bistable is differentiated and clamped so that a pulse is derived which occurs at t_m. This is amplified to provide a signal (12) which brightness-modulates a second beam on the A-scope display. This produces a bright spot at t_m, or at some other time if the system is not properly triggered.

The diagnostic value of time-position recording frequently depends upon accurate calibration. This is equally important with both photographic and analogue systems. Fixed targets can be used for distance calibration, and an

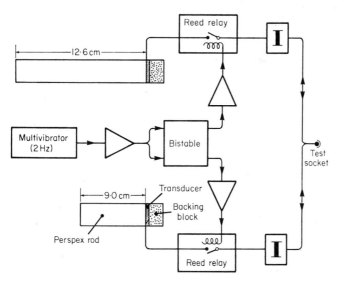

FIG. 4.43 Block diagram of system for distance and time calibration of time-position recorders. (After Fig. 3 of Wells and Ross, 1969.)

ordinary stop-watch, for time calibration. However, a convenient method which provides calibration of both distance and time has been described by Wells and Ross (1969). A block diagram of the arrangement is shown in Fig. 4.43. The multivibrator provides trigger pulses at a frequency of 2 Hz: the two outputs from the bistable are antiphase square waves with "on" times of 0·5 sec. These pulses switch reed relays which connect either one or the other of two transducers into circuit. One transducer provides an echo delayed by a time corresponding to 5 cm in blood, and the other, to 7 cm. Reed relays are used because of their fast switching time, long life and small open/closed signal ratio. The reflections from each of the two transducers are matched in amplitude by the preset attenuators.

Table 4.6 indicates many of the clinical applications of time-position recording. This Table, which is not comprehensive, is arranged for each diagnostic site in chronological order of recent articles, one from each

TABLE 4.6

Some clinical applications of time-position recording

Site	Applications	Reference	Note
Brain	Positional pulsation measurements (apparently related to various clinical conditions)	ter Braak and de Vlieger (1965) Avant (1966)	i
Cardio-vascular	Aortography	Goldberg et al. (1966) Evans et al. (1967)	ii
	Foetal heart movement	Bang and Holm (1968)	iii
	Heart valves: Aortic	Edler (1965)	v
	Mitral	Joyner (1966) Edler (1967) Effert (1967) Segal et ol. (1966) Zaky et al. (1968)	iv
	Prosthetic	Winters et al. (1967) Zaky et al. (1968)	v
	Pulmonary	Edler (1965)	v
	Tricuspic	Edler (1965) Effert and Bleifeld (1966) Joyner et al. (1967)	v
	Pericardial effusion	Feigenbaum et al. (1967)	vi

The Notes detailed in this Table appear as Subsections in Section 4.7.e.

particular group of investigators. Each of these articles contain bibliographies giving references to earlier relevant publications. Some of these applications are discussed in the following Subsections, the numbering of which corresponds to the Notes of Table 4.6.

(*i*) *Intracranial pulsations*

Time-position pulsation of intracranial echoes seems to be associated with variations in intracranial pressure. The pulsating shift is very small (around 0·01 cm (ter Braak and de Vlieger, 1965), and so quite sensitive equipment is needed for its measurement. On purely physical grounds, the measurement of so small a shift occurring synchronously with a variation in echo amplitude (see Section 4.7.a) is subject to relatively large errors due to the effect of the latter on the range resolution (see Section 4.1.b). Consequently it would be unrealistic to suggest that the method has been developed to a degree that is acceptable in clinical diagnosis.

(*ii*) *Aortography*

Aortography is chiefly used in the diagnosis of abdominal aortic aneurism. The accuracy of measurements of aortic size compares favourably with contrast aortography (Goldberg, Ostrum and Isard, 1966), and the movements of the opposite walls of the aorta can be studied by photographic time-position recordings (Segal *et al.* 1966; Evans *et al.* 1967).

(iii) Foetal heart movement

Bang and Holm (1968) have demonstrated the movement of the foetal heart as early as the 12th week of pregnancy, by means of photographic time-position recordings. However, this technique is considerably more complicated, and probably less reliable, than the Doppler method discussed in Section 5.5.c.

(iv) Mitral valve studies

There is no doubt that the principal application of ultrasonic time-position recording is, at the present time, in the diagnosis of abnormalities of the mitral valve of the heart. The method was first described by Edler and Hertz (1954), who considered that the structures the movements of which they observed were the left ventricle and left atrial walls. However, the actual origins of most of the echoes of interest in ultrasonic cardiology were demonstrated in the classic publication of Edler (1961). The diagnosis of mitral valve disease by ultrasound is nowadays a routine in several centres; for example, Joyner (1966) uses the method in preference to trans-septal left heart catheterization. The patient experiences no discomfort. The investigation can be completed in a few minutes, and may be repeated as often as necessary.

The ultrasonic probe is placed on the chest over an intercostal space (usually the third or fourth interspace) as shown in Fig. 4.44, so that

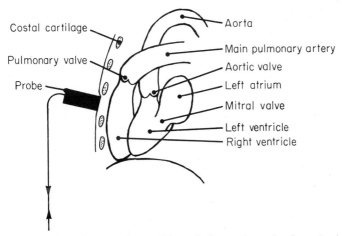

Costal cartilage
Pulmonary valve
Probe

Aorta
Main pulmonary artery
Aortic valve
Left atrium
Mitral valve
Left ventricle
Right ventricle

Fig. 4.44 Diagram showing the position of ultrasonic probe for mitral valvular investigations. (Adapted from Fig. 1 of Wells and Ross, 1969.)

echoes are received from the anterior cusp of the mitral valve. The position of the probe is controlled by the necessity to avoid underlying lung (which would almost completely reflect the ultrasound and give rise to multiple reflection artifacts), and to align the ultrasonic axis so that it is substantially normal to the valve cusp throughout the cardiac cycle. In an average normal adult, the anterior cusp lies between about 5·8 and 8·3 cm from the anterior surface of the chest, depending on several factors including the phase of the

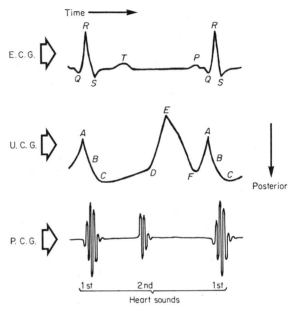

FIG. 4.45 Diagram illustrating the timing of the U.C.G. of a normal mitral valve. The annotation follows the scheme of Edler (1961). The *A*-wave is due to atrial activity. Point *C* represents the position of maximum closure of the valve on ventricular systole. The *E*-wave corresponds to the maximum opening of the valve in early ventricular diastole. The slope *EF* represents the motion of the valve towards closure during the rapid filling phase of early ventricular diastole. (After Fig. 7 of Wells and Ross, 1969.)

cardiac cycle (Edler, 1961). The ultrasonic recording of the movement of the anterior cusp of a normal mitral valve (the "ultrasoundcardiogram; U.C.G.") is shown diagrammatically in relation to the electrocardiogram (E.C.G.) and phonocardiogram (P.C.G.) in Fig. 4.45. This may be compared with the clinical recordings in Figs 4.46 and 4.47. These recordings were obtained using a 2·5 MHz probe with a diameter of 1·2 cm. The usual convention is that movements away from the probe produce downward deflections on the recording. The clinical diagnosis is made on the basis of criteria such as those listed in Table 4.7.

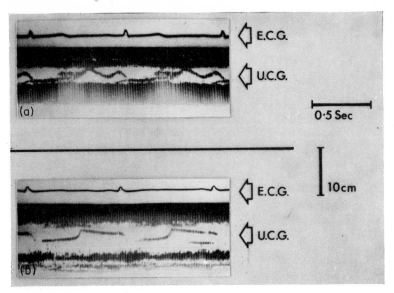

FIG. 4.46 Ultrasoundcardiograms of the mitral valve in some typical clinical conditions, obtained by photographic recording. The electrocardiograms were recorded synchronously for timing purposes, as explained in Fig. 4.45. (a) Normal valve. The slope EF is 135 mm sec^{-1}; the maximum amplitude CE is 30 mm; (b) Mitral stenosis in normal rhythm. The slope EF is 23 mm sec^{-1}; the maximum amplitude CE is 25 mm.

(v) Heart valve studies, other than of the mitral valve

Time-position recordings of the movements of the aortic, prosthetic, pulmonary and tricuspid valves have occasionally been described in the literature. It is considerably more difficult to obtain satisfactory recordings from these valves than from the mitral valve, and consequently the photographic method is often used. The most successful applications seem to be in the diagnosis of tricuspid stenosis (Joyner et al. 1967), and in the study of prosthetic replacements of the aortic, mitral and tricuspid valves (Winters et al. 1967).

The mitral valve U.C.G. is of value in estimating whether or not aortic valve diseases are combined with mitral stenosis (Edler, 1966).

(vi) Diagnosis of pericardial effusion

Edler (1955) described how the presence of pericardial fluid anterior to the anterior heart wall may be demonstrated by ultrasound. On the A-scope, the fluid appears as a transonic space in front of the pulsating echo from the heart. Feigenbaum et al. (1967) have developed the technique by the use of

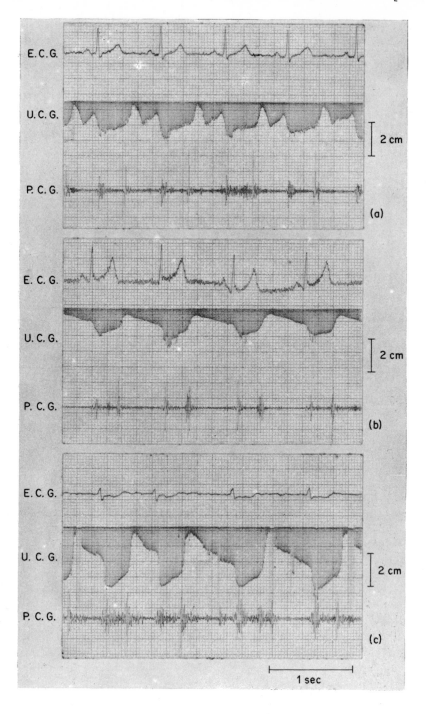

TABLE 4.7

Typical criteria for the analysis of mitral valve function from the U.C.G.

Clinical condition	Total amplitude CE, mm.		Slope EF, mm.sec^{-1}	
	Mean	Range	Mean	Range
Normal	27	20–33	140	90–190
Mitral stenosis	22	12–30	15	6–31
Mitral regurgitation	33	30–38	153	92–223
Combined mitral stenosis and regurgitation	24	17–32	41	9–78

Quantities defined according to the annotation in Figure 4.45.
From data of Edler (1966).

photographic time-position recording so that it is possible to demonstrate pericardial fluid both anterior and posterior to the heart. Time-position recording is helpful in deciding whether or not a particular space contains fluid, because the thickness of a fluid-filled space varies as the heart beats. This has been discussed by Pridie and Turnbull (1968). The method is not entirely satisfactory, and in particular the presence of pulmonary emphysema may make it impossible to obtain a satisfactory recording.

4.7.f Other Systems

(i) The C-scope

The C-scope is a brightness-modulated display in which the *x*-deflection corresponds to the bearing in azimuth, and the *y*-deflection, to the elevation. Kimoto *et al.* (1964) used a modified form of this display, in which the *y*-deflection is proportional to the vertical position of the probe, to demonstrate an atrial septal defect by means of a small ultrasonic probe inserted

---

Fig. 4.47 Ultrasoundcardiograms of the mitral valve in some typical clinical conditions, obtained by electronic analogue recording. The E.C.G. and P.C.G. recordings are shown for timing purposes, as explained in Fig. 4.44. (a) Normal valve. The slope *EF* is 100 mm sec^{-1}; the maximum amplitude *CE* is 22 mm; (b) Mitral stenosis in normal rhythm. The slope *EF* is 16 mm sec^{-1}; the maximum amplitude *CE* is 14 mm; (c) Mitral stenosis with dominant mitral regurgitation. The initial slope *EF* is 70 mm sec^{-1}, and this is followed by a plateau during ventricular diastole (the *A*-wave is absent); the maximum amplitude *CE* is 33 mm. (Adapted from Figs 8, 9 and 10 of Wells and Ross, 1969.)

under X-ray control into the right atrium. The scan resembles an X-radiograph, because it presents the data as a plan, rather than as a section. The ultrasonic pulse generator is synchronized to the cardiac cycle by means of a circuit which is triggered from the R-wave of the electrocardiogram. A signal gate is arranged so that the transmission pulse and echoes from beyond the septum do not appear on the display: this is necessary because the display does not give an indication of range. Using this method, Omoto (1967) demonstrated atrial septal defects in 6 out of 7 patients.

(ii) Highly focussed arrays

The lateral resolution of a pulse-echo system may be improved over a limited part of its range by the use of a highly-focussed ultrasonic beam. The focussing need not necessarily be applied to both the transmitting and receiving transducers.

The method was proposed by von Ardenne and Millner (1962). Their system employs a curved 5 MHz transducer. The transducer is mounted at one end of a water-filled column, which also contains an aperture and a lens, so arranged that the focal region is at a convenient distance from the other end of the column. The echo information is presented on a linear B-scope. The display is time-gated by means of a slit-mask placed in front of the screen of the cathode ray tube. This mask is moved in synchronism with the transducer, so that only echoes which return from the focus appear on the scan.

Thurstone and McKinney (1966a) have developed the system (apparently without knowledge of M. von Ardenne's earlier work). They use reflectors instead of a lens (see Section 3.2), and an electronic system for gating out echoes which do not originate from the focus. The frequency is 2·25 MHz; and the gate-time is 1 μsec, which corresponds to a target volume of 0·075 cm diameter. The improvement in resolution in comparison with conventional B-scanning is obtained at the expense of an increased scan time. As an example, Thurstone and McKinney (1966b) have shown a scan of a brain removed from the skull.

4.7.g Three-dimensional Display of Pulse-echo Information

Conventional two-dimensional scans, such as those described in Section 4.7.c, contain only information about single planes. This represents a substantial improvement in comparison with a single A-scan (Section 4.7.a), and in many situations the information contained in such a scan is adequate for an accurate diagnosis to be made. However, it often happens that a satisfactory diagnosis cannot be made from a single two-dimensional scan, and it is then necessary for several scans to be made, each in a different plane. The most usual method is to scan in parallel planes, either in transverse or in longitudinal section. An experienced observer can form a three-dimensional impression of the structures visualized in such a series of two-dimensional scans, and so be helped in making a diagnosis.

Baum and Greenwood (1961) prepared a series of photographically reversed scans on transparent plates, and by stacking these plates with the appropriate spacing constructed a three-dimensional model. Such a model enables even a relatively unskilled observer to appreciate the ultrasonic information in a three-dimensional form. However, the deeper areas tend to be only poorly visible because they are obscured by the structures closer to the edge of the model. Redman *et al.* (1969) have to some extent overcome this difficulty by making a hologram in which the serial scans are recorded in sequence. When the hologram is reconstructed, each scan is more clearly visible because it seems to be self-illuminated. This method is a development of the holographic multiplexing technique of Leith *et al.* (1966). The principles of optical holography, which was invented by Gabor (1948, 1949), have been explained in relatively simple terms by Leith and Upatnieks (1965).

It has been demonstrated that a three-dimensional impression is experienced if serial scans are photographed in sequence and projected like an ordinary ciné film ("Ultrasonic scanning in medical diagnosis" by P. N. T. Wells. Lecture to Joint I.E.R.E.-I.E.E. Medical and Biological Electronics Group; 11th October 1967). The effect is similar to that experienced when travelling through a fog-filled tunnel in which there is only a limited visibility: structures seem to emerge through the fog, become clearer and then disappear again. The film can be arranged in a loop, with reverse and forward sequences in alternation, so that the motion is continuously in and out of the three-dimensional volume. The scanning time required to obtain a very large number of scans situated close together renders the method impracticable as a routine with most current scanners. If only a limited number of scans is projected in strict sequence, the result is both jerky and rapid. Under such circumstances, the best effect is achieved by projecting in a sequence which contains several frames of the same scan. A suitable sequence is ....1112122232333....; this arrangement is satisfactory if about 20 separate scans are available.

Brown (1967) discussed the various factors which are important in three-dimensional scanning. He pointed out that compound scanning in any practical number of single planes does not solve the general problem of visualizing specularly reflecting interfaces of random orientation. In order to construct an absolutely complete two-dimensional scan, it is necessary to examine every point in the scan plane from every direction in space. Brown (1967) proposed several systems, including a method of conical scanning, the performances of which would approach the ideal. The three-dimensional information obtained with such systems could be presented not only in the form of complete serial two-dimensional scans, but it would be possible, for example, to generate a three-dimensional image by means of a stereoscopic cathode-ray tube display (Schmitt, 1947; Berkley, 1948; and Iams *et al.* 1948). Unfortunately, not everyone has the ability to appreciate the images of such stereoscopic displays in three dimensions. An alternative and somewhat simpler display has been demonstrated by Howry *et al.* (1956), in which a view of variable projection is presented on a single cathode ray tube.

Stereoscopic systems, although theoretically feasible, are likely to be rather disappointing when used to display information about complicated body structures. The most attractive possibility seems to be a system in which three-dimensional information of wide dynamic range is recorded, to be subsequently retrieved by a computer in the form of suitably processed images in any desired two-dimensional planes.

4.8 MEASUREMENT OF SYSTEM PERFORMANCE

The performance of a pulse-echo system depends on many factors. Some of these are concerned with the registration accuracy and scanning method, and are discussed elsewhere in this chapter. This section is concerned only with the performance of the ultrasonic signal path, which consists of the transmitter, the transducer, the receiver and the display. The information which is necessary to define the performance of the signal path is discussed in the following subsections.

The overall sensitivity of an ultrasonic pulse-echo system is determined by the performance of each of the many individual components in the signal path. It is already often necessary to be able to maintain the overall sensitivity of a particular instrument at a constant level, so that the comparison of different scans can have a diagnostic significance. In the future, it will become increasingly important for uniform standards of calibration to be adopted so that the results of different investigators may be freely interchanged and compared.

(*i*) *Ultrasonic frequency*

The ultrasonic frequency is determined by the thickness of the transducer (unless it is deliberately driven at an odd harmonic). This frequency is most easily determined by measuring the time-position of the zeroes in a received echo pulse displayed on a calibrated oscilloscope. It is important to realize that it is not strictly correct to describe the pulse as having any particular frequency, because the pulse energy is actually distributed over quite a wide frequency spectrum (see Section 2.7).

(*ii*) *Transmitted pulse amplitude and shape*

These quantities are rather difficult to measure. The pulse energy may be calculated by dividing the time-averaged power (measured, for example, by radiation pressure: see Section 3.5) by the pulse repetition frequency. Alternatively, the transmitted pulse may be observed by a capacitor microphone (Section 3.5), which can be calibrated absolutely in terms of displacement amplitude.

(iii) Overall voltage transfer function of the transducer

This quantity depends on the bandwidth and sensitivity of the transducer. Its importance and measurement are discussed in Section 2.8.

(iv) Transducer diameter and beam shape

The diameter of the transducer can be directly measured, but the beam shape depends upon many factors. Most plane transducers operating with pulses generate beams which are similar in shape to those which can be calculated for continuous wave excitation (see Section 3.1), but the distribution of focussed beams are more complicated (Section 3.2). For most purposes, it is best to plot the beam distribution by measuring the echo amplitudes received from a small spherical target as it is moved about in the field (Section 3.4.c).

(v) Pulse repetition frequency

This quantity may be measured by means of a calibrated oscilloscope.

(vi) Receiver bandwidth

The receiver bandwidth may be measured by means of a variable frequency oscillator, a calibrated attenuator, and an oscilloscope. It is usually best for the input to the receiver to be varied so that the output remains constant as the frequency band is covered, so that the demodulator nonlinearity does not introduce any error (see Section 4.4.e).

(vii) Maximum receiver gain

This quantity may be determined under pulse conditions by means of a calibrated attenuator at the input to the receiver, and a calibrated oscilloscope at its output, using an echo signal obtained from a convenient target with the transmitter and transducer normally used in the equipment.

(viii) Swept gain rate

The swept gain is usually controlled by a time-varying voltage (see Section 4.4.d). It is possible to measure the receiver gain using the apparatus described in subsection (vii) of this section, for several values of d.c. control voltage applied to the swept gain input of the receiver. The dynamic swept gain can then be estimated from measurements made on a calibrated oscilloscope of the voltage function actually used to control the gain.

A more direct method of measurement, which has the advantage that the gain is measured under conditions of dynamic control, is as follows. A target, such as a flat Perspex sheet, is arranged in a water bath in such a way that its distance from the transducer can be altered and measured. With no swept gain, the displayed amplitude is kept constant by appropriate electrical attenuation in the receiver input whilst the range is altered, to give a result such as that shown in Fig. 4.8. A similar set of measurements is then made, with the swept gain in operation. The difference between any pair of measurements made at the same range is due to the effect of swept gain.

A somewhat similar method employs an electrical pulse generator triggered by a variable delay. The variation in pulse amplitude necessary to maintain constant amplitude at the display as the delay is altered corresponds to the swept gain characteristic. Figure 4.48 is a diagram of a suitable pulse generator. This could be triggered from a delay generator such as a phantastron, and the control of the delay could be calibrated for convenience in centimetres. The output from the delay circuit consists of a negative-going pulse of about 20 V amplitude. This triggers the monostable $T_1 T_2$, which produces a pulse which is fed through T_3 to the base of T_4. T_4 is normally switched on; the arrival of the negative-going pulse at the base of T_4 switches it off. Whilst T_4 is switched on, a current flows through L_1; this current is interrupted when T_4 is switched off, and oscillation occurs in the resonant circuit formed by L_1 and C_1. However, the first positive-going oscillation to occur after T_4 has been switched on is rapidly damped. A proportion of the voltage developed across L_1 is fed to T_7, which is asymmetrically loaded by D_1 so that the positive and negative half cycles at the output of T_6 are of equal amplitudes. The output impedance is adjusted to be equal to 75 Ω, so that an ordinary calibrated attenuator may be used to apply the pulse to the input of the ultrasonic system. The circuit shown in Fig. 4.48 generates a pulse corresponding to 1·5 MHz; it is designed to provide an output of 1 V peak into a 75 Ω load. T_6 may be protected from damage by the transmitter pulse by arranging for the minimum attenuation to be, for example, 20 dB.

(ix) Signal processing arrangements

An accurate specification of the signal processing arrangements may be very complicated. The suppression level, and the amplitude and frequency characteristics of the receiver, are of particular importance.

(x) Overall dynamic range

This quantity may be measured using the equipment described in subsection (vii) of this section. The attenuation is decreased from a large value until a registration is just visible on the display. The difference between the

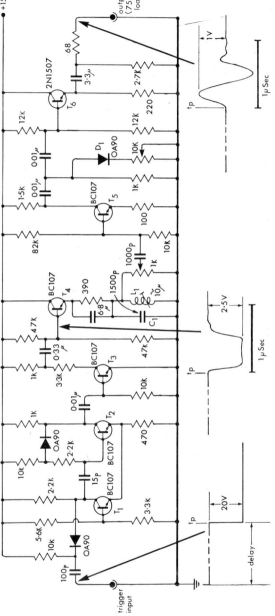

FIG. 4.48 Circuit diagram of a pulse generator for gain and swept gain calibrations.

value of this attenuation and the attenuation below which further decrease produces no increase in registration is equal to the overall dynamic range.

(xi) Overall paralysis time

Buschmann (1965) has described how the paralysis time may be measured by moving the transducer towards a flat target until the undisturbed part of the display time-base between the transmission pulse and the echo signal just disappears. The time interval corresponding to this distance is equal to the paralysis time at the particular settings of transmitter power and receiver gain used for the measurement.

It is a formidable task to make all the measurements necessary to define the complete specification of an ultrasonic system. Fortunately, the performance of a system can be quite quickly checked by a few measurements involving the use of simple targets. For example, Buschmann (1965) has described a method of sensitivity calibration based on the measurement of the range of penetration in an oil bath. Again, Holmes (1967b) has devised a method in which several spherical targets are fixed in an oil-filled tube at various distances from the transducer: this enables the swept gain and the overall sensitivity to be checked simultaneously. Yet another method is based on measurements of the echo amplitudes received from the flat surfaces of Perspex blocks of various thicknesses.

5. DOPPLER TECHNIQUES

5.1 TRANSMISSION TECHNIQUES

The Doppler effect is described in Section 1.12. The earliest use of the ultrasonic Doppler effect in medical diagnosis seems to have been for the measurement of flow velocity, particularly in intact blood vessels. The original flowmeters developed for this purpose were based on the measurement of the effective ultrasonic velocity between two transducers arranged at a fixed distance apart on the outside of the vessel. The difference between the measured velocity and the velocity in the same system but with no flow is equal to the flow velocity. In biological systems, the flow velocities are much less than the ultrasonic propagation velocity, and so a balanced system is used which is sensitive to the small difference in the transit times of signals travelling up and down stream. The original instrument of Kalmus (1954) was not developed specifically for biomedical applications, but Baldes *et al.* (1957) described an experimental system for blood flow velocity measurement. The best transducer arrangement for this application seems to be that of Franklin *et al.* (1959), illustrated in Fig. 5.1. The assembly is constructed in two halves, which can be clamped together to form a collar around the blood vessel. Neglecting the effect of the part of the ultrasonic path which does not lie in the moving liquid, the difference Δ_t between the up and down stream transit times is given by—

$$\Delta_t = d \left[\frac{1}{c-v} - \frac{1}{c+v} \right] \cos \theta, \qquad (5.1)$$

where $c =$ ultrasonic propagation velocity,

and $v =$ flow velocity.

In practice, $c \gg v$, and Equation 5.1 can be simplified to give—

$$v = \frac{\Delta_t c^2}{2d \cos \theta}. \qquad (5.2)$$

In a typical transducer assembly, $d = 2 \cdot 5$ cm and $\theta = 15°$. The ultrasonic velocity in blood is about 1570 msec^{-1} (see Table 1.2). Substitution of these values in Equation 5.2 indicates that $\Delta_t = 0 \cdot 2$ nsec per cm sec^{-1} of flow velocity. The transit time with no flow is equal to 15 μsec. Thus, a

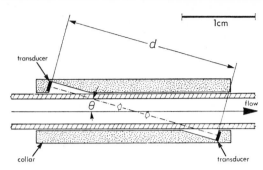

Fig. 5.1 Arrangement of transducers for measurement of flow velocity by transit time difference in up and down stream paths.

flow velocity of 1 cm sec^{-1} causes a difference of 0·0013% between the up and down stream transit times. In the system of Franklin *et al.* (1959), the up and down stream transit times of 3 MHz ultrasonic pulses are compared by the comparison of the amplitudes of corresponding ramps generated by a time-to-voltage analogue converter.

Farrall (1959) has described improvements to the earlier system of Baldes *et al.* (1957). Two transmitters and two receivers are used, but only one pair is in operation at any particular time. A reference signal from the transmitter is compared with the received signal by a phasemeter. The phasemeter gives a direct current output which is proportional to the transit time. The ultrasonic frequency is 380 kHz, and the transducer pairs are switched at a frequency of 100 Hz to provide up and down stream measurements. The difference between the outputs of the two phasemeters is proportional to the flow velocity. The phase difference is about 0·03° per cm sec^{-1} of flow velocity.

Measurements of the flow velocity based on the transit time difference determined either by direct or phase comparison require complicated equipment and are not very accurate. For example, drifts in zero calibration make both methods unsatisfactory at velocities below about 10 cm sec^{-1}. Consequently, the performance of the transmission type of ultrasonic flowmeter is no better than that of the electromagnetic flowmeter (Wetterer, 1962).

5.2 REFLECTION TECHNIQUES

5.2.a Basic Principles

The Doppler shift in the frequency of reflected ultrasound may be used as a measure of the velocity of movement of the reflecting surface. The relationship between the Doppler shift frequency f_D, the transmitted ultrasonic frequency f, the vector component v_i of the interface velocity along the direction of the ultrasonic axis, and the ultrasonic propagation velocity c, is given by Equation 1.33. If $c \gg v_i$, Equation 1.33 can be simplified to give—

$$v_i = -\frac{f_D c}{2f} \tag{5.3}$$

In cases where the various velocities do not all act along the same straight line, the appropriate velocity vectors must be used for the calculation of f_D. Thus, if γ is the angle of attack (defined as the angle between the direction of movement and the effective ultrasonic beam direction), Equation 5.3 can be modified to give—

$$v = -\frac{f_D c}{2f \cos \gamma}, \tag{5.4}$$

where v = absolute velocity of the reflector along the
              direction of flow.

The algebraic sign of f_D is not important in a simple system because the Doppler shift detector is sensitive only to the magnitude of f_D. The nomogram in Fig. 5.2 enables the relationships between v, f_D, f and γ to be found for the range of values which commonly occur in medical applications.

The effective direction of the ultrasonic beam lies along the central axis of the transducer assembly in the case of a coaxial transmitting and receiving system. The effective directions in other transducer arrangements are discussed in Section 5.2.b.

The reflected Doppler frequency shift method for measuring velocity is free from a number of the difficulties experienced with velocity meters based on the measurement of transit time (Section 5.1). In particular, there is no zero drift in the Doppler frequency shift method, and no error due to uncertainty in the path length in the moving liquid. However, it is important to realize that, in the case of blood flowing in a vessel, the velocity does not have a single value. This is because the blood at the centre flows faster than that nearer to the walls of the vessel. Consequently, the Doppler shift frequency extends over a spectrum, and its measurement may not be a simple matter. The tendency is for the estimate of flow velocity based on the Doppler frequency shift to be somewhat higher (around 20% for stream-lined flow in a tube of 0·7 cm diameter) than the true velocity (from data of Franklin et al. 1963). Green (1964) has discussed some other factors which contribute to spectral broadening in Doppler shift flowmeters which depend on ultrasound backscattered from small reflectors suspended in the moving liquid. For example, he considered the effects of the Brownian movement of the reflecting particles (the blood cells in a blood flowmeter), and the finite angular beamwidths of the transducers. With most practical

Doppler shift flowmeters, the spectral broadening produced by these and other effects is negligible.

A disadvantage of the reflected Doppler frequency shift method is that simple detectors do not differentiate between movements towards and away from the transducer assembly. The directional informaton is available in the form of the algebraic sign of f_D (see Equation 5.4), but it is difficult to determine whether f_r is greater or less than f. This is because f_D is only a very small fraction of f. Yoshitoshi et $al.$ (1966) attempted to develop a directionally sensitive Doppler flowmeter in which the reflected signals are

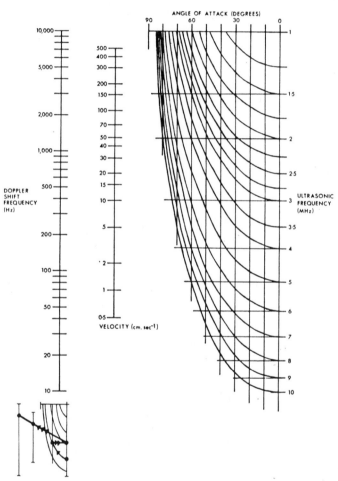

FIG. 5.2 Nomogram showing relationships between the reflector velocity, the Doppler shift frequency and the ultrasonic frequency for various angles of attack. Values calculated from Equation 5.3 for blood (velocity = 1570 m sec^{-1}, see Table 1.2). (After Wells, 1969.)

mixed both with the transmitter frequency, and with another frequency of 6 kHz below that of the transmitter. The dominant 6 kHz signal is attenuated by a differential amplifier before recording. It was expected that the output frequency would be greater than 6 kHz for movements towards the transducers, and below 6 kHz for the reverse direction. Unfortunately, the recording is confused by the presence of a mirror image. It has been suggested that this might be avoided by suppressing the 3 MHz carrier frequency, but this proposal does not seem to have been tested in practice.

Another method for detecting the direction of movement from the information in the Doppler signal has been described by McLeod (1964). The signal from the receiving transducer is fed into two separate filters. One of these filters is tuned so that its output increases with increasing frequency; the other gives a decreasing output with increasing frequency. Each of the filters is followed by a diode demodulator. The difference between the outputs of the two detectors is proportional to the flow velocity.

5.2.b Transducer Arrangements

Some of the transducer arrangements which have been described in the literature for the application of the reflection Doppler technique to medical diagnosis are shown in Fig. 5.3. The coaxial arrangement illustrated in Fig. 5.3.a has been used mainly in cardiology (see Section 5.5.a). In the design of Satomura (1957), a single 3 MHz disc of 1 cm diameter is used. The silvering of the front face forms a common electrode, but that of the rear face is divided into two zones: the central disc of 0·3 cm diameter acts as the transmitting electrode, whilst the outer ring serves as the receiver. In the design of Lubé et al. (1967), the 2 MHz transmitting and receiving transducers are similarly arranged but acoustically isolated. The use of separate transmitting and receiving transducers improves the performance of the system in the detection of weak signals. This is because the weakest signal may be 120 dB (a factor of 10^6 times in amplitude) less than the transmitted signal. In the case of a common transducer acting both as transmitter and receiver, the amplitude modulation of the transmitter would have to be less than 1 part in 10^6 to be unobstrusive. This would certainly be difficult to achieve, although perhaps not impossible.

The first application of the method to the measurement of blood flow by the Doppler shift in frequency of ultrasound backscattered from blood cells within an intact vessel (see Section 5.5.b) was reported in considerable detail by Satomura and Kaneko (1961). Their transcutaneous flowmeter, the transducer arrangement of which is illustrated in Fig. 5.3.b, operates at a frequency of 5 MHz. A somewhat similar transducer arrangement was described by Rushmer et al. (1966), and is illustrated in Fig. 5.3.d. This now seems to have been abandoned for routine application in favour of a system similar to that of Satomura and Kaneko (1961), but in which the two halves of the transducer are set at an angle so that the transmitting and receiving beams cross at a range of about 2–3 cm. An earlier system described by Franklin *et al.* (1961) is designed for use on an exposed vessel (in a manner similar to the method of Franklin *et al.* (1959), explained in Section 5.1): this arrangement is shown in Fig. 5.3.c.

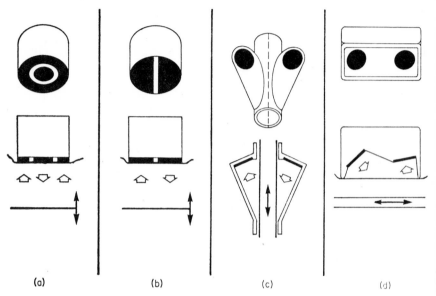

(a)   (b)   (c)   (d)

FIG. 5.3 Typical transducer arrangements for the measurement of reflector velocity by the Doppler shift in ultrasonic frequency. (a) Coaxial system of Satomura (1957); (b) Split disc transducer system of Satomura and Kaneko (1961); (c) Implantable system of Franklin, Schlegel and Rushmer (1961); (d) Transcutaneous flowmeter of Rushmer, Baker and Stegall (1966).

Transducer arrangements in which a disc is cut in half to form a separate transmitter and receiver (similar to the system of Satomura and Kaneko, 1961), illustrated in Fig. 5.3.b) are also used in some of the probes designed for use in obstetrics (Section 5.5.c), such as the 2·5 cm diameter assembly of Fielder (1968). The transducers are set at an angle, so that the transmitting and receiving beams cross at some convenient distance from the probe. The distribution of sensitivity of such an arrangement does not yet seem to have been measured. At the present time, probes for obstetrics usually have frequencies of around 2–3 MHz, which gives a greater penetration than that obtainable at higher frequencies, but a broader beam, and a lower Doppler shift frequency for a given reflector velocity.

The transcutaneous Doppler technique is a relatively recent development, and for this reason only rather scanty information on transducer design has been given in the literature. For example, details of the degree of transducer damping (see Section 2.6.a) required to give an adequate performance have not been revealed. However, it is certainly not necessary to employ such heavy damping as is required in pulse-echo transducers, because the Doppler systems operate with a relatively narrow bandwidth. The narrow bandwidth makes it possible to use a plastic matching layer to improve the efficiency of the transducer coupling (see Section 2.8); this has been mentioned by Lubé *et al.* (1967).

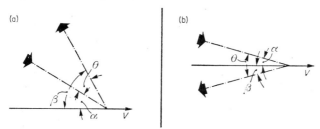

Fig. 5.4 Diagrams illustrating the calculation of the angle of attack in a system employing convergent transmitting and receiving ultrasonic beams. See text, Section 5.2.b.

It has been stated in Section 5.2.a that the effective direction of the ultrasonic beam in transducer arrangements which are coaxial lies along the central axis of the transducer assembly. However, the situation requires further analysis in the case of a system in which the transmitting and receiving beams converge in the region of the moving reflector.

Consider the examples illustrated in Fig. 5.4. It has been shown in Section 1.12 (Equation 1.32) that—

$$f_D = \left(\frac{c - v_r}{c - v_s} - 1 \right) f,$$

where v_r = velocity of receiver away from the source,

and v_s = velocity of the source in the same direction as v_r.

When both the source and the receiver are stationary, a moving reflector may be considered to act as a moving receiver which behaves as a virtual source moving with respect to the receiver. Substitution of the appropriate vector components of v for v_r and v_s gives—

$$f_D = \left(\frac{c - v \cos \alpha}{c + v \cos \beta} - 1 \right) f,$$

and hence, if $c \gg v$,

$$f_D = -\frac{fv}{c} (\cos \alpha + \cos \beta).$$

This can be rearranged to give—

$$v = - \frac{f_D c}{2f \left(\cos \tfrac{1}{2}(\alpha + \beta) \cos \tfrac{1}{2}(\alpha - \beta)\right)} \qquad (5.5)$$

Comparison of Equations 5.4 and 5.5 shows that—

$$\cos \gamma = \cos \tfrac{1}{2}(\alpha + \beta) \cos \tfrac{1}{2}(\alpha - \beta) \qquad (5.6)$$

In Equation 5.6, the angle $[\tfrac{1}{2}(\alpha + \beta)]$ is the angle between the direction of movement and the line which bisects the angle between the transmitting and receiving beams. The angle $(\alpha - \beta)$ has a value which lies between the angle of convergence θ of the transmitting and receiving beams (as in Fig. 5.4.a), and zero (Fig. 5.4.b). The angle θ is typically about $10°$ in foetal blood-flow detectors, and about $30°$ in peripheral blood-flow detectors. The errors introduced by assuming that $\gamma = \tfrac{1}{2}(\alpha + \beta)$ in calculating f_D from the nomogram in Fig. 5.2 for these two types of transducer arrangement have maximum values of about 0.5% and 3.5% respectively. These errors lead to underestimations in the calculated values of reflector velocity for a given Doppler shift frequency.

5.3 TRANSMITTERS AND RECEIVERS

Figure 5.5 is a block diagram showing a typical electronic system for an ultrasonic Doppler frequency shift detector. The receiver may be considered as a single sideband superheterodyne with zero intermediate frequency, the leakage from the transmitter providing the local oscillator power, and the modulation frequency being the Doppler shift frequency. Unfortunately, only rather brief descriptions of the characteristics of the various components have been given in the literature: some of this information is summarized in Table 5.1.

The design of the transmitter presents no special problems if separate transmitting and receiving transducers are used (see Section 5.2.b), and a circuit employing one or two transistors is usually satisfactory. The short-term frequency stability of the transmitter needs to correspond to less than the minimum detectable Doppler frequency shift which occurs during the transit time. Thus, a stability of better than 1 part in 10^5 over 500 μsec is normally adequate.

The receiver is required to accept a dynamic range which is in the order of 100 dB (Fielder (1968)). Because the simple Doppler method employs continuous waves, no range information is available in the signal. Consequently, it is not possible to compress the dynamic range by swept gain compensation as can be done in pulse-echo systems (see Section 4.1.b). In practice, the Doppler signals are often analysed by ear. The dynamic range of the ear extends from about 120 dB at around 2 kHz, to about 40 dB at

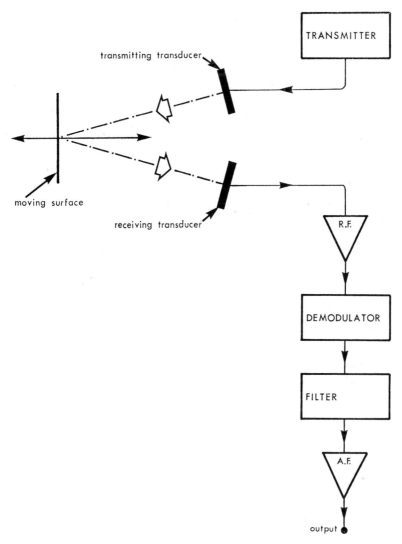

FIG. 5.5 Block diagram of an ultrasonic Doppler frequency shift system.

30 Hz and 17 kHz. However, these dynamic ranges are for monotonic sounds, and the presence of masking sounds of differing frequencies and intensities substantially reduces the dynamic range at any particular

TABLE 5.1

Data on electronic systems used in ultrasonic Doppler frequency shift detectors

Clinical application	Frequency MHz	Ultrasonic intensity mW cm^{-2}	Receiver circuit	Filter	Reference
Cardiology	3	20–50	Receiving transducer direct to demodulator; 60–80 dB a.f. gain.	200 Hz lowpass; 500–1000 Hz bandpass.	Satomura (1957) Yoshida et al. (1961)
	2	<50	R.f. amplifier, demodulator and a.f. amplifier.	300 Hz lowpass; 400 Hz highpass.	Lubé et al. (1967)
Blood flow studies	5	2000	Receiving transducer direct to demodulator; a.f. amplifier.	15 kHz lowpass.	Franklin et al. (1961)
	5	—	R.f. amplifier, demodulator and a.f. amplifier.	—	Franklin et al. (1963)
	5	10–100	Differential r.f. amplifier, demodulator and a.f. amplifier.	50 or 200 Hz highpass; 5 kHz lowpass.	Stegall et al. (1966)
Obstetrics	2–2·5	12·5	60 dB r.f. amplifier, demodulator and a.f. amplifier.	100 Hz highpass.	Fielder (1968)

frequency. Therefore, electronic dynamic range compression is necessary. The amplitudes of the Doppler signals are usually of much less importance than their frequencies, and so the performance requirements for electronic dynamic range compression are not severe. Simple limiting is usually employed; but this tends to reduce the sensitivity to signals of low amplitude. An amplifier with a logarithmic response (see Section 4.5.c) would no doubt give an improved performance in this respect.

A receiving arrangement which consists of a r.f. amplifier with a gain of about 60 dB, followed by a demodulator and an a.f. amplifier, seems to be satisfactory for most applications. The mixing which results in the detection of the Doppler shift frequency occurs in the demodulator, and it is unnecessary to inject the transmitter frequency at this point because it is already present as the result of stray coupling from the transmitter and ultrasonic reflections from stationary interfaces.

Noise in Doppler systems arise from a number of sources. The most important of these are:

(i) The equivalent input noise of the r.f. amplifier. Although the frequency spectrum of the Doppler signal generally extends over less than about 10 kHz, a somewhat broader receiver bandwidth is necessary in practice to accommodate drifts in the transmitter frequency and the receiver passband. For example, the receiver passband might typically be 1 MHz wide in a system centred on 2·5 MHz.

(ii) The demodulator acting as a mixer.

(iii) Reflections from other moving structures apart from those of primary interest, and movements of the probe. These are often the most important noise sources in biomedical applications, and are analogous to "clutter" in Radar.

The output from the demodulator covers a frequency spectrum which extends from very low frequencies up to about 10 kHz. Some of the frequency components carry useful information; others do not. It is usual to arrange for unwanted signals to be filtered out whenever this is possible without the loss of useful information. This matter is considered in greater detail in Sections 5.4 and 5.5.

An attractive development of the Doppler method in medical diagnosis may be possible. Range-measuring Doppler systems ("moving target indicators") have been used for many years in Radar (Ridenour (1947), pp. 139–157 and 626–676). Thus, a range-gated ultrasonic system could employ a transmitted wave-train of, say, 10 μsec duration (occupying a 1·5 cm length of soft tissue), repeated 1000 times per sec. A gated receiver could be switched on for 10 μsec at a time after transmission appropriate to the range of the moving structure being investigated. Several other similar systems also appear to be feasible.

5.4 METHODS OF DOPPLER SIGNAL ANALYSIS

5.4.a The Ear

In many kinds of clinical examinations, a diagnosis can be made by listening to the Doppler shift frequency. This is often made easier by electrically filtering out the components of frequency below about 100 Hz, which otherwise obscure the more important frequencies in the range 200–1000 Hz. Aural analysis is generally not satisfactory in cardiological investigations, because of the rapid rate of change of information. However, Strandness et al. (1967) considered that audible information is more useful than the recording of a sound spectroscope (Section 5.4.d) in the diagnosis of peripheral vascular disease. In obstetrics, almost all clinical investigations at the present time are made by ear, without the use of other analysing systems.

Although a trained investigator can obtain a great deal of clinical information by listening to the Doppler signals, there are some situations in which a quantitative analysis is helpful. The various methods which have been used to obtain such analyses are discussed in the following sections.

5.4.b Ratemeters

The simplest form of Doppler information consists of a single frequency component. Such a signal may be analysed by measuring its frequency with a ratemeter. Thus, Franklin et al. (1963) used the type 500 B ratemeter of the Hewlett-Packard Co. for measuring flow rate. Other investigators, for example Strandness et al. (1966) have obtained analogue signals similar to the output of a ratemeter by differentiating, rectifying and filtering the audio frequencies. This method has been used not only in blood flow studies, but also in obstetrics (Rushmer et al. 1967).

5.4.c Bandpass Filters

If several reflectors moving at differing velocities lie in the ultrasonic beam, the Doppler signal contains several principal components of frequency, one for each reflector. Each of these frequency components may extend over a spectrum, as discussed in Section 5.2.a.

Some separation of the Doppler information can be achieved by frequency selective filtering. In cardiology, both Satomura (1957) and Lubé et al. (1967) separate the Doppler signals into two frequency channels, the division being made at between 200 and 500 Hz. Signals in the lower frequency channel are identified primarily with movements of the heart muscles, whilst those in the higher frequency channel arise from the heart valves.

Bandpass filters seem to have been little used in the analysis of Doppler signals in other clinical investigations apart from cardiology. However, the sound spectroscope (Section 5.4.d) is in reality a multichannel bandpass system, and this instrument has considerable value in many other applications.

5.4.d Sound Spectroscopes

The principle of the sound spectroscope was proposed by R. K. Potter. The sound is analysed to produce a chart in which time and frequency are represented on the x and y axes respectively, and the corresponding amplitudes are represented by the degree of blackening of the recording.

Koenig et al. (1946) have described the construction of the first practical sound spectroscope. The basic principles are as follows. The sound to be analysed is recorded in such a way that it can be replayed over and over again. The continuously replayed sound is then analysed by means of a modulator and variable frequency oscillator which shifts each part of the recorded spectrum in sequence to the passband of a fixed frequency filter. The output from the filter is arranged to control the degree of blackening of the write-out recording. The write-out paper and the recording of the sound move in synchronism so that the x-axis represents time. The position on the y-axis of the write-out is arranged to correspond to the instantaneous value of the frequency being analysed. Electrically sensitive paper is used, and the dynamic range of the write-out is about 12 dB. An input of greater dynamic range can be accommodated by compressing the output dynamic range, for example by means of a thermistor with a rapid response included at a suitable point in the amplifier.

Electrically sensitive paper has certain disadvantages when used as the write-out material in a simple sound spectroscope: in particular, it is difficult to estimate the amplitude of any part of the spectrum from the degree of blackening of the recording. Koenig and Ruppel (1948) have described two methods of reducing this difficulty. In one method, different shades of gray are represented by dots of varying size. In the other method, which is nowadays quite commonly used in commercial spectroscopes, iso-amplitude curves are traced by means of an amplitude-gated write-out.

Mathes, Norwine and Davis (1949) have described a method for generating sound spectrograms on a brightness-modulated cathode ray tube display. The principle is similar to that of Koenig et al.'s (1946) spectroscope, but the recording is speeded up 200 times on playback, and the frequency analysis is performed by a relatively broadband high-frequency system with a filter centred on 1·2 MHz. The frequency of the beating oscillator is changed from 1·22 to 2·00 MHz in 190 equal increments. The patterns are scanned at a rate of 2 per sec. The dynamic range of the display is limited to about 20 dB (see Sections 4.6.a), and dynamic range compression is normally required in the analysing amplifier.

Commercially available sound spectroscopes are rather expensive instruments, and consequently their use may not be justified in some investigations. However, Ramaswamy and Ramakrishna (1962) have described one method for obtaining sound spectrograms using common laboratory equipment, and no doubt other methods could be devised which would be equally satisfactory.

Sound spectroscopes have been mainly used in the analysis of Doppler information on blood flow (see Section 5.5.b).

5.5 CLINICAL APPLICATIONS

5.5.a Cardiology

The Doppler method of investigating cardiac function requires apparatus which is less complicated than that necessary for time-position pulse-echo recording (see Section 4.7.e). For this reason alone the method would deserve attention, but it seems likely that the two techniques used together will eventually become complementary to other cardiac investigations.

An important use of the Doppler technique in cardiology is for the detection of the timing of the operations of the heart valves (Yoshida *et al.* 1961). Selected frequency bands of the Doppler signal can be recorded synchronously with the electrocardiogram and other conventional measurements of cardiac function. The timing of the valve movements is related to the clinical condition of the valve. The method is considerably more sensitive, and less subject to artifacts, than phonocardiography. Microphones for phonocardiography are not very directional, and so the sounds which they detect are only partly related to the movements of any particular structure. On the other hand, the ultrasonic beam of a Doppler system is highly directional, and so (within the limitations of transmission through ribs and lung) the structure being studied can be located with precision.

Analysis of the Doppler signals by sound spectroscope (Section 5.4.d) enables the velocities of the more rapid movements of the valves to be estimated with greater accuracy than is possible from pulse-echo measurements. These rapid movements give rise to Doppler shift frequencies which are considerably higher than those occurring simultaneously due to muscle and blood movements, and so they can be easily distinguished on the spectrogram. For example, Yoshitoshi *et al.* (1966) have measured the maximum velocity of closure of the mitral valve. This velocity corresponds to the slope AB in Fig. 4.45. In a normal valve the velocity is 200–400 mm sec^{-1} (mean 270 mm sec^{-1}), compared with a velocity of 300–800 mm sec^{-1} (mean 520 mm sec^{-1}) in mitral stenosis. It is expected that similar diagnostic information could also be obtained from other cardiac valves.

McLeod (1964) has described a transducer arrangement mounted at the tip of a 0·25 cm diameter catheter for intracardiac investigations. This method does not yet seem to have been used in man.

Another possible application of the Doppler effect in cardiology is in the study of prosthetic ball-valve function in experimental animals by means of the shift in frequency of the signal received from an ultrasonic source built into the ball. The study of such prostheses by pulse-echo methods is made difficult by the relatively strong echoes which return from the valve cage. This problem should not arise in the case of an active Doppler system.

5.5.b Blood Flow Studies

The Doppler method has been used for a number of studies of blood flow, some of which are listed in Table 5.2. All these investigations were made using ultrasonic frequencies of 5 or 6 MHz. In the diagnosis of occlusions, the method is generally more sensitive and specific than clinical appraisal; and in this application, the diagnosis is more conveniently and accurately made by listening to the Doppler signals, than from recordings made on ratemeters or spectroscopes (Strandness *et al.* 1967).

5.5.c Obstetrics

The use of the ultrasonic Doppler frequency shift method for the detection of the movement of the foetal heart seems to have been first reported by Callagan *et al.* (1964). Johnson *et al.* (1965), using the 5 MHz transcutaneous flowmeter described in Section 5.2.b, noticed two types of foetal sound. One of these is biphasic, and is presumed to arise from within the foetal heart. The other is monophasic and is probably due to movements within foetal blood vessels: flow within a maternal vessel sounds similar except for the striking difference in rate. In a series of 25 patients, the foetal heart was heard in 17, all of whom were more than 12 weeks pregnant. It was not detected in 5 patients who were less than 12 weeks pregnant, nor in 3 patients in whom intrauterine foetal death had occurred. Fielder and Pocock (1968) have pointed out that the uterus is more easily accessible in early pregnancy to ultrasonic examination if the patient's bladder is first allowed to fill with urine (this is also useful in similar pulse-echo examinations: see Section 4.7.d). They have reported that the foetus can be detected after 9–10 weeks gestation in the majority of cases.

Rushmer *et al.* (1966) demonstrated that it is possible to locate the placenta if it lies on the anterior or lateral walls of the uterus. The placental sounds are at the foetal rate and have characteristics which distinguish them from other signals. Fielder and Pocock (1968) have reported that it is also often possible to locate a posterior placenta if sufficient care is taken in the examination.

The Doppler technique has a number of additional uses in obstetrics.

TABLE 5.2

Some clinical applications of the reflected ultrasonic Doppler flowmeter in the study of blood flow

Site of application	Method of analysis	Information obtained	Reference
Various blood vessels: implanted transducers	Ratemeter	Blood flow rate	Franklin *et al.* (1963)
Common, internal and external carotid arteries	Spectroscope	Diagnosis of arterioschlerosis	Kaneko *et al.* (1966)
Brachial, common femoral, popliteal and pedal arteries	Ear Ratemeter Spectroscope	Localization of occlusions	Strandness *et al.* (1966, 1967)
Deep venous system	Ear Spectroscope	Localization of occlusions	Strandness *et al.* (1967) Sigel *et al.* (1968)

Thus, it is valuable in the diagnosis of intrauterine foetal death throughout the last six months of pregnancy, particularly in obese patients and those with hydramnios where the foetal stethoscope is not always satisfactory. It is also useful in the diagnosis of multiple pregnancies, and in the detection of foetal distress during labour. Finally, it is sometimes valuable to be able to give audible evidence to the mother that her pregnancy is continuing satisfactorily.

5.5.d Other Applications

The ultrasonic Doppler flowmeter has a number of applications in biomedicine apart from those already discussed in this Section. For example Kelsey (1968) has described a method for locating the scan plane in a water bath scanner by holding the Doppler probe on the patient's skin to detect the pulses from the scanning probe. A similar method can be used to identify "dead" areas in the scan plane due to the presence of gas.

Minifie et al. (1968) have used a 6 MHz Doppler flowmeter to measure the movements of the vocal fold during speech. The displacement patterns derived in this way are in good agreement with those obtained using high-speed cinématography.

Doppler techniques do not seem to have been used in the study of gas flow in biomedicine. For example, it may be possible to devise a system capable of measuring gas velocity in the trachea, using a transcutaneous flowmeter. Such a method might be valuable in anaesthesiology.

6. MISCELLANEOUS TECHNIQUES

6.1 INTRODUCTION

Ultrasound may be used in medical diagnosis in a number of ways in addition to the pulse-echo and Doppler techniques described in Chapters 4 and 5. Some of these methods are of historical interest, and others are either already well developed or seem likely to become important in the future. It is appropriate that such techniques should be at least mentioned in a book which aims to review the whole field of ultrasonic diagnosis; and for convenience, they are considered in separate sections in this chapter.

6.2 UNSCANNED TRANSMISSION TECHNIQUES

Ultrasonic transmission techniques give diagnostic information based either on transit time or on attenuation. Refraction is another effect which could be measured by transmission, but this does not yet seem to have been used in diagnosis.

In the simpler transmission techniques, the transmitting and receiving transducers are placed one on each side of the specimen, and the ultrasonic information is processed without regard to the positions of the transducers. More complicated data processing may employ scanning techniques, as described in Sections 6.3, 6.4 and 6.5.

Unscanned ultrasonic techniques have been devised for several diagnostic and experimental procedures. Their descriptions are rather scattered in the literature; a few typical examples are discussed here.

Rushmer *et al.* (1956) used an early version of their transit time flowmeter (see Section 5.1) to measure the left ventricular size of the heart. Two transducers, one for transmitting and the other for receiving, are sutured one on each side of the ventricle in an experimental animal. The transit time is measured by a time-to-voltage analogue converter somewhat similar to that described in Section 4.7.e. The pulse repetition frequency is between 1 and 2·5 kHz.

Crawford *et al.* (1959) reported a correlation between the transmission of continuous 1 MHz ultrasound through the thorax in man, and the movement of the intrathoracic structures. The method does not seem to have been used for any diagnostic purpose.

Horn and Robinson (1965) have proposed a method for the assessment of fracture union in bone, in which both longitudinal and transverse waves are transmitted simultaneously. Using a brass bar, they demonstrated that the shear waves are attenuated if a fracture is present, whereas the longitudinal waves are substantially unaffected. The method does not seem to have been tested in bone, the relatively high absorption of which may be an insuperable difficulty.

Mullins and Guntheroth (1966) have developed a method for measuring changes in mesenteric blood volume. A small sample of intact mesentery is inserted between two transducers held by a rigid frame so that their axes are in line, the ultrasonic beam passing through the sample. Mesentery consists mainly of fat and blood vessels: the fat is forced in and out of the frame by volume changes in the blood contained by the frame. The ultrasonic velocity in blood is about 8% greater than that in fat (see Table 1.2), and so changes in the volume of blood in the sample can be estimated from changes in the transit time between the two transducers. An ultrasonic frequency of 3 MHz is used, with a pulse repetition frequency of 400 Hz. It is possible to detect changes in blood volume of 0·2% with a transducer spacing of 1·5 cm.

Kossoff and Sharpe (1966) have used a transmission technique to detect the presence of gas within the pulp chamber of the tooth in degenerative pulpitis. They consider that the technique is simpler to use than the pulse-echo method, particularly as it is not affected by the inclined surfaces which occur in the pulp chamber. Ultrasonic transducers of 14–18 MHz, and diameters of 0·1–0·15 cm, are used.

6.3 MECHANICALLY SCANNED TRANSMISSION TECHNIQUES

The first attempts to use ultrasound for medical diagnosis were based on the expectation that it would be possible to demonstrate various tissue masses by differential absorption. Thus, the method is analogous to that used in X-radiology. In X-radiology, the whole of the transmitted beam can be recorded by the exposure of a photographic plate. However, no detector of sufficient sensitivity and size has been developed for direct ultrasonic recording (with the possible exception in a few applications of the ultrasonic image converter described in Section 6.4), and so it is usually necessary to employ scanning techniques which visualize the transmission characteristics of many separate small areas.

The early investigators hoped in particular that the method might be used to visualize abnormalities of the brain. The demonstration of such abnormalities by means of X-rays is usually only possible by deduction based on observations which may carry a significant risk for the patient.

Dussik et al. (1947) constructed an ultrasonic scanner, based on the original proposal of K. T. Dussik, in which a beam of ultrasound is directed through the patient's head, and detected by a receiver placed in line with the transmitter. This instrument produces a recording in the form of a plan in which the degree of blackening is related to the received intensity.

As a result of the encouraging results produced by this instrument, Ballantine et al. (1950) constructed a similar scanner. This instrument is described in detail by Hueter and Bolt (1951). It operates at a frequency of 2·5 MHz, with a transmitted power of about 1 Wcm^{-2}. In brain scanning, the attenuation amounts to about 70 dB in the thicker parts of the skull, and to 40 dB in the brain. The receiver bandwidth is quite narrow; the equivalent input noise is 2 μV. Hueter and Bolt (1951) concluded that "a preliminary evaluation indicates that the echo-reflection method is considerably less promising (than the transmission method) for general ventriculography, mainly because of the small amount of reflection at the interface between tissue and ventricular fluid".

Güttner et al. (1952) carried out a critical analysis of the transmission technique as a method for outlining the ventricles of the brain. They pointed out that the attenuation due to the ventricles is small compared with that of the brain and the skull, and that the curved shape of the skull produces refraction which distorts the ultrasonic scan. Variation in the thickness of the skull is associated with a variation in attenuation which masks the changes due to the presence or absence of the ventricles. These factors combine to make it impossible to outline the ventricles by the transmission technique. Ballantine et al. (1954) reached a similar conclusion, and the method has fallen into disuse.

It is unlikely that refraction and the small degree of differential absorption are the only factors which cause difficulty in transmission techniques. Important effects also occur because such methods usually employ continuous waves, or at least rather long pulse trains. Multiple reflections and standing waves occur both in the specimen and in the water used for coupling, and these give rise to artifacts which may lead to an unacceptable confusion of the scan.

Despite the difficulties associated with transmission techniques, Dunn and Fry (1959) have constructed an ultrasonic microscope in which the differential ultrasonic absorption of a complex specimen is scanned by means of a small thermocouple. They demonstrated that a structure with a diameter of 25 μ can be recorded using 0·1 sec duration pulses at a frequency of 12 MHz, and a thermocouple of about 13 μ diameter. They concluded that, under specified conditions, it should be possible to detect a structure with a radius of 0·4 μ by the use of 1 μsec pulses of 1000 MHz ultrasound at an intensity of 1000 Wcm^{-2}, with a thermocouple of 0·1 μ diameter and a pulse repetition frequency of 1000 Hz.

Another transmission technique which involves scanning has been described by Rich *et al.* (1966). Differences in transit time are used to give a measure of bone mass, for example by scanning across a limb. The transit time of 3 MHz pulses is measured by means of a time-to-voltage analogue converter. The transmitting and receiving transducers are mounted in line so that they can be scanned together across the specimen. The recorder is coupled to the position of the transducer assembly, so that the results are presented in the form of a graph showing the variation in transit time with position. The results of preliminary experiments on samples of cortical bone and humerus of rabbit (either intact or stripped of soft tissues) showed good agreement between the predicted mass of calcium and that subsequently determined chemically.

6.4 ELECTRICALLY SCANNED TRANSMISSION TECHNIQUES

The ultrasonic image converter is a detector which provides a C-scan display (Section 4.7.f) of the ultrasonic transmission characteristics of an object, and is thus analogous to the fluoroscopic image converter used in X-radiology.

Ultrasonic to electronic image conversion was first proposed in the 1930's by the Russian S. Ya. Sokolov. The most common form of converter is based on the property of a piezoelectric plate which allows it to resonate point by point in sympathy with an incident ultrasonic distribution, with negligible lateral spread in the thickness mode. The method has been developed in Russia (Semennikov, 1958), in Germany (Freitag *et al.* 1960), in Great Britain (Smyth *et al.* 1963), and in the U.S.A. (Jacobs *et al.* 1963).

The basic principles of a typical system are illustrated in Fig. 6.1. The ultrasonic transmitting transducer irradiates the specimen with continuous ultrasonic waves, producing a "shadow" image on the transducer of the image converter. The acoustic image is thus converted to an electrical charge pattern on the inside surface of the transducer. The electron beam scans the charge pattern in a raster. If the scanning beam is of high energy (around 1000 V), the instantaneous current of secondary emission electrons which flows into the collector is proportional to the charge on each element of the transducer. In the design of Jacobs (1965), the performance is improved by the use of an electron multiplier which is integral with the converter. The secondary electrons from the transducer are collected by the multiplier, the output of which is fed to the video amplifier.

The converter of Smyth *et al.* (1963) uses a low energy scanning beam (around 200 V), which cannot generate secondary electrons. A sequential process is necessary in normal operation. The transducer is first scanned once, with no incident ultrasound. This depresses the inside surface of the transducer to the electron gun potential. The ultrasound is switched on during the next scanning process, and more electrons can arrive at the transducer only during positive half-cycles at those points which are in vibration: the charging current is proportional to the corresponding ultrasonic amplitude. The transducer is prepared for the next sequence by allowing positive ions to be drawn to it until it is again at cathode potential. The signal-to-noise ratio is larger with low voltage than with high voltage scanning.

A large source-to-specimen distance is necessary to avoid the inhomogeneity of the ultrasonic field in the Frésnel zone (see Section 3.1). The specimen is placed close to the image converter to obtain the best

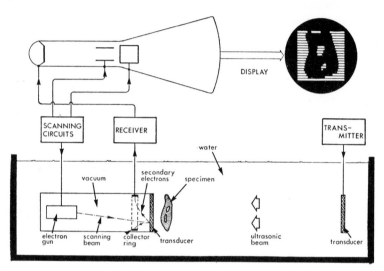

FIG. 6.1 Basic principles of ultrasonic image conversion. This system uses continuous wave ultrasound, and high energy electron scanning.

resolution and the minimum effects from the scattering and refraction within the specimen. Alternatively, a lens can be used to focus the image on the transducer (Smyth *et al.* 1963). However, Jacobs (1967) has pointed out that a lens system involves oblique incidence on the transducer, and that optimum resolution is only obtained if the incidence is normal. At normal incidence, the resolution is limited by the thickness of the transducer. The smallest resolvable detail is a cylindrical volume whose depth and diameter are both equal to the thickness of the transducer (Jacobs, 1965).

The sensitivity of a practical ultrasonic image converter is in the order of 10^{-7} to 10^{-8} Wcm^{-2} (Freitag, Martin and Schellbach, 1960; Smyth *et al.* 1963). The maximum sensitivity occurs when the transducer is of half-wavelength thickness. In principle, the resolution may be improved by using a thinner transducer operating at a higher frequency: but in practice, the transducer cannot be made both large in diameter and thin in section, because it forms one of the walls of a vacuum enclosure. Consequently, most converters operate at frequencies below about 5 MHz, and have transducer diameters of less than 5 cm. Several methods have been suggested for mechanically supporting very thin transducers (Jacobs, 1965). However, the potentially improved resolution would be obtained at the expense of greater absorption in the specimen, and the necessity for an increased source-to-converter distance because of the extension of the Frésnel zone at higher frequencies (see Section 3.1).

Most converters employ quartz transducers. The limiting sensitivity with quartz is about 100 times worse than that with lead zirconate titanate (Smyth et al. 1963). Another disdvantage of quartz is that it has a greater lateral mechanical coupling than the ferroelectrics, and so has an inferior limiting resolution. Quartz has been used in the past because it is the only transducer that has been found to be sufficiently uniform in piezoelectric properties, and sufficiently gas-tight and strong, to allow commercial production of image converter tubes.

Unfortunately, continuous wave operation of the converter is not entirely satisfactory because the image is degraded by standing waves and multiple reflections within the specimen and the water bath. It is possible to use a pulsed system in which a separate pulse is used for each position of the scanning beam. This arrangement would require 2 sec for 2000 resolution elements to be scanned at a rate of 1000 per sec, which is probably about the maximum which could be achieved in practice. As one of the attractive features of the image converter is its potentially high speed, so slow a rate is most unsatisfactory; in any event, a similar performance could probably be obtained by mechanical scanning.

In order to maintain fast display rates with pulsed ultrasound, it is necessary to arrange for the entire image to be stored on some kind of sensitized plate, so that this plate can be scanned completely during the intervals between ultrasonic pulses. The stored pattern is erased after it has been scanned, just before the arrival of the next pulse. Two storage systems have been described by Goldman (1962), both of which could operate with 10 μsec pulses of 1 MHz ultrasound. In the converter illustrated in Fig. 6.2.a, the flood gun is turned on at the instant that the leading edge of the pulse arrives at the transducer. If the outer surface of the transducer is at earth potential, the potential of the inner surface begins to alternate with respect to earth at the ultrasonic frequency. Each point on this surface exhibits a self-rectifying action and so stores an electron charge proportional to the corresponding ultrasonic amplitude. The flood gun is turned off at the end of the ultrasonic pulse, leaving a negative charge pattern on the inside of the transducer. This charge pattern is then scanned in a raster in the same way that a high energy continuous wave converter is scanned, the secondary electrons being collected by the mesh. When the scanning process has been completed, the charge pattern is erased by turning on the flood gun to that the inside surface of the transducer goes positive until it reaches earth potential. The converter is then ready to store the image of the next pulse.

The converter illustrated in Fig. 6.2.b is both easier to manufacture and electronically simpler to operate than the secondary emission storage type.

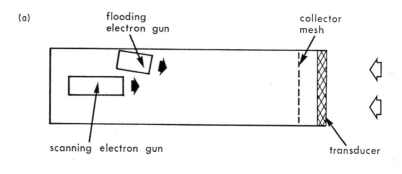

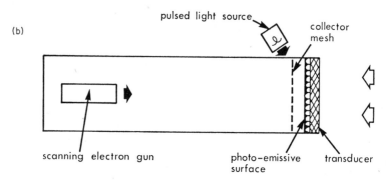

FIG. 6.2 Two types of pulsed ultrasonic image converters. (a) Secondary emission storage type; (b) Photo-emission storage type.

Goldman's (1962) design uses magnetic deflection and focussing. The inside surface of the transducer is coated with a photoemissive layer of high lateral resistivity. The light source is turned on during the time that the ultrasonic pulse is arriving: this causes electrons to be emitted in proportion to the maximum negative voltage developed at each point on the transducer. Therefore a stored charge pattern is formed which is positive with respect to earth. Scanning at high energy not only provides the video signal, but also neutralizes the charge pattern to that no erasing process is necessary before the arrival of the next pulse.

Although the ultrasonic image converter was originally expected to have a number of applications in biomedicine, it has been little used in this or any other field. The reasons for this are the small screen size and lack of storage in most of the converters available at the present time. If these limitations could be overcome, a few practical applications might be possible. One such possibility is in the study of cardiovascular flow patterns within intact animals (Jacobs, 1965).

Jacobs (1968a) has described how the sensitivity of an ultrasonic image converter to acoustic impedance changes may be increased by a factor of 20 to 40 times by the use of a colour television display system. The ability to detect changes in acoustic impedance in the order of one part in 10^8 may be of value in biomedical investigations.

Another development of the ultrasonic image converter with possible biomedical applications is in microscopy. Thus, Jacobs (1967) has discussed the factors which would affect the performance of an image converter operating at a frequency of 3000 MHz. New transducers would be required, and other formidable problems would need to be solved, before such a converter could be constructed. A resolution in the order of 20 μ seems to be feasible in a system in which the specimen is in contact with the transducer.

Although the likely biomedical application of the ultrasonic microscope (another form of which is described in Section 6.3) seems to be rather limited, it might be useful as a complementary technique to light micro-scopy. This is because the ultrasonic microscope visualizes discontinuities in the absorption coefficient of biological structures, and these discontinu-ities may not coincide with discontinuities in refractive index or light absorption.

6.5 ULTRASONIC HOLOGRAPHY

Ultrasonic holography is a two-stage process in which the diffraction pattern of an object irradiated by ultrasound is biassed by a coherent reference wave and recorded to generate an ultrasonic hologram. A three-dimensional image of the original object is created when the ultrasonic hologram is illuminated by a coherent light source. Thus, the principles are the same as those of optical holography (mentioned in Section 4.7.g). The method has a number of potential advantages in comparison with other forms of ultrasonic visualization. Metherell et al. (1967) consider that these advantages are those of simplicity, the reconstruction of the image in three-dimensional form, the large depth of field, the insensitivity to turbulence and turbidity of the medium, and the capability of retrieving the informa-tion about the target from discrete sampling points. In addition, Thurstone (1967) expects that the ultimate resolution should be comparable to the ultrasonic wavelength.

The basis of the method is illustrated in Fig. 6.3. This diagram shows one possible arrangement for the generation of acoustical holograms. The transmitting transducer is in the form of part of a spherical shell radiating from its convex surface. The receiving transducer is mounted on an *x-y* scanner which enables it to sample the utrasound scattered from the patient over a wide area. The receiver is essentially non-directional, so that scattered signals are received from every point within the object at any position in the scan.

The occurrence of standing waves and multiple reflections may make ultrasonic holography impossible with continuous waves (Halstead, 1968). In such a situation, it is necessary to pulse the transmitter and to gate the receiver. The ultrasonic pulse duration, and the timing and duration of the receiver gate, need to be chosen carefully so that the received signal

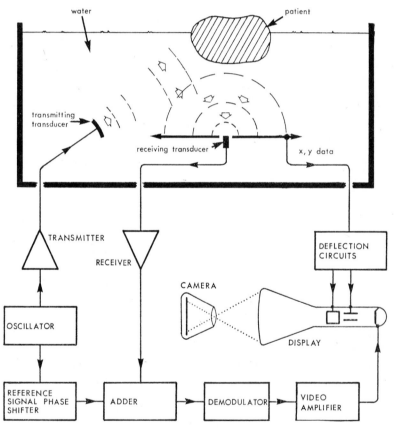

FIG. 6.3 Basic system for generating ultrasonic holograms. A mechanically scanned non-directional receiving transducer and an electrical reference signal are used.

contains the maximum amount of complete information with respect to both the phase and the amplitude of the entire scattered field.

In optical holography, it is necessary for the addition of the scattered and the reference fields to occur before the hologram is recorded. This is because most optical detectors (such as photographic film) are sensitive only to intensity, and not to phase. On the other hand, many types of ultrasonic detector are sensitive to both amplitude and phase. If such a detector is used as the receiver, an electrical signal derived from the transmitting oscillator may be used as the phase reference in the recording process. An electrical reference signal has two important advantages. Firstly, it behaves like a perfectly plane wave, which would be difficult to generate ultrasonically. Secondly, the effective position of the reference source can be varied by altering the phase of the reference signal with respect to that of the transmitter, as the receiver is being scanned.

If the ultrasonic frequency is, for example, 1 MHz, then the ratio of the ultrasonic wavelength used to generate the hologram, to that of the light wavelength used to reconstruct the image, is about 2300 to 1 (Metherell, 1968). This causes longitudinal distortion of the image along the reference axis, so that the limited depth-of-field of the observer may permit the observation of only one plane in two dimensions (at any time) in the three dimensional image. Some improvement can be obtained by demagnifying the ultrasonic hologram before reconstruction. However, this does not completely solve the problem, because the reconstructed image of a greatly demagnified hologram is so small that it requires magnification which simply reintroduces the distortion.

A number of difficulties are associated with the generation of a hologram by means of a scanned receiving transducer. A complete hologram can only be generated by scanning the scattered field from every possible direction. The scanning process is a compromise which allows the hologram to be generated by sampling the field from a number of discrete positions. If the sampling points are too far apart, the reconstructed image is unacceptable. If, for example, 10^6 sampling points were to be necessary to generate a satisfactory hologram, and each sampling process occupied 1 msec, then the total scanning time would be 1000 sec. Sampling at so great a rate as 1000 per sec would be extremely difficult.

It has been suggested that it might be possible to reduce the total scanning time by using an ultrasonic image converter (Section 6.4) as the detector, but these devices have several disadvantages in this application. Firstly, it is necessary for incidence to be within $3°$ of normal for optimum performance (Jacobs, 1968b), and this would severely restrict the holographic detection aperture. Secondly, the storage type of converter has no phase information in its output, and so it could not be used with an electrical phase reference. It would be necessary to use a non-storage type of converter, and information would only be available during the relatively short time that the receiver was gated on, if an electrical phase reference were to be used. Thirdly, it is impossible at the present time to construct large-area converters, and so it might still be necessary to use some kind of mechanical scanner to cover the required area.

Quite satisfactory images reconstructed from ultrasonic holograms have already been demonstrated (see, for example, Preston and Kruezer, 1967). However, such demonstrations seem to have been confined to the visualization of simple, highly reflective structures in water. The extension of the method to the visualization of tissue structures presents formidable problems, some of which do not seem to have been considered in detail by those who have suggested that ultrasonic holography may become a useful diagnostic technique. These difficulties are discussed in the following paragraphs.

In a practical system, the minimum ultrasonic intensity for satisfactory detection by a receiving transducer with a 1 MHz bandwidth is in the order of 10^{-7} Wcm^{-2}. A bandwidth of between 10 to 100 kHz might be satisfactory in holography; assuming that the gain-bandwidth product of the receiving system is constant (see Section 4.4.a), the maximum sensitivity would be between 10^{-9} to 10^{-8} Wcm^{-2}. The maximum echo amplitude from the skin surface might be about 20 dB below the incident intensity. A dynamic range of 50 dB would give marginally satisfactory visualization in a pulse-echo system for abdominal scanning at 1·5 MHz, allowing 30 dB for absorption and 20 dB reflectivity variation. Thus, the minimum incident intensity would be 70 dB above 10^{-9} Wcm^{-2}; this is equal to 0·01 Wcm^{-2}.

A marginally satisfactory abdominal investigation by ultrasonic holography would require the uniform irradiation of an area of perhaps 30 × 30 cm at an intensity of 0·01 Wcm^{-2}. This corresponds to a total power of 9 W. Such conditions approach the level which would be considered to place the patient at risk (see Chapter 7), but the dangers would be reduced by pulsed operation.

A more serious problem is due to the largely specular nature of the reflection of ultrasonic waves by the body. The objects which have been visualized with almost unbelievably high fidelity by optical holography have surfaces which are excellent light scatterers. However, in ultrasonic holography, it is to be expected that the reconstructed image would be spoilt by what is equivalent to "glare" in photography. In effect, the reflection from the body surface would mask the much weaker reflections from within. Thus, if the reflection from the skin was 20 dB below 0·01 Wcm^{-2}, and the weakest reflection from within the patient was a further 50 dB down, then the holographic information would consist of a signal of 10^{-4} Wcm^{-2}, varying by a minimum of 10^{-9} Wcm^{-2}. This would correspond to a variation of 1 part in 10^5, and its detection would almost certainly be impossible in the presence of other variations such as those due to movement of the patient. A variation of 1 part in 10^3 might be detectable, but this would correspond to a dynamic range of only 30 dB.

The problem of glare cannot be eliminated by the use of swept gain, such as is used in pulse-echo techniques to compress the dynamic range. This is because the holographic process is based on the propagation of what are essentially continuous waves.

Progress in the development of ultrasonic holography has been extremely rapid. The feasibility of the method in medical applications has been demonstrated by Greguss (1968), who has generated ultrasonic holograms of the eye; but he has not yet found a satisfactory method for reconstructing the image. Thus, although new techniques will first have to be devised, it seems reasonable to expect that ultrasonic holography will eventually be improved so that it has at least a limited application in medical diagnosis.

7. THE POSSIBILITY OF HAZARD IN ULTRASONIC DIAGNOSIS

7.1 INTRODUCTION

Ultrasonic diagnosis involves the exposure of the patient to ultrasonic radiation. Ultrasonic radiation affects biological systems, and so ultrasonic diagnosis is a potentially hazardous technique. The likelihood that an undesirable effect will result from an ultrasonic diagnostic investigation depends upon a large number of factors. In order to assess the possibility of such a hazard in any particular situation, it is necessary to consider both the parameters of the ultrasonic field and the nature of its interactions with the biological system.

7.2 ULTRASONIC FIELD PARAMETERS

It is a simple matter to calculate the parameters of a plane wave ultrasonic field in a homogeneous lossless medium. The various relationships are given in Equations 1.1, 1.2, 1.3, 1.9, 1.10, 1.11, 1.14, 1.17 and 1.34. Values which correspond to an intensity of 1 Wcm^{-2} at a frequency of 1 MHz in water are given in Table 7.1. The Table also shows the dependence of each parameter on the intensity and the frequency.

TABLE 7.1

Field parameters for plane waves in water. Values for 1 Wcm^{-2} at 1 MHz.

Parameter	Value	Dependence
Propagation velocity	1500 m sec^{-1}	
Wavelength	0·15 cm	$(frequency)^{-1}$
Peak particle displacement	0·018 μ	$(intensity)^{1/2}$, $(frequency)^{-1}$
Peak particle acceleration	71,000 gravity	$(intensity)^{1/2}$, $(frequency)$
Peak particle velocity	12 cm sec^{-1}	$(intensity)^{1/2}$
Peak particle pressure	1·8 atmosphere	$(intensity)^{1/2}$
Radiation pressure (complete absorption)	0·069 g cm^{-2}	$(intensity)$
Heat equivalent	0·24 cal sec^{-1} cm^{-2}	$(intensity)$

Soft tissues are quasi-liquids which in many respects resemble water. However, an important difference is the striking contrast in absorption (see Section 1.16). For example, at a frequency of 1 MHz, the absorption coefficients differ by a factor of about 500. In the consideration of ultrasonic fields in water at frequencies in the order of a few megahertz, the absorption may usually be neglected without introducing any serious error. This is not the case in soft tissues, in which absorption not only reduces the amplitudes of the field parameters as the distance from the source increases, but also results in a local heating effect.

Both pulsed and continuous wave fields are used in ultrasonic diagnosis, according to the particular application. The calculation of the field parameters in the case of a pulsed field requires a knowledge of the pulse shape. In a typical pulse-echo diagnostic procedure (McCarthy $et\ al.$ 1967), the maximum mean ultrasonic power is about 100 μW. Allowing for the intensity distribution of the beam, the maximum intensity is about 500 μWcm^{-2}. Taking account of the pulse repetition frequency and the pulse shape, the maximum instantaneous pulse intensity is in the order of 5 Wcm^{-2}. The highest estimate of pulse intensity in a diagnostic procedure seems to be that of Edler (1961), who calculated a value of 80 Wcm^{-2}.

7.3 INTERACTIONS OF ULTRASONIC WAVES WITH BIOLOGICAL TISSUES

7.3.a Mechanisms

The mechanisms of the various biological effects of ultrasound are still, to some extent, the subject of speculation. Three biophysical effects seem to occur when ultrasonic waves interact with biological tissues. These are—

(i) Thermal effects

The heat produced when ultrasound is absorbed may lead to an increase in temperature to a level at which irreversible tissue damage occurs. The damaging effects of heat on biological systems have not yet been systematically investigated. However, it seems likely that many human tissues are irreversibly damaged by heating to temperatures in excess of about 50°C.

(ii) Cavitational effects

The term "cavitation" is used to describe the situation which exists when gas-filled cavities occur in the ultrasonic field. Stable cavitation is associated with vibration amplitude magnification around stable microbubbles: the bubbles act as resilient cavities which resonate at the ultrasonic frequency, allowing neighbouring liquid particles to vibrate with increased amplitude. Unstable cavitation occurs when the pressure variations in the ultrasonic field are of such large amplitude that unstable cavities grow during the negative pressure changes, but collapse completely during the compression phase.

Stable cavitation is accompanied by small-scale circulation, or micro-eddying (Nyborg, 1965). Such streaming can damage biological systems (Nyborg and Dyer, 1960). The investigations of this phenomenon have been made using rather low ultrasonic frequencies (around 20 kHz), and the magnitudes of the corresponding effects at megahertz frequencies are uncertain.

Unstable cavitation does not occur unless the intensity exceeds a threshold value. Data quoted by Hueter and Bolt (1955), p. 230, indicate that the threshold level in water is about $300 \mathrm{Wcm}^{-2}$ at 1 MHz, and that the threshold increases with increasing frequency. The threshold level in soft tissues is presumably higher than that in water at the same frequency. Therefore, it is unlikely that unstable cavitation is a significant factor contributing hazard in diagnostic ultrasonic techniques.

Hill (1968) has pointed out that cavitation, particularly in the stable form, is a resonance phenomenon, and may not occur with very short ultrasonic pulses.

(iii) "Direct" effects

Hill (1968) considered that certain biological effects which have been reported in the literature cannot be explained in terms of either thermal or cavitational mechanisms. He proposed the term "direct" to indicate ignorance of the nature of any possible intermediate steps between the vibration of the ultrasonic field and the observed biological response.

7.3.b Biological Effects

There is no end to the speculation which is possible concerning the biological effects of the mechanisms discussed in Section 7.3.a. In the consideration of possible hazards, the biological effect is of more importance than the mechanism by which it occurs. Unfortunately, adequately detailed experimental results are not commonly found in the literature. There are three reasons for this deficiency. Firstly, it is difficult to devise experiments in which every important quantity is properly controlled and recorded. Secondly, it is only recently that the importance of defining and measuring the ultrasonic field has been realized. Thirdly, adequate methods for defining and recording the ultrasonic field have only recently been developed.

A study of the literature does reveal some data on the relationship between the ultrasonic conditions and their biological effects. In particular, it is instructive to consider the relationship between the ultrasonic intensity and the biological effect. Table 7.2 is designed to facilitate such a comparison. The data in this Table are not comprehensive, but they have been

TABLE 7.2

Results of some experiments in which biological effects are related to ultrasonic intensity

Intensity, Wcm^{-2}	Frequency, MHz	Duration of irradiation, min	Biological effect investigated	Result	Reference
<1050	2·7	~0·1	Brain damage	+	Basauri and Lele (1962)
1000	1	0·5	Permeability changes in frog moscle	+	Hughes et al. (1963)
~400	0·6–2·7	~0·1	Nerve block	+	Lele (1963)
7–120	1–3	~0·3	Changes in nervous conduction	+	Takagi et al. (1960)
60	1	~0·5	Non-thermal damage in liver	+	Curtis (1965)
30–40	1	<0·7	Nerve block	+	Fry et al. (1950)
30	1	<8	DNA degradation	+	Hawley et al. (1963)
~25	3	2	Non-thermal damage in *Daphnia*	+	Wells (1968)
20	3	10	Permeability changes in inner ear	+	James et al. (1963)
~10	0·3	1–2	Mortality in *Spirogyra*	+	Wood and Loomis (1927)
0·4–4	0·8	0·1–20	Developmental abnormalities in *Drosophila*	+	Fritz-Niggli and Böni (1950)
~2	0·8	<10	Nerve block	+	Herrick (1953)
<1·5	1–3	~10	Damage in physiotherapy	–	Patrick (1966)
0·1–1	3·6	~5	Tissue regeneration rate	+	Pond and Dyson (1967)
~0·05	15	15–30	Brain damage	–	French et al. (1951)
~0·01	2·25	~20	Genetic and other damage in mice	–	Smyth (1966)
~0·005	~2	?	Developmental abnormalities in rabbit	–	Holmes and Howry (1963)
~0·0015	2·5	60	Brain damage in young kittens	–	Donald et al. (1958)
~0·0015	~2	1440	Developmental abnormalities in frog and perch	–	Andrew (1964)
~0·001	2	30–90	Brain damage	–	Garg and Taylor (1967)

chosen to cover a wide range of intensities within the range of frequencies of importance in medical diagnosis. The biological changes for which the different investigators were searching are certainly rather varied: but one conclusion at least is quite clear. Biological effects have been observed at intensities above $0{\cdot}1$ Wcm^{-2}, but not at intensities below $0{\cdot}1$ Wcm^{-2}. In many of the experiments in which no effect was observed, the irradiation was carried out using pulses of ultrasound from pulse-echo systems designed for diagnostic applications.

Two factors tend to reduce the risk of biological damage in ultrasonic diagnosis. Firstly, the absorption of the tissues being examined reduces the intensity which reaches the deeper structures. Secondly, in scanning, any particular volume of tissue is irradiated only for a relatively short time.

7.4 CONCLUSIONS

There is not sufficient evidence available at the present time to be able to state that the ultrasonic intensities currently used in diagnosis are safe. However, it seems rather unlikely that any hazard does exist. There is a remote possibility that genetic damage may occur: the results of no experiment sensitive enough for the detection of such damage have yet been reported.

Until the safety of ultrasonic techniques has been established, the continued use of the method is justified not only by the value of the diagnostic data which it supplies, but also by the frequent reports in the literature that the technique seems to be free from hazard. Such reports, which individually have little significance, combine to represent an informed body of opinion which cannot be neglected. However, until safety levels have been defined, it is undesirable either to use greater ultrasonic intensities than those which are currently being employed, or to subject patients (particularly pregnant women and young children) to unnecessarily lengthy investigations.

REFERENCES

1.1 Wave motion

1.2 Velocity of propagation

Greenspan, M. and Tschiegg, C. E. (1959). Tables of the speed of sound in water, *J. acoust. Soc. Am.*, **31**, 75–76.

Kaye, G. W. C. and Laby, T. H. (1959). "Tables of Physical and Chemical Constants" 12th edn. Longmans, Green and Co. Ltd., London.

Wood, A. B. (1932). "A Textbook of Sound", G. Bell and Sons Ltd., London.

1.3 Wavelength and frequency

1.4 Velocity in biological materials

Begui, Z. E. (1954). Acoustic properties of the refractive media of the eye, *J. acoust. Soc. Am.*, **26**, 365–368.

Frucht, A. H. (1953). Die schallgeschwindigkeit in menschlichen und tierischen geweben, *Z. ges. exp. Med.*, **120**, 526–557.

Goldman, D. E. and Richards, J. R. (1954). Measurement of high-frequency sound velocity in mammalian soft tissues, *J. acoust. Soc. Am.*, **26**, 981–983.

Ludwig, G. D. (1950). The velocity of sound through tissues and the acoustic impedance of tissues, *J. acoust. Soc. Am.*, **22**, 862–866.

Theisman, H. and Pfander, F. (1949). Uber die durchlässigkeit des knochens für ultraschall, *Strahlentherapie*, **80**, 607–610.

Urick, R. J. (1947). A sound velocity method for determining the compressibility of finely divided substances. *J. appl. Phys.*, **18**, 983–987.

Wells, P. N. T. (1966a). Ultrasonics in clinical diagnosis, pp. 38–53. *In* "Scientific Basis of Medicine—Annual Reviews", The Athlone Press, London.

1.5 Intensity and the decibel notation

1.6 Particle pressure

Blitz, J. (1963). "Fundamentals of Ultrasonics", Butterworths, London.

1.7 Characteristic impedance

Kossoff, G. (1966). The effects of backing and matching on the performance of piezoelectric ceramic transducers, *I.E.E.E. Trans. Sonics Ultrason.*, **SU-13**, 20–30.

Ludwig, G. D. (1950). The velocity of sound through tissues and acoustic impedance of tissues, *J. acoust. Soc. Am.*, **22**, 862–866.

1.8 Reflection and refraction at plane surfaces

1.9 Reflection at rough interfaces and small obstacles

LaCasce, E. O. (1961). Some notes on the reflection of sound from a rigid corrugated surface, *J. acoust. Soc. Am.*, **33**, 1772–1777.

Rayleigh, J. W. Strutt, 3rd Baron (1878): "The Theory of Sound", Macmillan, London.

Tamarkin, P. (1949). Scattering of an underwater ultrasonic beam from liquid cylindrical obstacles, *J. acoust. Soc. Am.*, **21**, 612–616.

1.10 Standing waves

1.11 Transmission through layers

Kinsler, L. E. and Frey, P. (1962). "Fundamentals of Acoustics", 2nd edn. John Wiley and Sons Inc., New York.

1.12 The Doppler effect

Stephens, R. W. B. and Bate, A. E. (1950). "Wave Motion and Sound", Arnold, London.

1.13 Radiation pressure

Blitz, J. (1963). "Fundamentals of Ultrasonics", Butterworths, London.

Borgnis, F. E. (1953). Acoustic radiation pressure of plane compressional waves, *Rev. mod. Phys.*, **25**, 653–664.

Hueter, T. F. and Bolt, R. H. (1955). "Sonics", John Wiley and Sons Inc., New York.

Seegall, M. I. (1961). Acoustic radiation pressure bearing, *J. acoust. Soc. Am.*, **33**, 566–574.

Stephens, R. W. B. and Bate, A. E. (1950). "Wave Motion and Sound", Arnold, London.

Wood, A. B. (1932). "A Textbook of Sound", G. Bell and Sons Ltd., London.

1.14 Non-planar waves

1.15 Attenuation mechanisms

Hueter, T. F. and Bolt, R. H. (1955). "Sonics", John Wiley and Sons Inc., New York.

Kaye, G. W. C. and Laby, T. H. (1959). "Tables of Physical and Chemical Constants", 12th edn. Longmans, Green and Co. Ltd., London.

Kossoff, G. (1966). The effects of backing and matching on the performance of piezoelectric ceramic transducers, *I.E.E.E. Trans. Sonics Ultrason.*, **SU-13**, 20–30.

Litovitz, T. A. (1959). Ultrasonic spectroscopy in liquids, *J. acoust. Soc. Am.*, **31**, 681–691.

1.16 Absorption in biological materials

Begui, Z. E. (1954). Acoustic properties of the refractive media of the eye, *J. acoust. Soc. Am.*, **26**, 365–368

Carstensen, E. L., Li, K. and Schwann, H. P. (1953). Determination of the acoustic properties of blood and its components, *J. acoust. Soc. Am.*, **25**, 286–289.

Carstensen, E. L. and Schwann, H. P. (1959a). Absorption of sound arising from the presence of intact cells in blood, *J. acoust. Soc. Am.*, **31**, 185–189.

Carstensen, E. L. and Schwann, H. P. (1959b). Acoustic properties of hemoglobin solutions, *J. acoust. Soc. Am.*, **31**, 305–311.

Colombati, S. and Petralia, S. (1950). Assorbimento di ultrasuoni in tessuti animali, *Ricerca scient.*, **20**, 71–78.

Dunn, F. (1962). Temperature and amplitude dependence of acoustic absorption in tissue, *J. acoust. Soc. Am.*, **34**, 1545–1547.

Dunn, F. (1965). Ultrasonic absorption by biological materials, pp. 51–65. *In* "Ultrasonic Energy" (ed. E. Kelly), University of Illinois Press, Urbana.

Dunn, F. and Fry, W. J. (1961). Ultrasonic absorption and reflection by lung tissue, *Physics Med. Biol.*, **5**, 401–410.

Esche, R. (1952). Untersuchungen zur ultraschallabsorption in tierischen geweben und kuntstoffen, *Akust. Beih.*, **2**, 71–74.

Filipčzynski, L., Etienne, J., Lypacewicz, G. and Salkowski, J. (1967). Visualising internal structures of the eye by means of ultrasonics, *Proc. Vibr. Probl.*, **4**, 357–368.

Fry, W. J. (1952). Mechanism of acoustic absorption in tissue, *J. acoust. Soc. Am.*, **24**, 412–415.

Fry, W. J. and Dunn, F. (1962). Ultrasound: analysis and experimental methods in biological research, pp. 261–394. *In* "Physical Techniques in Biological Research", Vol. 4 (ed. W. L. Nastuk), Academic Press, London.

Goldman, D. E. and Hueter, T. F. (1956). Tabular data of the velocity and absorption of high-frequency sound in mammalian tissues, *J. acoust. Soc. Am.*, **28**, 35–37.

Goldman, D. E. and Hueter, T. F. (1957). Tabular data of the velocity and absorption of high-frequency sound in mammalian tissues—errata, *J. acoust. Soc. Am.*, **29**, 655.

Hueter, T. F. (1948). Messung der ultraschallabsorption in tierischen geweben und ihre abhängigkeit von der frequenz, *Naturwissenschaften*, **35**, 285–286.

Hueter, T. F. (1952). Messung der ultraschallabsorption im menschlichen schädelknochen und ihre abhängigkeit von der frequenz *Naturwissenschaften*, **39**, 21–22.

Hueter, T. F. and Bolt, R. H. (1951). An ultrasonic method for outlining the cerebral ventricles, *J. acoust. Soc. Am.*, **23**, 160–167.

Kossoff, G. (1966). The effects of backing and matching on the performance of piezoelectric ceramic transducers, *I.E.E.E. Trans. Sonics Ultrason.*, **SU-13**, 20–30.

Pohlman, R. (1939). Über die absorption des ultraschalls im menschlichen gewebe und ihre abhängigkeit von der frequenz, *Phys. Z.*, **40**, 159–161.

1.17 Non-linear effects with waves of finite amplitude

Dunn, F. (1962). Temperature and amplitude dependence of acoustic absorption in tissue, *J. acoust. Soc. Am.*, **34**, 1545–1547.

Fox, F. E. (1950). Dependence of ultrasonic absorption on intensity and the phenomenon of cavitation, *Nuovo cim.*, **7**, ser. ix, suppl. 2, 198–203.

Fox, F. E. and Wallace, W. A. (1954). Absorption of finite amplitude sound waves, *J. acoust. Soc. Am.*, **26**, 994–1006.

Ryan, R. P., Lutsch, A. G. and Beyer, R. T. (1962). Measurement of the distortion of finite ultrasonic waves in liquids by a pulse method, *J. acoust. Soc. Am.*, **34**, 31–35.

Zarembo, L. K. and Krasil'nikov, V. A. (1959). Some problems in the propagation of ultrasonic waves of finite amplitude in liquids, *Soviet Phys. Usp.*, **2**, 580–599.

2.1 Piezoelectricity

Berlincourt, D. A., Cmolik, C. and Jaffe, H. (1960). Piezoelectric properties of polycrystalline lead titanate zirconate compositions, *Proc. I.R.E.* **48**, 220–229.

Berlincourt, D., Jaffe, B., Jaffe, H. and Krueger, H. H. A. (1960). Transducer properties of lead titanate zirconate ceramics, *I.R.E. Trans. Ultrason. Engng.*, **UE-7**, 1–6.

Brown, C. S., Kell, R. C., Taylor, R. and Thomas, L. A. (1962). Piezo-electric materials, *Proc. I.E.E.*, **109** (pt. B), 99–114.

Crawford, A. E. (1961). Lead zirconate-titanate piezoelectric ceramics, *Br. J. appl. Phys.*, **12**, 529–534.

Jaffe, B., Roth, R. S. and Marzullo, S. (1955). Properties of piezoelectric ceramics in solid-solution series lead titanate-lead zirconate-lead oxide: tin oxide and lead titanate-lead hafnate, *J. Res. natn. Bur. Stand.*, **55**, 239–254.

2.2 Piezoelectric constants

Mason, W. P. (1950). "Piezoelectric Crystals and their Application to Ultrasonics", Van Nostrand, Princetown, New Jersey, U.S.A.

2.2.a Piezoelectric coefficients

2.2.b Dielectric constant

2.2.c Electromechanical coupling coefficient

2.3 Piezoelectric transducers for ultrasonic diagnosis

Bechman, R. (1958). Elastic and piezoelectric constants of alpha-quartz, *Phys. Rev,.* 2, **110**, 1060–1061.

Cady, W. G. (1946), "Piezoelectricity", McGraw-Hill Book Co. Inc., New York.

Crawford, A. E. (1961). Lead zirconate-titanate piezoelectric ceramics, *Br. J. appl. Phys.*, **12**, 529–534.

Mason, W. P. (1950). "Piezoelectric crystals and their application to ultrasonics", Van Nostrand, Princetown, N. J.

Walker, D. C. B. and Lumb, R. F. (1964). Piezoelectric probes for immersion ultrasonic testing, *Appl. mater. Res.*, **3**, 176–183.

2.4 Resonance

2.5 Q-factor

Blitz, J. (1963). "Fundamentals of Ultrasonics", Butterworths, London.

Hueter, T. F. and Bolt, R. H. (1955). "Sonics", John Wiley and Sons Inc., New York.

Millman, J. and Taub, H. (1956). "Pulse and Digital Circuits", McGraw-Hill Book Co. Inc., New York.

2.6 Short pulses

2.6.a Basic principles

Carome, E. F., Parks, P. E. and Mraz, S. J. (1964). Propagation of acoustic transients in water, *J. acoust. Soc. Am.*, **36**, 946–952.

Cook, E. G. (1956). Transient and steady-state response of ultrasonic piezo-electric transducers, *I.R.E. Conv. Rec.*, **4**, pt. 9, 61–69.

Jacobsen, E. H. (1960). Sources of sound in piezoelectric crystals, *J. acoust. Soc. Am.*, **32**, 949–953.

Lutsch, A. (1962). Solid mixtures with specified impedances and high attenuation for ultrasonic waves, *J. acoust. Soc. Am.*, **34**, 131–132.

Petersen, R. G. and Rosen, M. (1967). Use of thick transducers to generate short-duration stress pulses in thin specimens, *J. acoust. Soc. Am.*, **41**, 336–345.

Ponomarev, P. V. (1957). Transients in piezoelectric resonators, *Soviet Phys. Acoust.*, **3**, 260–271.

Redwood, M. (1963). A study of waveforms in the generation and detection of short ultrasonic pulses, *Appl. mater. Res.*, **2**, 76–84.

Van der Pauw, L. J. (1966). The planar transducer—a new type of transducer for exciting longitudinal acoustic waves, *Appl. Phys. Letters*, **9**, 129–131.

Washington, A. B. G. (1961). The design of piezoelectric ultrasonic probes, *Br. J. non-destr. Test.*, **3**, 56–63.

2.6.b Detailed analysis

Beveridge, H. N. and Keith, W. W. (1952). Piezoelectric transducers for ultrasonic delay lines, *Proc. I.R.E. Aust.*, **40**, 828–835.

Cook, E. G. (1956). Transient and steady-state response of ultrasonic piezo-electric transducers, *I.R.E. Conv. Rec.*, **4**, pt. 9, 61–69.

Redwood, M. (1961). Transient performance of a piezoelectric transducer, *J. acoust. Soc. Am.*, **33**, 527–536.

Redwood, M. (1963). A study of waveforms in the generation and detection of short ultrasonic pulses, *Appl. mater. Res.*, **2**, 76–84.

Redwood, M. (1964). Experiments with the electrical analog of a piezoelectric transducer, *J. acoust. Soc. Am.*, **36**, 1872–1881.

2.7 Pulse frequency spectrum

Kolsky, H. (1956). The propagation of stress pulses in viscoelastic solids, *Phil. Mag.*, *8th. ser.*, **1**, 693–710.

Markham, M. F. (1963). Scattering of elastic stress pulses in a polycrystalline solid, *Appl. mater. Res.*, **2**, 109–114.

Merkulova, V. M. (1967). Accuracy of the pulse method for measuring the attenuation and velocity of ultrasound, *Soviet Phys. Acoust.*, **12**, 411–414.

Pellam, J. R. and Galt, J. K. (1946). Ultrasonic propagation in liquids. 1. Application of the pulse technique to velocity and absorption measurements at 15 Mc/s. *J. chem. Phys.*, **14**, 608–614.

Redwood, M. (1963). A study of waveforms in the generation and detection of short ultrasonic pulses, *Appl. mater. Res.*, **2**, 76–84.

Serabian, S. (1967). Influence of attenuation upon the frequency content of a stress wave packet in graphite. *J. acoust. Soc. Am.*, **42**, 1052–1059.

2.8 Mechanical impedance matching

Gericke, O. R. (1966). Experimental determination of ultrasonic transducer frequency response, *Mater. Eval.*, **24**, 409–411.

Kossoff, G. (1966). The effects of backing and matching on the performance of piezoelectric ceramic transducers, *I.E.E.E. Trans. Sonics Ultrason.*, **SU-13**, 20–30.

McSkimin, H. J. (1955). Transducer design for ultrasonic delay lines, *J. acoust. Soc. Am.*, **27**, 302–309.

Walker, D. C. B. and Lumb, R. F. (1964). Piezoelectric probes for immersion ultrasonic testing, *Appl. mater. Res.*, **3**, 176–183.

2.9 Electrical impedance matching

Walker, D. C. B. and Lumb, R. F. (1964). Piezoelectric probes for immersion ultrasonic testing, *Appl. mater. Res.*, **3**, 176–183.

2.10 Dynamic range

Kossoff, G., Robinson, D. E. and Garrett, W. J. (1965). Ultrasonic two dimensional visualisation techniques, *I.E.E.E. Trans. Sonics Ultrason.*, **SU-12**, 31–37.

3.1 Steady state conditions

Bradfield, G. (1960). The use of radially graded ultrasonic radiators to improve the uniformity of the near field, pp. 367–372. *In* "Proc. 2nd Int. Conf. Med. Electron" (ed. C. N. Smyth), Iliffe and Sons Ltd., London.

Carter, A. H. and Williams, A. O. (1951). A new expansion for the velocity potential of a piston source, *J. acoust. Soc. Am.*, **23**, 179–184.

Deferrari, H. A., Darby, R. A. and Andrews, F. A. (1967). Vibrational displacement and mode-shape measurement by a laser interferometer, *J. acoust. Soc. Am.*, **42**, 982–990.

Dehn, J. T. (1960). Interference patterns in the near field of a circular piston, *J. acoust. Soc. Am.*, **32**, 1692–1696.

Dye, W. D. (1932). The modes of vibration of quartz piezo-electric plates as revealed by an interferometer, *Proc. R. Soc.*, A138, 1–16.

Haselberg, K. von, and Krautkramer, J. (1959). Ein ultraschall-strahler für die werkstoffprüfung mit verbessertum nahfeld, *Acustica*, **9**, 359–364.

Hueter, T. F. and Bolt, R. H. (1955). "Sonics", John Wiley and Sons Inc., New York.

Kinsler, L. E. and Frey, P. (1962). "Fundamentals of Acoustics", 2nd edn. John Wiley and Sons Inc., New York.

Lord, A. E. (1966). Changes in velocity of an elastic pulse owing to geometrical diffraction, *J. acoust. Soc. Am.*, **40**, 163–169.

McSkimin, H. J. (1960). Empirical study of the effect of diffraction on velocity of propagation of high frequency ultrasonic waves, *J. acoust. Soc. Am.*, **32**, 1401–1404.

Papadakis, E. P. (1966). Ultrasonic diffraction loss and phase change in anisotropic materials, *J. acoust. Soc. Am.*, **40**, 863–876.

Seki, H., Granato, A. and Truell, R. (1956). Diffraction effects in the ultrasonic field of a piston source and their importance in the accurate measurement of attenuation, *J. acoust. Soc. Am.*, **28**, 230–238.

Sharaf, H. F. (1954). A non-contact micro-displacement meter, *I.R.E. Trans. Ultrason. Engng.*, **UE-1**, 14–23.

Tjaden, K. (1961). Absorption longitudinaler ultraschallwellen in aluminium bei hohen temperaturen, *Acustica*, **11**, 127–136.

Tolansky, S. (1960). "Surface Microtopography," Longmans, Green and Co. Ltd., London.

3.2 Focussing systems

Belle, T. S. (1968). Analysis of a double-mirror focussing system, *Soviet Phys. Acoust.*, **13**, 290–294.

Fox, F. E. and Griffing, V. (1949). Experimental investigation of ultrasonic intensity gain in water due to concave reflectors, *J. acoust. Soc. Am.*, **21**, 352–359.

Griffing, V. and Fox, F. E. (1949). Theory of ultrasonic intensity gain due to concave reflectors, *J. acoust. Soc. Am.*, **21**, 348–351.

Hertz, C. H. and Olofsson, S. (1965). A mirror system for ultrasonic visualisation of soft tissues, pp. 322–326. *In* "Ultrasonic Energy" (ed. E. Kelly), University of Illinois Press, Urbana.

Horton, C. W. and Naral, F. C. (1950). On the diffraction of a plane sound wave by a parabaloid of revolution, *J. acoust. Soc. Am.*, **22**, 855–856.

Kossoff, G. (1963). Design of narrow-beamwidth transducers, *J. acoust. Soc. Am.*, **35**, 905–912.

Kossoff, G., Robinson, D. E. and Garrett, W. J. (1965). Ultrasonic two dimensional visualization techniques, *I.E.E.E. Trans. Sonics Ultrason.*, **SU-12**, 31–37.

Kossoff, G., Robinson, D. E., Liu, C. N. and Garrett, W. J. (1964). Design criteria for ultrasonic visualisation systems, *Ultrasonics*, **2**, 29–38.

Olofsson, S. (1963). An ultrasonic optical mirror system, *Acustica*, **13**, 361–367.

O'Neil, H. T. (1949). Theory of focusing radiators, *J. acoust. Soc. Am.*, **21**, 516–526.

Sette, D. (1949). Ultrasonic lenses of plastic materials, *J. acoust. Soc. Am.*, **21**, 375–381.

Tarnóczy, T. (1965). Sound focussing lenses and waveguides, *Ultrasonics*, **3**, 115–127.

Thurstone, F. L. and McKinney, W. M. (1966a). Resolution enhancement in scanning tissues, *Ultrasonics*, **4**, 25–27.

Thurstone, F. L. and McKinney, W. M. (1966b). Focused transducer arrays in an ultrasonic scanning system for biologic tissue, pp. 191–194. *In* "Diagnostic Ultrasound" (ed. C. C. Grossman *et al.*), Plenum Press, New York.

Willard, G. W. (1949). Focusing ultrasonic radiators, *J. acoust. Soc. Am.*, **21**, 360–375.

3.3 Transient condition

Christie, D. G. (1962). The distribution of pressure in the sound beams from probes used with ultrasonic flaw detection, *App. mater. Res.*, **1**, 86–97.

Farn, C. L. S. and Huang, H. (1968). Transient acoustic fields generated by a body of arbitrary shape, *J. acoust. Soc. Am.*, **43**, 252–257.

Filipčzynski, L. (1956). Radiation of acoustic waves for pulse ultrasonic flaw detection purposes, pp. 29–34. *In* "Proc. 2nd Conf. Ultrason., Polish Acad. Sci., Inst. Basic Tech. Probl., Warsaw".

Kaspar'yants, A. A. (1960). Non-stationary radiation of sound by a piston, *Soviet Phys. Accoust.*, **6**, 52–56.

Kossoff, G. (1963). Design of narrow-beamwidth transducers, *J. acoust. Soc. Am.*, **35**, 905–912.

Oberhettinger, F. (1961). On transient solutions of the "baffled piston" problem, *J. Res. natn. Bur. Stand.*, **65B**, 1–6.

3.4 Methods of observation

3.4.a Schlieren method

Aldridge, E. E. (1967). A study of the ultrasonic micrometer, *I.E.E.E. Trans. Sonics Ultrason.*, **SU-14**, 89–99.

Barnes, N. F. and Bellinger, J. L. (1945). Schlieren and shadowgraph equipment for air flow analysis, *J. opt. Soc. Am.*, **35**, 497–509.

Barnes, R. S. and Burton, C. S. (1949). Visual methods of studying ultrasonic phenomena, *J. appl. Phys.*, **20**, 286–294.

Debye, R. and Sears, F. W. (1932). On the scattering of light by supersonic waves, *Proc. natn. Acad. Sci. U.S.A.*, **18**, 409–414.

Foucault, L. (1859). Mémoire sur la construction des télescopes en verre argenté, *Anns Obs. Paris*, **5**, 197–237.

Hunter, H. H., Ensminger, D., Stutz, D. E. and Ullrich, O. A. (1964). Stroboscopic schlieren system for the visual observation of pulsed ultrasonic waves, *Proc. I.E.E.E.*, **52**, 744–745.

James, J. A., Dalton, G. A., Bullen, M. A., Freundlich, H. F. and Wells, P. N. T. (1961). The effect of ultrasonics on the temporal bone, *Acta oto-lar.*, **53**, 168–181.

Lester, W. W. and Hiedemann, E. A. (1962). Optical measurement of the sound-pressure amplitude and waveform of ultrasonic pulses, *J. acoust. Soc. Am.*, **34**, 265–268.

Lucas, R. and Biquard, P. (1932). Nouvelles propriétés optiques des liquides soumis à des ondes ultrasonores, *C.r. hebd. Séanc. Acad. Sci., Paris*, **194**, 2132–2134.

Sjöberg, A., Stahle, J., Johnson, S. and Sahl, R. (1963). Treatment of Menière's Disease by ultrasonic irradiation, *Acta oto-lar.*, Suppl. **178**.

Töpler, A. (1867). Optische studien nach der methode der schlierenbeobachtung, *Annln Phys.*, **131**, 33–35.

Willard, G W (1947) Ultrasound waves made visible, *Bell Labs. Rec.*, **25**, 194–200.

3.4.b Microphones

Aveyard, S. (1962). Radiation patterns from ultrasonic probes, *Brit. J. non-destr. Test.*, **4**, 120–124.

Christie, D. G. (1962). The distribution of pressure in the sound beams from probes used with ultrasonic flaw detectors, *Appl. mater. Res.*, **1**, 86–97.

Hodgkinson, W. L. (1966). Isosonography, *Ultrasonics*, **4**, 138–142.

Hueter, T. F. and Bolt, R. H. (1955). "Sonics", John Wiley and Sons Inc., New York.

Koppelmann, J. (1952). Beiträge zur ultraschallmesstechnik in flüssigkeiten, *Acustica*, **2**, 92–95.

Mellen, R. H. (1956). An experimental study of the collapse of a spherical cavity in water, *J. acoust. Soc. Am.*, **28**, 447–454.

Romanenko, E. V. (1957). Miniature piezoelectric ultrasonic receivers, *Soviet Phys. Acoust.*, **3**, 364–370.

Saneyoshi, J., Okujima, M. and Ide, M. (1966). Wide frequency calibrated probe microphones for ultrasound in liquid, *Ultrasonics*, **4**, 64–66.

Schmitt, H. J. (1961). Ceramic capacitors as sound probes in liquids, *Rev. scient. Instrum.*, **32**, 215–217.

3.4.c Pulse-echo methods

Gordon, D. (1964). Comparison of ultrasonic pulse-echo apparatus used in medicine, *Ultrasonics*, **2**, 199–202.

Panian, F. C. and van Valkenburg, H. E. (1961). Development of ASTM standard reference blocks for ultrasonic inspection, *Non-destruct. Test.*, **19**, 45–57.

Wells, P. N. T. (1966a). Ultrasonics in clinical diagnosis, pp. 38–53. *In* "Scientific Basis of Medicine—Annual Reviews", The Athlone Press, London.

Wells, P. N. T. (1966b). Some physical limitations in ultrasonic diagnosis, *Bio-med. Engng.*, **1**, 390–394.

3.4.d Other methods

Barnes, N. F. and Bellinger, J. L. (1945). Schlieren and shadowgraph equipment for air flow analysis, *J. opt. Soc. Am.*, **35**, 497–509.

Ernst, P. J. and Hoffman, C. W. (1952). New methods of ultrasonoscopy and ultrasonography, *J. acoust. Soc. Am.*, **24**, 207–211.

Fry, W. J. and Fry, R. B. (1954a). Determination of absolute sound levels and acoustic absorption coefficients by thermocouple probes—theory, *J. acoust. Soc. Am.*, **26**, 294–310.

Fry, W. J. and Fry, R. B. (1954b). Determination of absolute sound levels and acoustic absorption coefficients by thermocouple probes—experiment, *J. acoust. Soc. Am.*, **26**, 311–317.

Gessert, W. L. and Hiedemann, E. A. (1956). Ultrasonic stroboscopes for the study of ultrasonic fields, *J. acoust. Soc. Am.*, **28**, 944–950.

Nomoto, O. (1954a). Theory of the visualization of ultrasonic waves. (I) Theory of the schlieren method for visualizing ultrasonic waves, *J. phys. Soc. Japan*, **9**, 267–278.

Nomoto, O. (1954b). Theory of the visualization of ultrasonic waves. (II) Theory of the phase-shift method for visualizing ultrasonic waves, *J. phys. Soc. Japan*, **9**, 279–286.

3.5 Power measurement

Arnold, R. T., MacKey, J. E. and Meeks, E. L. (1967). Capacitance microphone for measurement of small attenuation coefficients, *J. acoust. Soc. Am.*, **42**, 677–678.

Blitz, J. and Warren, D. G. (1968). Absolute measurements of the intensity of pulsed ultrasonic waves in solids and liquids with a capacitor microphone at megahertz frequencies, *Ultrasonics*, **6**, 235–239.

Filipćzynski, L. (1966). Measuring pulse intensity of ultrasonic longitudinal and transverse waves in solids, *Proc.Vibr. Probl.*, **7**, 31–46.

Filipćzynski, L. (1967). The absolute method for intensity measurements of liquid-borne ultrasonic pulses with the electrodynamic transducer, *Proc. Vibr. Probl.*, **8**, 21–26.

Filipćzynski, L. and Groniowski, J. T. (1967). Visualization of the inside of the abdomen by means of ultrasonics, and two methods for measuring ultrasonic doses, p. 320. *In* "Dig. 7th Int. Conf. Med. Biol. Engng., Stockholm".

Gauster, W. B. and Breazeale, M. A. (1966). Detector for measurement of ultrasonic strain amplitudes in solids, *Rev. scient. Instrum.*, **37**, 1544–1548.

Kolsky, H. (1956). The propagation of stress pulses in viscoelastic solids, *Phil. Mag.*, 8th. ser., **1**, 693–710.

Kossoff, G. (1965). Balance technique for the measurement of very low ultrasonic power outputs, *J. acoust. Soc. Am.*, **38**, 880–881.

Newell, J. A. (1963). A radiation pressure balance for absolute measurement of ultrasonic power, *Physics Med. Biol.*, **8**, 215–221.

Wells, P. N. T., Bullen, M. A., Follett, D. H., Freundlich, H. F. and James, J. A. (1963). The dosimetry of small ultrasonic beams, *Ultrasonics*, **1**, 106–110.

Wells, P. N. T., Bullen, M. A. and Freundlich, H. F. (1964). Milliwatt ultrasonic radiometry, *Ultrasonics*, **2**, 124–128.

4.1 Introduction

4.1.a Basic principles

Firestone, F. A. (1945). The supersonic reflectoscope for interior inspection, *Metal Prog.*, **48**, 505–512.

4.1.b Dynamic range, swept gain and resolution

Kossoff, G. (1966). The effects of backing and matching on the performance of piezoelectric ceramic transducers, *I.E.E.E. Trans. Sonics Ultrason.*, **SU-13**, 20–30.

Wells, P. N. T. (1966b). Some physical limitations in ultrasonic diagnosis, *Bio-med. Engng.*, **1**, 390–394.

4.1.c Interface characteristics

Wells, P. N. T. (1966a). Ultrasonics in clinical diagnosis, pp. 38–53. *In* "Scientific Basis of Medicine—Annual Reviews", The Athlone Press, London.

4.1.d Multiple reflection artifacts

Robinson, D. E., Kossoff, G. and Garrett, W. J. (1966). Artefacts in ultrasonic echoscopic visualisation, *Ultrasonics*, **4**, 186–194.

Wells, P. N. T. (1965). Resonance artifacts, *Ultrasonics*, **3**, 154.

4.1.e Ultrasonic frequency

Donald, I., MacVicar, J. and Brown, T. G. (1958). Investigation of abdominal masses by pulsed ultrasound, *Lancet*, i, 1188–1194.

4.2 Timing circuits

Davies, J. G. and Mitchell, M. (1960). Timing of injections for angiocardiography: description of an automatic device, *Clin. Radiol.*, **11**, 214–218.

Millman, J. and Taub, H. (1956). "Pulse and Digital Circuits", McGraw-Hill Book Co. Inc., New York.

4.3 The transmitter

Kossoff, G., Robinson, D. E. and Garrett, W. J. (1965). Ultrasonic two dimensional visualization techniques, *I.E.E.E. Trans. Sonics Ultrason.*, **SU-12**, 31–37.

Kossoff, G., Robinson, D. E., Liu, C. N. and Garrett, W. J. (1964). Design criteria for ultrasonic visualisation systems, *Ultrasonics*, **2**, 29–38.

Wells, P. N. T., Bullen, M. A. and Freundlich, H. F. (1964). Milliwatt ultrasonic radiometry, *Ultrasonics*, **2**, 124–128.

4.4 Radio frequency amplifiers

4.4.a General considerations

Valley, G. E. and Wallman, H. (eds.) (1948). Vacuum tube amplifiers, M.I.T. Radiation Lab. ser. no. 18, McGraw-Hill Book Co. Inc., New York.

4.4.b Linear r.f. amplifiers

Gay, M. J., Moore, A. D. and Skingley, J. A. (1967). Monolithic circuits for r.f. communications systems, pp. 258–266. *In* "Integrated Circuits", I.E.E., London.

Larsen, F. J. (1946). Ultrasonic trainer circuits, *Electronics*, **19**, 6, 126–129.

Reid, J. M. and Wild, J. J. (1952). Ultrasonic ranging for cancer diagnosis. *Electronics*, **25**, 7, 136–138.

Valley, G. E. and Wallman, H. (eds.) (1948). Vacuum tube amplifiers. M.I.T. Radiation Lab. ser. no. 18, McGraw-Hill Book Co. Inc., New York.

Wells, P. N. T. and Evans, K. T. (1968). An immersion scanner for two-dimensional ultrasonic examination of the human breast. *Ultrasonics*, **6**, 220–228.

Wood, M. D. (1964a). Gain controlled band-pass amplifiers (part 1). *Electron. Engng.*, **36**, 150–153.

Wood, M. D. (1964b). Gain controlled band-pass amplifiers (part 2). *Electron. Engng.*, **36**, 234–237.

4.4.c Electronically controlled attenuators

Bilotti, A. (1966). Operation of an MOS transistor as a variable resistor. *Proc. I.E.E.E.*, **54**, 1093–1094.

Bilotti, A. (1967). A distributed MOS attenuator. *Proc. I.E.E.E.*, **55**, 562–563.

Heller, R. E. (1963). The *pin* diode: versatile microwave component. *Electronics*, **36**, 10, 40–43.

Martin, T. B. (1962). Circuit applications of the field-effect transistor: part 2. *Semicond. Prod.*, **5**, 3, 30–38.

Morris, A. G. (1965). A constant volume amplifier covering a wide dynamic range. *Electron. Engng.*, **37**, 502–507.

Sah, C. T. (1962). Effect of surface recombination and channel on P–N junction and transistor characteristics, *I.R.E. Trans. electronic Devices*, **ED-9**, 94–108.

Sevin, L. J. (1965), "Field-Effect Transistors", Texas Instruments Electronics Series, McGraw-Hill Book Co. Inc., New York.

Shockley, W. (1950). "Electrons and Holes in Semiconductors", D. van Nostrand Inc., New York.

4.4.d Swept gain function generators

Korn, G. A. and Korn, T. M. (1956). "Electronic Analog Computers", 2nd. edn. McGraw-Hill Book Co. Inc., New York.

Sunstein, D. E. (1949). Photoelectric waveform generator, *Electronics*, **22**, 2, 100–103.

Wells, P. N. T. and Evans, K. T. (1968). An immersion scanner for two-dimensional ultrasonic examination of the human breast, *Ultrasonics*, **6**, 220–228.

4.4.e Demodulation and suppression

4.5 Video amplifiers

4.5.a General considerations

Brinker, R. A. (1966). Ultrasound brain scanning utilizing the contact method, pp. 186–190. *In* "Diagnostic Ultrasound" (ed. C. C. Grossman *et al.*), Plenum Press, New York.

Brinker, R. A. and Taveras, J. A. (1966). Ultrasound cross-sectional pictures of the head, *Acta Radiol.* (Diagnosis), **5**, 2, 745–753.

4.5.b Linear video amplifiers

Kossoff, G., Robinson, D. E. and Garrett, W. J. (1965). Ultrasonic two dimensional visualization techniques, *I.E.E.E. Trans. Sonics Ultrason.*, **SU-12**, 31–37.

Millman, J. and Taub, H. (1956). "Pulse and Digital Circuits", McGraw-Hill Book Co. Inc., New York.

Reid, J. M. and Wild, J. J. (1952). Ultrasonic ranging for cancer diagnosis, *Electronics*, **25**, 7, 136–138.

Wells, P. N. T. (1967). Signal processing in two-dimensional ultrasonography, *Bio-med. Engng.*, **2**, 165–167.

Wells, P. N. T. and Evans, K. T. (1968). An immersion scanner for two-dimensional ultrasonic examination of the human breast, *Ultrasonics*, **6**, 220–228.

4.5.c Logarithmic video amplifiers

Alcock, R. N. (1962). A wide-band transistor logarithmic amplifier at 45 Mc/s, *Electron. Engng.*, **34**, 444–449.

Alred, R. V. and Reiss, A. (1948). An anti-clutter Radar receiver, *J.I.E.E.*, **95**, pt. 3, 459–465.

Croney, J. (1951). A simple logarithmic amplifier, *Proc. I.R.E.*, **39**, 807–813.

Kossoff, G., Liu, C. N. and Robinson, D. E. (1965). A video logarithmic amplifier with quick recovery, *Electron. Engng.*, **37**, 306–310.

Lunsford, J. S. (1965). Logarithmic pulse amplifier, *Rev. scient. Instrum.*, **36**, 461–464.

Ophir, D. and Galil, U. (1961). Zener diodes create logarithmic pulse amplifier, *Electronics*, **34**, 28, 68–70.

Paterson, W. L. (1963). Multiplication and logarithmic conversion by operational amplifier-transistor circuits, *Rev. scient. Instrum.*, **34**, 1311–1316.

4.5.d First echo swept gain trigger circuits

Wells, P. N. T. and Evans, K. T. (1968). An immersion scanner for two-dimensional ultrasonic examination of the human breast, *Ultrasonics*, **6**, 220–228.

4.6 Cathode ray tube displays

4.6.a Conventional cathode ray tubes

Soller, T., Starr, M. A. and Valley, G. E. (eds.) (1948). "Cathode Ray Tube Displays", M.I.T. Radiation Lab. ser. no. 22, McGraw-Hill Book Co. Inc., New York.

4.6.b Electronic storage tubes

Anderson, R. H. (1967). A simplified direct-viewing bistable storage tube, *I.E.E.E. Trans. electronic Devices*, **ED-14**, 838–844.

Knoll, M. and Kazan, B. (1956). Viewing storage tubes, pp. 447–501. *In* "Advances in Electronics and Electron Physics", Vol. 8 (ed. L. Marton), Academic Press Inc., New York.

4.6.c Photographic recording

Land, E. H. (1947). A new one-step photographic process, *J. opt. Soc. Am.*, **37**, 61–77.

4.7 Data presentation systems and clinical applications

4.7.a The A-scope

An, S., Tao-Hsin, W., Shih-Yuan, A., Shih-Liang, C., Hsiang-Huei, W., Chih-Chang, H. and Kuo-Juei, Y. (1962). The use of pulsed ultrasound in clinical diagnosis, *Chin. med. J.*, **81**, 315–325.

Bang, J. and Holm, H. H. (1968). Ultrasonic examination by means of A-presentation and scanning in gynaecology and obstetrics, *Dan. med. Bull.*, **15**, 101–106.

Braak, J. W. G. ter, and Vlieger, M. de, (1965). Cerebral pulsations in echoencephalography, *Acta. neurochir.*, **12**, 678–694.

Brinker, R. A. (1967). Simultaneous presentation in echoencephalography, *Radiology*, **88**, 360–361.

Brinker, R. A., King, D. L. and Taveras, J. M. (1965). Echoencephalography, *Am. J. Roentg.*, **93**, 781–790.

Bronson, N. R. (1965). Techniques of ultrasonic localisation and extraction of intra- and extra-ocular foreign bodies. *Am. J. Ophthal.*, **60**, 596–603.

Buschmann, W. (1965). New equipment and transducers for ophthalmic diagnosis, *Ultrasonics*, **3**, 18–21.

Campbell, S. (1968). An improved method of foetal cephalometry by ultrasound, *J. Obstet. Gynaec. Br. Commonw.*, **75**, 568–576.

Coleman, D. J. and Carlin, B. (1967). Transducer alignment and electronic measurement of visual axis dimensions in the human eye using time-amplitude ultrasound, pp. 207–214. *In* "Ultrasonics in Ophthalmology, Symp. Münster", Karger, Basel.

Donald, I. (1968). Ultrasonics in obstetrics, *Brit. med. Bull.*, **24**, 71–75.

Freeman, M. H. (1963). Ultrasonic pulse-echo techniques in ophthalmic examination and diagnosis, *Ultrasonics*, **1**, 152–160.

Feigenbaum, H., Zaky, A. and Waldhausen, J. A. (1967). Use of reflected ultrasound in detecting pericardial effusion, *Am. J. Cardiol.*, **19**, 84–90.

Ford, R. and Ambrose, J. (1963). Echoencephalography; measurement of position of mid-line structures in skull with high frequency pulsed ultrasound, *Brain*, **86**, 189–196.

Ford, R. and McRae, D. L. (1966). Echoencephalography—a standardized technique for the measurement of the width of the third and lateral ventricles, pp. 117–129. *In* "Diagnostic Ultrasound" (ed. C. C. Grossman *et al.*), Plenum Press, New York.

French, L. A., Wild, J. J. and Neal, D. (1950). Detection of cerebral tumours by ultrasonic pulses, *Cancer, N.Y.*, **3**, 705–708.

Gordon, D. (1959). Echoencephalography: ultrasonic rays in diagnostic radiology, *Br. Med. J.*, i, 1500–1504.

Holmes, J. H. (1966a). Ultrasonic diagnosis of liver disease, pp. 249–263. *In* "Diagnostic Ultrasound" (ed. C. C. Grossman *et al.*), Plenum Press, New York.

Holmes, J. H. (1967a). Ultrasonic studies of the bladder, *J. Urol.*, **97**, 654–663.

Jansson, F. (1963). Determination of the axis length of the eye roentgenologically and by ultrasound, *Acta ophthal.*, **41**, 236–246.

Jeppsson, S. (1961). Echoencephalography IV. The mid-line-echo; an evaluation of its usefulness for diagnosing intracranial expansivities and an investigation into its sources, *Acta chir. scand.*, Suppl. 272.

Jeppsson, S. (1964). Echoencephalography V. A method for recording the intracranial pressure with the aid of the echoencephalographic technique. A preliminary report, *Acta chir. scand.*, **128**, 218–224.

Kimoto, S., Omoto, R., Tsunemoto, M., Moroi, T., Atsumi, K. and Uchida, R. (1964). Ultrasonic tomography of the liver and detection of heart atrial septal defect with the aid of ultrasonic intravenous probes, *Ultrasonics*, **2**, 82–86.

Knight, P. R. and Newell, J. A. (1963). Operative use of ultrasonics in cholelithiasis, *Lancet*, i, 1023–1025.

Kossoff, G. and Sharpe, C. J. (1966). Examination of the contents of the pulp cavity in teeth, *Ultrasonics*, **4**, 77–83.

Leary, G. A. (1967). Basic techniques for applying ultrasonics to ophthalmic measurement and diagnosis, *Ultrasonics*, **6**, 84–87.

Leksell, L. (1956). Echo-encephalography. 1. Detection of intracranial complications following brain injury, *Acta chir. scand.*, **110**, 301–315.

Lithander, B. (1960). A control method for echo-encephalography, *Acta psychiat. neurol. scand.*, **35**, 235–240.

Ludwig, J. and Struthers, F. (1950). Detecting gall-stones with ultrasonic echoes, *Electronics*, **23**, 2, 172–178.

Miller, L. D., Joyner, C. R., Dudrick, S. J. and Eskin, D. J. (1967). Clinical use of ultrasound in the early diagnosis of pulmonary embolism, *Ann. Surg.*, **166**, 381–392.

Oksala, A. (1967). Development and significance of ultrasonic diagnosis in eye diseases (review), pp. 1–21. *In* "Ultrasonics in Ophthalmology, Symp. Münster", Karger, Basel.

Ostrum, B. J., Goldberg, B. B. and Isard, H. J. (1967). A-mode ultrasound differentiation of soft tissue masses, *Radiology*, **88**, 745–749.

Pätzold, J., Güttner, W. and Bastir, R. (1951). Beitrag zum dosiproblem in der ultraschall-therapie, *Strahlentherapie*, **86**, 298–305.

Pell, R. L. (1964). Ultrasound for routine clinical investigations, *Ultrasonics*, **2**, 87–89.

Ramsden, D., Peabody, C. O. and Speight, R. G. (1967). The use of ultrasonics to investigate soft tissue thickness on the human chest, U.K.A.E.A. Reactor Group Report A.E.E.W.-R493, H.M.S.O.

Robinson, D. E. and Kossoff, G. (1966). An ultrasonic echo-encephaloscope for the examination of the human brain, *Proc. I.R.E.*, **27**, 39–44.

Segal, B. L., Likoff, W., Asperger, Z. and Kingsley, B. (1966). Ultrasound diagnosis of abdominal aortic aneurism, *Am. J. Cardiol.*, **17**, 101–103.

Schentke, K. U. and Renger, F. (1966). Über die diagnostische verwertbarkeit des ultraschallhepatograms, *Z. ges. inn. Med.*, **21**, 239–240.

Schlegal, J. V., Diggdon, P. and Cuellar, J. (1961). The use of ultrasound for localising renal calculi, *J. Urol.*, **86**, 367–369.

Sorsby, A., Leary, G. A., Richards, M. J. and Chaston, J. (1963). Ultrasonic measurement of the components of occular refraction in life, *Vision Res.*, ?, 499–505.

Thompson, H. E. (1966). Studies of fetal growth by ultrasound, pp. 416–427. *In* "Diagnostic Ultrasound" (ed. C. C. Grossman *et al.*), Plenum Press, New York.

Thompson, H. E., Holmes, J. H., Gottesfeld, K. R. and Taylor, E. S. (1965). Fetal development as determined by ultrasonic pulse echo techniques, *Am. J. Obstet. Gynec.*, **92**, 44–50.

Vlieger, M. de (1967). Evolution of echo-encephalography in neurology—a review, *Ultrasonics*, **6**, 91–97.

Wagai, T., Miyazawa, R., Ito, K. and Kikuchi, Y. (1965). Ultrasonic diagnosis of intracranial disease, breast tumours and abdominal diseases, pp. 346–360. *In* "Ultrasonic Energy" (ed. E. Kelly), University of Illinois Press, Urbana.

Wang, H. F., Wang, C. E., Chang, C. P., Kao, J. Y., Yü, L. and Chiang, Y. N. (1964). The application and value of ultrasonic diagnosis of liver abscess: a report of 218 cases, *Chin. med. J.*, **83**, 133–140.

White, D. N. (1966). Studies in ultrasonic echoencephalography VI. A critical analysis of the amplitude-averaging, A-scan technique, *Neurology*, **16**, 358–366.

White, D. N. (1967). The limitations of echo-encephalography, *Ultrasonics*, **5**, 88–90.

White, D. N. and Blanchard, J. B. (1966). Studies in echo-encephalography II. An objective technique for the A-scan presentation of the cerebral mid-line structures, *Acta Radiol.* (Diagnosis), **5**, 936–952.

Wild, J. J. (1950). The use of ultrasonic pulses for the measurement of biologic tissues and the detection of tissue density changes, *Surgery, St. Louis*, **27**, 183–188.

Wild, J. J. and Reid, J. M. (1952b). Further pilot echographic studies on the histologic structure of the living intact human breast, *Am. J. Path.*, **28**, 839–861.

Willocks, J., Donald, I., Duggan, T. C. and Day, N. J. (1964). Foetal cephalometry by ultrasound, *J. Obstet. Gynaec. Br. Commonw.*, **71**, 11–20.

4.7.b The B-scope

4.7.c The two-dimensional scanned B-scope

Baum, G. and Greenwood, I. (1958). The application of ultrasonic locating techniques to ophthalmology, *A.M.A. Archs. Ophthal.*, **60**, 263–279.

Brown, T. G. (1960). Direct contact ultrasonic scanning techniques for the visualization of abdominal masses, pp. 358–366. *In* "Proc. 2nd Int. Conf. Med. Electron" (ed. C. N. Smyth), Illiffe and Sons Ltd., London.

Donald, I. and Brown, T. G. (1961). Demonstration of tissue interfaces within the body by ultrasonic echo sounding, *Br. J. Radiol.*, **34**, 539–546.

Evans, G. C., Lehman, J. S., Brady, L. W., Smyth, M. G. and Hart, D. J. (1966). Ultrasonic scanning of abdominal and pelvic organs using the B-scan display, pp. 369–415. *In* "Diagnostic ultrasound" (ed. C. C. Grossman *et al.*), Plenum Press, New York.

Filipćzynski, L., Etienne, J., Lypacewicz, G. and Salkowski, J. (1967). Visualising internal structures of the eye by means of ultrasonics, *Proc. Vibr. Probl.*, **4**, 357–368.

Filipćzynski, L. and Groniowski, J. T. (1967). Visualization of the inside of the abdomen by means of ultrasonics, and two methods for measuring ultrasonic doses, p. 320. *In* "Dig. 7th. Int. Conf. Med. Biol. Engng., Stockholm".

Fleming, J. E. and Hall, A. J. (1968). Two dimensional compound scanning—effects of maladjustment and calibration, *Ultrasonics*, **6**, 160–166.

Gordon, D. (1962). An ultrasonic tomograph for medical diagnosis, *Proc. San Diego Symp. Biomed. Engng.*, **2**, 20–22.

Greatorex, C. A. and Ireland, H. J. D. (1964). An experimental scanner for use with ultrasound, *Br. J. Radiol.*, **37**, 179–184.

Hertz, C. H. and Olofsson, S. (1963). A mirror system for ultrasonic visualization of soft tissues, pp. 322–326. *In* "Ultrasonic energy" (ed. E. Kelly), University of Illinois Press, Urbana.

Holm, H. H. and Northeved, A. (1968). An ultrasonic scanning apparatus for use in medical diagnosis, *Acta. chir. scand.*, **134**, 177–181.

Holmes, J. H., Wright, W., Meyer, E. P., Posakony, G. J. and Howry, D. H. (1965). Ultrasonic contact scanner for diagnostic applications, *Am. J. med. Electron.*, **4**, 147–152.

Howry, D. H. (1955). Techniques used in ultrasonic visualization of soft tissue structures of the body, *I.R.E. Conv. Rec.*, pt. 9, 75–81.

Howry, D. H. (1957). Techniques used in ultrasonic visualization of soft tissues, pp. 49–63. *In* "Ultrasound in Biology and Medicine" (ed. E. Kelly), A.I.B.S., Washington.

Howry, D. H. (1965). A brief atlas of diagnostic ultrasonic radiologic results, *Radiol. Clin. N. Am.*, **3**, 433–452.

Howry, D. H. and Bliss, W. R. (1952). Ultrasonic visualization of soft tissue structures of the body, *J. Lab. clin. Med.*, **40**, 579–592.

Kikuchi, Y., Uchida, R., Tanaka, K. and Wagai, T. (1957). Early cancer diagnosis through ultrasonics, *J. acoust. Soc. Am.*, **29**, 824–833.

Kimoto, S., Omoto, R., Tsunemoto, M., Moroi, T., Atsumi, K. and Uchida, R. (1964). Ultrasonic tomography of the liver and detection of heart atrial septal defect with the aid of ultrasonic intravenous probe, *Ultrasonics*, **2**, 82–86.

Kossoff, G. (1966). The effects of backing and matching on the performance of piezoelectric ceramic transducers, *I.E.E.E. Trans. Sonics Ultrason.*, **SU-13**, 20–30.

Kossoff, G., Garrett, W. J. and Robinson, D. E. (1965). An ultrasonic echoscope for visualizing the pregnant uterus, pp. 365–376. *In* "Ultrasonic Energy" (ed. E. Kelly), University of Illinois Press, Urbana.

Kossoff, G., Robinson, D. E. and Garrett, W. J. (1965). Ultrasonic two dimensional visualization techniques, *I.E.E.E. Trans. Sonics Ultrason.*, **SU-12**, 31–37.

Kossoff, G., Robinson, D. E., Liu, C. N. and Garrett, W. J. (1964). Design criteria for ultrasonic visualization systems, *Ultrasonics*, **2**, 29–38.

Krause, W. E. E. and Soldner, R. E. (1967). Ultrasonic imaging technique (B-scan) with high image rate for medical diagnosis—principle and technique of method, p. 315. *In* "Dig. 7th Int. Conf. Med. & Biol. Engng., Stockholm".

Makow, D. M. and Real, R. R. (1966). Development of a 360° compound immersion head scanner, pp. 166–185. *In* "Diagnostic Ultrasound" (ed. C. C. Grossman *et al.*), Plenum Press, New York.

Somer, J. C. (1968). Electronic sector scanning for ultrasonic diagnosis, *Ultrasonics*, **6**, 153–159.

Vlieger, M. de, Sterke, A. de, Molin, C. E. and Ven, C. van der, (1963). Ultrasound for two-dimensional echoencephalography, *Ultrasonics*, **1**, 148–151.

Wells, P. N. T. (1966c). Developments in medical ultrasonics, *Wld. med. Electron.*, **4**, 272–277.

Wells, P. N. T. and Evans, K. T. (1968). An immersion scanner for two-dimensional ultrasonic examination of the human breast, *Ultrasonics*, **6**, 220–228.

Wild, J. J. and Reid, J. M. (1952a). Application of echo-ranging techniques to the determination of structure of biological tissues, *Science, N.Y.*, **115**, 226–230.

Wild, J. J. and Reid, J. M. (1952b). Further pilot echographic studies on the histologic structure of the living intact human breast, *Am. J. Path.*, **28**, 839–861.

Wild, J. J. and Reid, J. M. (1954). Echographic visualization of lesions of the living intact human breast, *Cancer Res.*, **14**, 277–283.

4.7.d Clinical application of the two-dimensional scanned B-scope

Åsberg, A. (1967). Ultrasonic cinématography of the living heart, *Ultrasonics*, **5**, 113–117.

Bang, J. and Holm, H. H. (1968). Ultrasonic examination by means of A-presentation and scanning in gynaecology and obstetrics, *Dan. med. Bull.*, **15**, 101–106.

Baum, G. and Greenwood, I. (1965). Current status of ophthalmic ultrasonography, pp. 260–275. *In* "Ultrasonic Energy" (ed. E. Kelly), University of Illinois Press, Urbana.

Brinker, R. A. and Taveras, J. M. (1966). Ultrasound cross-sectional pictures of the head, *Acta Radiol.* (Diagnosis), **5**, pt. 2, 745–753.

Brown, T. G. (1960). Direct contact scanning techniques for the visualization of abdominal masses, pp. 358–366. *In* "Proc. 2nd Int. Conf. Med. Electron" (ed. C. N. Smyth), Illiffe and Sons Ltd., London.

Damascelli, B., Lattuada, A., Musumeci, R. and Severini, A. (1968). Two-dimensional ultrasonic investigations of the urinary tract, *Br. J. Radiol.*, **41**, 837–843.

Donald, I. (1963). Use of ultrasonics in diagnosis of abdominal swellings, *Br. med. J.*, **2**, 1154–1155.

Donald, I. (1968). Ultrasonics in obstetrics, *Br. med. Bull.*, **24**, 71–75.

Donald, I and Abdulla, U (1967). Ultrasonics in obstetrics and gynaecology, *Br. J. Radiol.*, **40**, 604–611.

Donald, I. and Brown, T. G. (1961). Demonstration of tissue interfaces within the body by ultrasonic echo sounding, *Br. J. Radiol.*, **34**, 539–546.

Fujimoto, Y., Oka, A., Omoto, R. and Hirose, M. (1967). Ultrasound scanning of the thyroid gland as a new diagnostic approach, *Ultrasonics*, **5**, 177–180.

Gottesfeld, K. R. (1966). The practical applications of ultrasound in obstetrics and gynaecology, pp. 428–451. *In* "Diagnostic Ultrasound" (ed. C. C. Grossman *et al.*), Plenum Press, New York.

Gottesfeld, M. D., Thompson, H. E., Holmes, J. H. and Taylor, E. S. (1966). Ultrasonic placentography—a new method for placental localization, *Am. J. Obstet. Gynec.*, **96**, 538–547.

Grossman, C. C. (1965). Acoustic phenomena in ultrasonic detection of brain tumours, *Ultrasonics*, **3**, 22–24.

Hayashi, S., Wagai, T., Miyazawa, R., Ito, K., Ishikawa, S., Uematsu, K., Kikuchi, Y. and Uchida, R. (1962). Ultrasonic diagnosis of breast tumour and cholelithiasis, *West. J. Surg. Obstet. Gynec.*, **70**, 34–40.

Holmes, J. H. (1966a). Ultrasonic diagnosis of liver disease, pp. 249–263. *In* "Diagnostic Ultrasound" (ed. C. C. Grossman *et al.*), Plenum Press, New York.

Holmes, J. H. (1966b). Ultrasonic studies of the bladder and kidney, pp. 465–480. *In* "Diagnostic Ultrasound" (ed. C. C. Grossman *et al.*), Plenum Press, New York.

Howry, D. H. (1955). Techniques used in ultrasonic visualization of soft tissue structures of the body, *I.R.E. Conv. Rec.*, pt. 9, 75–81.

Howry, D. H. (1957). Techniques used in ultrasonic visualization of soft tissues, pp. 49–63. *In* "Ultrasound in Biology and Medicine" (ed. E. Kelly), A.I.B.S. Washington.

Howry, D. H. (1965). A brief atlas of diagnostic ultrasonic radiologic results, *Radiol. Clin. N. Am.*, **3**, 433–452.

Howry, D. H. and Bliss, W. R. (1952). Ultrasonic visualization of soft tissue structures of the body, *J. Lab. clin. Med.* **40**, 579–592.

Kimoto, J., Omoto, R., Tsunemoto, M., Moroi, T., Atsumi, K. and Uchida, R. (1964). Ultrasonic tomography of the liver and detection of heart atrial septal defect with the aid of ultrasonic intravenous probes, *Ultrasonics*, **2**, 82–86.

Kossoff, G., Robinson, D. H. and Garrett, W. J. (1966). Two dimensional ultrasonography in obstetrics, pp. 333–347. *In* "Diagnostic Ultrasound" (ed. C. C. Grossman *et al.*), Plenum Press, New York.

Krause, W. E. E. and Soldner, R. E. (1967). Ultrasonic imaging technique (B-scan) with high image rate for medical diagnosis—principle and technique of method, p. 315. *In* "Dig. 7th Int. Conf. Med. Biol. Engng., Stockholm".

Lehman, J. S., Evans, G. C. and Brady, L. W. (1966). Ultrasound exploration of the spleen, pp. 264–295. *In* "Diagnostic Ultrasound" (ed. C. C. Grossman *et al.*), Plenum Press, New York.

MacVicar, J. and Donald, I. (1963). Sonar in the diagnosis of early pregnancy and its complications, *J. Obstet. Gynaec. Br. Commonw.*, **70**, 387–395.

Makow, D. M. and McRae, D. L. (1967). Horizontal scanning of the head with ultrasound, *Med. Biol. Engng.*, **5**, 33–39.

McCarthy, C. F., Read, A. E. A., Ross, F. G. M. and Wells, P. N. T. (1967). Ultrasonic scanning of the liver, *Quart. J. Med.*, **36**, 517–524.

Micsky, L. I. von (1966). Ultrasonic tomography in obstetrics and gynecology, pp. 348–368. *In* "Diagnostic ultrasound" (ed. C. C. Grossman *et al.*), Plenum Press, New York.

Sundén, B. (1964). On the diagnostic value of ultrasound in obstetrics and gynecology, *Acta obstet. gynec. scand.*, **43**, Suppl. 6.

Vlieger, M. de, Sterke, A. de, Molin, C. E. and Ven, C. van der (1963). Ultrasound for two-dimensional echoencephalography, *Ultrasonics*, **1**, 148–151.

Wagai, T., Miyazawa, R., Ito, K. and Kikuchi, Y. (1965). Ultrasonic diagnosis of intracranial disease, breast tumours and abdominal diseases, pp. 346–360. *In* "Ultrasonic Energy" (ed. E. Kelly), University of Illinois Press, Urbana.

Wang, H. F., Wang, C. E., Chang, C. P., Kao, J. Y., Yü, L. and Chiang, Y. N. (1964). The application and value of ultrasonic diagnosis of liver abscess: a report of 218 cases, *Chin. med. J.*, **83**, 133–140.

Wells, P. N. T. and Evans, K. T. (1968). An immersion scanner for two-dimensional ultrasonic examination of the human breast, *Ultrasonics*, **6**, 220–228.

Wild, J. J. and Reid, J. M. (1952a). Application of echo-ranging techniques to the determination of structure of biological tissues, *Science, N.Y.*, **115**, 226–230.

Wild, J. J. and Reid, J. M. (1952b). Further pilot echographic studies on the histologic structure of the living intact human breast, *Am. J. Path.*, **28**, 839–861.

Wild, J. J. and Reid, J. M. (1954). Echographic visualization of lesions of the living intact human breast, *Cancer Res.*, **14**, 277–283.

Wild, J. J. and Reid, J. M. (1957). Progress in the techniques of soft tissue examination by 15 MC pulsed ultrasound, pp. 30–45. *In* "Ultrasound in Biology and Medicine" (ed. E. Kelly), A.I.B.S., Washington.

4.7.e Time-position recording

Avant, W. S. (1966). Pulsatile echoencephalography, *Neurology*, **16**, 1033–1040.

Bang, J. and Holm, H. H. (1968). Ultrasonic examination by means of A-presentation and scanning in gynaecology and obstetrics, *Dan. med. Bull.*, **15**, 101–106.

Braak, J. W. G. ter, and Vlieger, M. de (1965). Cerebral pulsations in echoencephalography, *Acta neurochir.*, **12**, 678–694.

Edler, I. (1955). The diagnostic use of ultrasound in heart disease, *Acta med. scand.*, **152**, Suppl. 308, 32–36.

Edler, I. (1961). Ultrasoundcardiography, *Acta med. scand.*, **170**, Suppl. 370.

Edler, I. (1965). The diagnostic use of ultrasound in heart disease, pp. 303–321. *In* "Ultrasonic Energy" (ed. E. Kelly), University of Illinois Press, Urbana.

Edler, I. (1966). Mitral valve function studied by the ultrasound echo method, pp. 198–228. *In* "Diagnostic Ultrasound" (ed. C. C. Grossman *et al.*), Plenum Press, New York.

Edler, I. (1967). Ultrasoundcardiography in mitral valve stenosis, *Am. J. Cardiol.*, **19**, 18–31.

Edler, I. and Hertz, C. H. (1954). The use of the ultrasonic reflectoscope for the continuous recording of the movements of heart walls, *K. fysiogr. Sällsk. Lund Förh.*, **24**, 40–58.

Effert, S. (1967). Pre- and postoperative evaluation of mitral stenosis by ultrasound, *Am. J. Cardiol.*, **19**, 59–65.

Effert, S. and Bleifeld, W. (1966). Diagnostic value of ultrasound reflection procedures in cardiology, pp. 229–236. *In* "Diagnostic Ultrasound" (ed. C. C. Grossman *et al.*), Plenum Press, New York.

Effert, S., Hertz, C. H. and Böhme, W. (1959). Direkte registrierung des ultraschallkardiograms mit dem elektrokardiographen, *Z. Kreislaufforsch.*, **48**, 230–236.

Evans, G. C., Lehman, J. S., Segal, B. L., Likoff, W., Ziskin, M. and Kingsley, B. (1967). Echoaortography, *Am. J. Cardiol.*, **19**, 91–96.

Feigenbaum, H., Zaky, A. and Waldhausen, J. A. (1967). Use of reflected ultrasound in detecting pericardial effusion, *Am. J. Cardiol.*, **19**, 84–90.

Goldberg, B. B., Ostrum, B. J. and Isard, H. J. (1966). Ultrasonic aortography, *J. Am. med. Ass.*, **198**, 353–358.

Joyner, C. R. (1966). Experience with ultrasound in the study of heart disease and the production of intracardiac sound, pp. 237–248. *In* "Diagnostic Ultrasound" (ed. C. C. Grossman *et al.*), Plenum Press, New York.

Joyner, C. R., Hey, E. B., Johnson, J. and Reid, J. M. (1967). Reflected ultrasound in the diagnosis of tricuspid stenosis, *Am. J. Cardiol.*, **19**, 66–73.

Kossoff, G. and Wilcken, D. E. L. (1967). The C.A.L. ultrasonic cardioscope, *Med. Biol. Engng.*, **5**, 25–32.

Pridie, R. B. and Turnbull, T. A. (1968). Diagnosis of pericardial effusion by ultrasound, *Br. med. J.*, iii, 356–357.

Segal, B. L., Likoff, W., Asperger, Z. and Kingsley, B. (1966). Ultrasound diagnosis of abdominal aortic aneurism, *Am. J. Cardiol.*, **17**, 101–103.

Segal, B. L., Likoff, W. and Kingsley, B. (1967). Echocardiography. Clinical application in combined mitral stenosis and mitral regurgitation, *Am. J. Cardiol.*, **19**, 42–58.

Wells, P. N. T. and Ross, F. G. M. (1969). A time-to-voltage analogue converter for ultrasonic cardiology, *Ultrasonics*, **7**, 171–176.

Winters, W. L., Gimenez, J. and Soloff, L. A. (1967). Clinical applications of ultrasound in the analysis of prosthetic ball function, *Am. J. Cardiol.*, **19**, 97–107.

Zaky, A., Nasser, W. K. and Feigenbaum, H. (1968). A study of mitral valve action recorded by reflected ultrasound and its application in the diagnosis of mitral stenosis, *Circulation*, **37**, 789–799.

4.7.f Other systems

Ardenne, M. von and Millner, R. (1962). The US-Focoscan method, *I.R.E. Trans. med. Electron.*, **ME-9**, 145–149.

Kimoto, S., Omoto, R., Tsunemoto, M., Moroi, T., Atsumi, K. and Uchida, R. (1964). Ultrasonic tomography of the liver and detection of heart atrial septal defect with the aid of ultrasonic intravenous probe, *Ultrasonics*, **2**, 82–86.

Omoto, R. (1967). Intracardiac scanning of the heart with the aid of ultrasonic intravenous probe, *Jap. Heart J.*, **8**, 569–581.

Thurstone, F. L. and McKinney, W. M. (1966a). Resolution enhancement in scanning of tissue, *Ultrasonics*, **4**, 25–27.

Thurstone, F. L. and McKinney, W. M. (1966b). Focused transducer arrays in an ultrasonic scanning system for biologic tissue, pp. 191–194. *In* "Diagnostic Ultrasound" (ed. C. C. Grossman *et al.*), Plenum Press, New York.

4.7.g Three-dimensional display of pulse-echo information

Baum, G. and Greenwood, I. (1961). Orbital lesion localization by three dimensional ultrasonography, *N.Y. State J. Med.*, **61**, 4149–4157.

Berkley, C. (1948). Three-dimensional representation on cathode ray tubes, *Proc. I.R.E.*, **36**, 1530–1535.

Brown, T. G. (1967). Visualization of soft tissues in two and three dimensions—limitations and development, *Ultrasonics*, **5**, 118–124.

Gabor, D. (1948). A new microscopic principle. *Nature, Lond.*, **161**, 777–778.

Gabor, D. (1949). Microscopy by reconstructed wavefronts, *Proc. R. Soc.*, A197, 454–487.

Howry, D. H., Posakony, G. J., Cushman, C. R. and Holmes, J. H. (1956). Three-dimensional and stereoscopic observation of body structures by ultrasound, *J. appl. Physiol.*, **9**, 304–306.

Iams, H. A., Burtner, R. L. and Chandler, C. H. (1948). Stereoscopic viewing of cathode-ray tube presentations, *R.C.A. Rev.*, **9**, 149–158.

Leith, E. N. and Upatnieks, J. (1965). Photography by laser, *Scient. Am.*, **212**, 6, 24–35.

Leith, E. N. Upatnieks, J., Kozma, A. and Massey, N. (1966). Hologram visual displays, *J. Soc. Motion Pict. Telev. Engrs.*, **75**, 323–326.

Redman, J. D., Walton, W. P., Fleming, J. E. and Hall, A. J. (1969). Holographic display of data from ultrasonic scanning, *Ultrasonics*, **7**, 26–29.

Schmitt, O. H. (1947). Cathode ray presentation of three dimensional data, *J. appl. Phys.*, **18**, 819–829.

4.8 Measurement of system performance

Buschmann, W. (1965). New equipment and transducers for ophthalmic diagnosis, *Ultrasonics*, **3**, 18–21.

Holmes, J. H. (1967b). Standards for medical equipment, *Ultrasonics*, **5**, 189.

5.1 Transmission techniques

Baldes, E. J., Farral, W. R., Haugen, M. C. and Herrick, J. F. (1957). A forum on an ultrasonic method for measuring the velocity of blood, pp. 165–176. *In* "Ultrasound in Biology and Medicine" (ed. E. Kelly), A.I.B.S., Washington.

Farrall, W. R. (1959), Design considerations for ultrasonic flowmeters, *I.R.E. Trans. med. Electron.*, **ME-6**, 198–201.

Franklin, D. L., Baker, D. W., Ellis, R. M. and Rushmer, R. F. (1959). A pulsed ultrasonic flowmeter, *I.R.E. Trans. med. Electron.*, **ME-6**, 204–206.

Kalmus, H. P. (1954). Electronic flowmeter system, *Rev. scient. Instrum.*, **25**, 201–206.

Wetterer, E. (1962). A critical appraisal of methods of blood flow determination in animals and man, *I.R.E. Trans. med. Electron.*, **ME-9**, 165–173.

5.2.a Basic principles

Franklin, D. L., Schlegel, W. A. and Watson, N. W. (1963). Ultrasonic Doppler shift blood flowmeter, *Biomed. Scis. Instrum.*, **1**, 309–315.

Green, P. S. (1964). Spectral broadening of acoustic reverberation in Doppler-shift fluid flowmeters, *J. acoust. Soc. Am.*, **36**, 1383–1390.

McLeod, F. D. (1964). A Doppler ultrasonic physiological flowmeter, *Proc. 17th Ann. Conf. Engng. Med. Biol., Cleveland, Ohio*, **6**, 81.

Wells, P. N. T. (1969). A nomogram for the calculation of Doppler frequency shift, *Ultrasonics*, **7**, 18–19.

Yoshitoshi, Y., Machii, K., Sekiguchi, H., Mishina, Y., Ohta, S., Hanaoka, Y., Kohashi, Y., Shimuzu, S. and Kuno, H. (1966). Doppler measurement of mitral valve and ventricle wall velocities, *Ultrasonics*, **4**, 27–28.

5.2.b Transducer arrangements

Fielder, F. D. (1968). Ultrasonic foetal blood flow detector, *Bio-med. Engng.*, **3**, 262–264.

Franklin, D. L., Baker, D. W., Ellis, R. M. and Rushmer, R. F. (1959). A pulsed ultrasonic flowmeter, *I.R.E. Trans. med. Electron.*, **ME-6**, 204–206.

Franklin, D. L., Schlegel, W. and Rushmer, R. F. (1961). Blood flow measured by Doppler frequency shift of backscattered ultrasound, *Science, N.Y.*, **134**, 564–565.

Lubé, V. M., Safonov, Yu. D. and Yakiemenkov, L. I. (1967). Ultrasonic detection of the motions of cardiac valves and muscle, *Soviet Phys. Acoust.*, **13**, 59–65.

Rushmer, R. F., Baker, D. W. and Stegall, H. F. (1966). Transcutaneous Doppler flow detection as a nondestructive technique, *J. Appl. Physiol.*, **21**, 554–566.

Satomura, S. (1957). Ultrasonic Doppler method for the inspection of cardiac functions, *J. acoust. Soc. Am.*, **29**, 1181–1185.

Satomura, S. and Kaneko, Z. (1961). Ultrasonic blood rheograph, pp. 254–258. *In* "Proc. 3rd Int. Conf. Med. Electron", I.E.E., London.

5.3 Transmitters and receivers

Fielder, F. D. (1968). Ultrasonic foetal blood flow detector, *Bio-med. Engng.*, **3**, 262–264.

Franklin, D. L., Schlegel, W. A. and Rushmer, R. F. (1961). Blood flow measured by Doppler frequency shift of backscattered ultrasound, *Science, N.Y.*, **134**, 564–565.

Franklin, D. L., Schlegel, W. A. and Watson, N. W. (1963). Ultrasonic Doppler shift blood flowmeter, *Biomed. Scis. Instrum.*, **1**, 309–315.

Lubé, V. M., Safonov, Yu. D. and Yakimenkov, L. I. (1967). Ultrasonic detection of the motions of cardiac valves and muscle, *Soviet Phys. Acoust.*, **13**, 59–65.

Ridenour, L. N. (ed.) (1947). "Radar System Engineering", M.I.T. Radiation Lab. ser. no. 1, McGraw-Hill Book Co. Inc., New York.

Satomura, S. (1957). Ultrasonic Doppler method for the inspection of cardiac functions, *J. acoust. Soc. Am.*, **29**, 1181–1185.

Stegall, H. F., Rushmer, R. F. and Baker, D. W. (1966). A transcutaneous ultrasonic blood velocity meter, *J. appl. Physiol.*, **21**, 707–711.

Yoshida, T., Mori, M., Nimura, Y., Hikita, G., Takagishi, S., Nakanishi, K. and Satomura, S. (1961). Analysis of heart motion with ultrasonic Doppler method, and its clinical application, *Am. Heart J.*, **61**, 61–75.

5.4 Methods of Doppler signal analysis

5.4.a The ear

Strandness, D. E., Schultz, R. D., Sumner, D. S. and Rushmer, R. F. (1967). Ultrasonic flow detection. A useful technic in the evaluation of peripheral vascular disease, *Am. J. Surg.*, **113**, 311–320.

5.4.b Ratemeters

Franklin, D. L., Schlegel, W. A. and Watson, N. W. (1963). Ultrasonic Doppler shift blood flowmeter, *Biomed. Scis. Instrum.*, **1**, 309–315.
Rushmer, R. F., Baker, D. W., Johnson, W. L. and Strandness, D. E. (1967). Clinical applications of a transcutaneous ultrasonic flow detector, *J. Am. med. Ass.*, **199**, 326–328.
Strandness, D. E., McCutcheon, E. P. and Rushmer, R. F. (1966). Application of a transcutaneous Doppler flowmeter in evaluation of occlusive arterial disease, *Surg. Gynec. Obstet.*, **122**, 1039–1045.

5.4.c Bandpass filters

Lubé, V. M., Safonov, Yu. D. and Yakimenkov, L. I. (1967). Ultrasonic detection of the motions of cardiac valves and muscle, *Soviet Phys. Acoust.*, **13**, 59–65.
Satomura, S. (1957). Ultrasonic Doppler method for the inspection of cardiac functions, *J. acoust. Soc. Am.*, **29**, 1181–1185.

5.4.d Sound spectroscopes

Koenig, W., Dunn, H. K. and Lacy, L. Y. (1946). The sound spectrograph, *J. acoust. Soc. Am.*, **18**, 19–49.
Koenig, W. and Ruppel, A. E. (1948). Quantitative amplitude representation in sound spectrograms, *J. acoust. Soc. Am.*, **20**, 787–795.
Mathes, R. C., Norwine, A. C. and Davis, K. H. (1949). The cathode-ray sound spectroscope, *J. acoust. Soc. Am.*, **21**, 527–537.
Ramaswamy, T. K. and Ramakrishna, B. S. (1962). Simple laboratory setup for obtaining sound spectrograms, *J. acoust. Soc. Am.*, **34**, 515–517.

5.5 Clinical applications

5.5.a Cardiology

McLeod, F. D. (1964). A Doppler ultrasonic physiological flowmeter, *Proc. 17th Ann. Conf. Engng. Med. Biol. Cleveland, Ohio*, **6**, 81.
Yoshida, T., Mori, M. Nimura, Y., Hikita, G., Takagishi, S., Nakanishi, K. and Satomura, S. (1961). Analysis of heart motion with ultrasonic Doppler method, and its clinical application, *Am. Heart J.*, **61**, 61–75.
Yoshitoshi, Y., Machii, K., Sekiguchi, H., Mishina, Y., Ohta, S., Hanaoka, Y., Kohashi, Y., Shimizu, S. and Kuno, H. (1966). Doppler measurement of mitral valve and ventricle wall velocities, *Ultrasonics*, **4**, 27–28.

5.5.b Blood flow studies

Franklin, D. L., Schlegel, W. A. and Watson, N. W. (1963). Ultrasonic Doppler shift blood flowmeter, *Biomed. Scis. Instrum.*, **1**, 309–315.
Kaneko, Z., Shiraishi, J., Omizo, H., Kato, K., Motomiya, M., Izumi, T. and Okumura, T. (1966). Analysing blood flow with a sonagraph, *Ultrasonics*, **4**, 22–23.

Sigel, B., Popky, G. L., Wagner, D. K., Boland, J. P., Mapp, E. McD. and Feigl, P. (1968). Comparison of clinical and Doppler ultrasound evaluation of confirmed lower extremity venous disease, *Surgery, St. Louis*, **64**, 332–338.

Strandness, D. E., McCutcheon, E. P. and Rushmer, R. F. (1966). Application of a transcutaneous Doppler flowmeter in evaluation of occlusive arterial disease, *Surg. Gynec. Obstet.*, **122**, 1039–1045.

Strandness, D. E., Schultz, R. D., Sumner, D. S. and Rushmer, R. F. (1967). Ultrasonic flow detection. A useful technic in the evaluation of peripheral vascular disease, *Am. J. Surg.*, **113**, 311–320.

5.5.c Obstetrics

Callagan, D. A., Rowland, T. C. and Goldman, D. E. (1964). Ultrasonic Doppler observation of the fetal heart, *Obstet. Gynec.*, *N.Y.*, **23**, 637.

Fielder, F. D. and Pocock, P. (1968). Foetal blood flow detector, *Ultrasonics*, **6**, 240–241.

Johnson, W. L., Stegall, H. F., Lein, J. N. and Rushmer, R. F. (1965). Detection of fetal life in early pregnancy with an ultrasonic Doppler flowmeter, *Obstet. Gynec.*, *N.Y.*, **26**, 305–307.

Rushmer, R. F., Baker, D. W. and Stegall, H. F. (1966). Transcutaneous Doppler flow detection as a nondestructive technique, *J. appl. Physiol.*, **21**, 554–566.

5.5.d Other applications

Kelsey, C. A. (1968). Ultrasonic Doppler shift as an aid to diagnostic ultrasonic scanning, *J. acoust. Soc. Am.*, **43**, 171–172.

Minifie, F. D., Kelsey, C. A. and Hixon, T. J. (1968). Measurement of vocal fold motion using an ultrasonic Doppler monitor, *J. acoust. Soc. Am.*, **43**, 1165–1169.

6.1 Introduction

6.2 Unscanned transmission techniques

Crawford, H. D., Wild, J. J., Wolf, P. I. and Fink, J. S. (1959). Transmission of ultrasound through the living human thorax, *I.R.E. Trans. Med. Electron.*, **ME-6**, 141–146.

Horn, C. A. and Robinson, D. (1965). Assessment of fracture healing by ultrasonics, *J. Coll. Radiol. Aust.*, **9**, 165–167.

Kossoff, G. and Sharpe, C. J. (1966). Examination of the contents of the pulp cavity in teeth, *Ultrasonics*, **4**, 77–83.

Mullins, G. L. and Guntheroth, W. G. (1966). Continuous recording of changes in mesenteric blood volume, *Ultrasonics*, **4**, 24–25.

Rushmer, R. F., Franklin, D. L. and Ellis, R. M. (1956). Left ventricular dimensions recorded by sonocardiometry, *Circulation Res.*, **4**, 684–688.

6.3 Mechanically scanned transmission techniques

Ballantine, H. T., Bolt, R. H., Hueter, T. F. and Ludwig, G. D. (1950). On the detection of intracranial pathology by ultrasound, *Science*, *N.Y.*, **112**, 525–528.

Ballantine, H. T., Hueter, T. F. and Bolt, R. H. (1954). On the use of ultrasound for tumour detection, *J. acoust. Soc. Am.*, **26**, 581.

Dunn, F. and Fry, W. J. (1959). Ultrasonic absorption microscope, *J. acoust. Soc. Am.*, **31**, 632–633.

Dussik, K. T., Dussik, F. and Wyt, L. (1947). Auf dem wege zur hyperphonographie des gehirnes, *Wien. med. Wschr.*, **97**, 425–429.

Güttner, W., Fielder, G. and Pätzold, J. (1952). Über ultraschallabbildungem am menschlichen schädel, *Acustica*, **2**, 148–156.

Hueter, T. F. and Bolt, R. H. (1951). An ultrasonic method for outlining the cerebral ventricles, *J. acoust. Soc. Am.*, **23**, 160–167.

Rich, C., Klinik, E., Smith, R. and Graham, B. (1966). Measurement of bone mass from ultrasonic transmission time, *Proc. Soc. exp. Biol. Med.*, **123**, 282–285.

6.4 Electrically scanned transmission techniques

Freitag, W., Martin, H. J. and Schellbac, G. (1960). Descriptions and results of investigations of an electronic ultrasonic image converter, pp. 373–379. *In* "Proc. 2nd Int. Conf. Med. Electron" (ed. C. N. Smyth), Illiffe and Sons Ltd., London.

Goldman, R. G. (1962). Electronic acoustic image converter, *J. acoust. Soc. Am.*, **34**, 514–515.

Jacobs, J. E. (1965). The ultrasound camera, *Science J.*, **1**, 4, 60–65.

Jacobs, J. E. (1967). Performance of the ultrasound microscope, *Mater. Eval.*, **25**, 3, 41–45.

Jacobs, J. E. (1968a). Ultrasound image converter systems utilizing electron-scanning techniques, *I.E.E.E. Trans. Sonics Ultrason.*, **SU-15**, 146–152.

Jacobs, J. E., Berger, H. and Collis, W. J. (1963). An investigation of the limitations to the maximum attainable sensitivity in acoustical image converters, *I.E.E.E. Trans. Ultrason. Engng.*, **UE-10**, 83–88.

Semennikov, Iu. B. (1958). A study of acoustic image converters, *Soviet Phys. Acoust.*, **4**, 72–83.

Smyth, C. N., Poynton, F. Y. and Sayers, J. F. (1963). The ultrasound image camera, *Proc. I.E.E.*, **110**, 16–28.

6.5 Ultrasonic holography

Greguss, P. (1968). Ultrasonic holography in ophthalmology, *Optics Technology*, **1**, 40–41.

Halstead, J. (1968). Ultrasound holography, *Ultrasonics*, **6**, 79–87.

Jacobs, J. E. (1968b). Present status of ultrasound image converter systems, *Trans. N.Y. Acad. Sci.*, II, **30**, 444–456.

Metherell, A. F. (1968). Holography with sound, *Science J.*, **4**, 11, 57–62.

Metherell, A. F., El-Sum, H. M. A., Dreher, J. J. and Larmore, L. (1967). Introduction to acoustical holography, *J. acoust. Soc. Am.*, **42**, 733–742.

Preston, H. and Kruezer, J. L. (1967). Ultrasonic imaging using a synthetic holographic technique, *Appl. Phys. Letters*, **10**, 150–152.

Thurstone, F. L. (1967). Three-dimensional imaging by ultrasound holography, p. 313. *In* "Dig. 7th Int. Conf. Med. Biol. Engng., Stockholm".

7.1 Introduction

7.2 Ultrasonic field parameters

Edler, I. (1961). Ultrasoundcardiography, *Acta. med. scand.*, **170**, Suppl. 370.

McCarthy, C. F., Read, A. E. A., Ross, F. G. M. and Wells, P. N. T. (1967). Ultrasonic scanning of the liver, *Quart. J. Med.*, **36**, 517–524.

7.3 Interactions of ultrasonic waves with biological tissues

7.3.a Mechanisms

Hill, C. R. (1968). The possibility of hazard in medical and industrial applications of ultrasound, *Br. J. Radiol.*, **41**, 561–569.

Hueter, T. F. and Bolt, R. H. (1955). "Sonics", John Wiley and Sons Inc., New York.

Nyborg, W. L. (1965). Physical principles involved in the action of weak ultrasound, pp. 1–5. *In* "Ultrasonic Energy" (ed. E. Kelly), University of Illinois Press, Urbana.

Nyborg, W. L. and Dyer, H. J. (1960). Ultrasonically induced motions in single plant cells, pp. 391–396. *In* "Proc. 2nd Int. Conf. Med. Electron" (ed. C. N. Smyth), Illiffe and Sons Ltd., London.

7.3.b Biological effects

Andrew, D. S. (1964). Ultrasonography in pregnancy—an enquiry into its safety, *Br. J. Radiol.*, **37**, 185–186.

Basauri, L. and Lele, P. P. (1962). A simple method for production of trackless focal lesions with focussed ultrasound: statistical evaluation of the effects of irradiation on the central nervous system of the cat, *J. Physiol., Lond.*, **160**, 513–534.

Curtis, J. C. (1965). Action of intense ultrasound on the intact mouse liver, pp. 85–109. *In* "Ultrasonic Energy" (ed. E. Kelly), University of Illinois Press, Urbana.

Donald, I., MacVicar, J. and Brown, T. G. (1958). Investigation of abdominal masses by pulsed ultrasound, *Lancet*, i, 1188–1194.

Fry, W. J., Wulff, V. J., Tucker, D. and Fry, F. J. (1950). Physical factors involved in ultrasonically induced changes in living systems. I. Identification of non-temperature effects, *J. acoust. Soc. Am.*, **22**, 867–876.

French, L. A., Wild, J. J. and Neal, D. (1951). Attempts to determine harmful effects of pulsed ultrasonic vibrations, *Cancer, N.Y.*, **4**, 342–344.

Fritz-Niggli, H. and Böni, A. (1950). Biological experiments on *Drosophila melanogaster* with supersonic vibrations, *Science, N.Y.*, **112**, 120–122.

Garg, A. G. and Taylor, A. R. (1967). An investigation into the effect of pulsed ultrasound on the brain, *Ultrasonics*, **5**, 208–212.

Hawley, S. A., MacLeod, R. M. and Dunn, F. (1963). Degradation of DNA by intense, noncavitating ultrasound, *J. acoust. Soc. Am.*, **35**, 1285–1287.

Herrick, J. F. (1953). Temperatures produced in tissues by ultrasound: experimental study using various technics, *J. acoust. Soc. Am.*, **25**, 12–16.

Holmes, J. H. and Howry, D. H. (1963). Ultrasonic diagnosis of abdominal disease, *Am. J. dig. Dis.*, **8**, 12–32.

Hughes, D. E., Chou, J. T. Y., Warwick, R. and Pond, J. (1963). The effect of focussed ultrasound on the permeability of frog muscle, *Biochim. biophys. Acta*, **75**, 137–139.

James, J. A., Dalton, G. A., Freundlich, H. F., Bullen, M. A., Wells, P. N. T., Hughes, D. E. and Chou, J. T. Y. (1963). Histological, thermal and bio-chemical effects of ultrasound on the labyrinth and temporal bone, *Acta oto-lar.*, **57**, 306–311.

Lele, P. P. (1963). Effects of focussed ultrasonic radiation on peripheral nerve, with observations on local heating, *Expl. Neurol.*, **8**, 47–83.

Patrick, M. K. (1966). Ultrasound in physiotherapy, *Ultrasonics*, **4**, 10–14.

Pond, J. and Dyson, M. (1967). A device for the study of the effects of ultrasound in tissue growth in rabbit's ears, *J. scient. Instrum.*, **44**, 165–166.

Smyth, M. G. (1966). Animal toxicity studies with ultrasound at diagnostic power levels, pp. 296–299. *In* "Diagnostic Ultrasound" (ed. C. C. Grossman *et al.*), Plenum Press, New York.

Takagi, S. F., Higashino, S., Shikurya, T. and Osawa, N. (1960). The actions of ultrasound on the myelinated nerve, the spinal cord, and the brain, *Jap. J Physiol.*, **10**, 183–193.

Wells, P. N. T. (1968). The effect of ultrasonic irradiation on the survival of *Daphnia magna*, *J. exp. Biol.*, **49**, 61–70.

Wood, R. W. and Loomis, A. L. (1927). The physical and biological effects of high-frequency sound waves of great intensity, *Phil. Mag.*, *7th. series*, **4**, 417–436.

7.4 Conclusions

GLOSSARY

Abortion: the expulsion of the foetus before the infant is sufficiently mature to survive.

Abscess: a localized collection of pus.

Absorption: loss of energy during propagation by conversion into another form, usually heat. The absorption coefficient of a material describes the rate at which absorption occurs, usually in dB cm^{-1}.

Aneurism: a permanent dilatation of an artery.

Anisotropic: having a directional orientation.

Aortic valve: the valve which guards the entrance from the left ventricle to the aorta.

Aortography: the process of producing a graphic representation of the aorta.

A–P dimension: the distance between the anterior and posterior surfaces of a structure.

Arterioschlerosis: degeneration of an artery resulting in the hardening of its walls.

Artifact: a representation corresponding to a structure which does not in fact exist.

Ascites: an effusion of watery fluid into the abdominal cavity.

A-scope: a display in which structures are represented by deflection modulation of a time-base which represents range.

Atrial septal defect (a.s.d.): a defect in the septum between the right and left atria of the heart.

Attenuation: reduction in intensity during propagation, not necessarily resulting from absorption.

Attenuator: a device which introduces attenuation. In the case of an electrical attenuator, the calibration may be in dB.

Blighted ovum: an abortus in which the membrane which normally protects the embryo is present, but from which the embryo has disappeared.

Brachial artery: the main artery of the arm.

B-scope: a display in which structures are represented by brightness modulation of a time-base which represents range.

Calculus: a solid mass composed chiefly of inorganic salts.

Carcinoma: a type of cancer growing from epithelial tissue, which is spread by the lymph channels.

Cardiology: the study of the heart.

Cardiovascular: pertaining to the heart and the blood vessels.

Carotid artery: the principal large artery on each side of the neck.

Catheter: a hollow tube designed to be introduced into a cavity through a narrow canal.

Cephalometry: the measurement of the distance between the parietal bones of the skull.

Cerebro-spinal fluid: the clear watery fluid which surrounds the bain and the spinal cord.

Cholelithiasis: the formation of gall-stones.

Cirrhosis: the contracted granular state of an organ.

Clutter: those signals, due to noise and other sources, which confuse the information.

Conformity: a term used to describe the manufacturing tolerance of a sine/cosine potentiometer; equal to the maximum deviation between the ideal and actual outputs of the potentiometer.

Costal margin: the border at the base of the rib-cage.

C-scope: a brightness-modulated display in which the x-deflection corresponds to the bearing in azimuth, and the y-deflection, to the elevation.

Curie point: temperature above which residual polarization is not possible.

Cyst: a tumour containing fluid or semifluid in a membranous sac.

Degenerative pulpitis: degeneration of the soft vascular tissue which fills the pulp chamber and the root canal of the tooth.

Delay line: a system in which the output is delayed in time from the input.

Demodulation: the process by which the modulating signal is separated from its carrier.

Diastole: the period of relaxation during which a chamber of the heart fills with blood.

Differentiation: a process in which the output is equal to the rate of change of the input, with respect to a third quantity (often time).

Diffraction: the tendency of waves to bend around an obstacle which is small in size in relation to the wavelength. Geometrical diffraction is the term used to describe the excess attenuation and velocity associated with propagation in the Frésnel zone.

Dispersion: the variation of any property with frequency.

DNA: deoxyribonucleic acid, a non-protein constituent of nucleoproteins.

Duty cycle: the ratio of on to off times during a repetitive sequence.

Dynamic range: the difference in amplitude between the largest and the smallest signals in a complex. Usually expressed in dB.

Echoencephalography: the process of producing a graphic representation of the brain by an echo technique.

Ectopic gestation: fertilization of the ovum and growth of the foetus outside the uterus.

Effusion: an abnormal outpouring of fluid into the tissues or cavities of the body.

Electrocardiogram: a graphic recording of electrical changes associated with the cardiac cycle.

Embolism: the blocking of a blood vessel by a mass, often a clot of blood.

Emphysema: the formation in the lung of spaces containing air, often associated with lung distension.

Epoxy resin: a polymer derived from two components, used as a structural plastic, surface coating or adhesive.

Femoral artery: the main artery of the thigh.

Ferroelectricity: the piezoelectric phenomenon analogous to ferromagnetism.

Fibroadenoma: a tumour composed of mixed fibrous and glandular elements.

Fibroids: the uterine tumour composed of mixed muscular and fibrous tissue.

Fluoroscopic image converter: a device in which ionizing radiation is converted to form a visible image by means of a fluorescent screen.

Fraunhofer zone: the region of a wave field which lies beyond the last axial maximum, moving away from the source.

Frésnel zone: the region of a wave field which lies between the source and the last axial maximum.

Gall-stone: a calculus in the gall-bladder.

Gastroenterology: the study of the stomach and the intestine.

Gate: an arrangement which can be switched electronically to control the transmission of a signal.

Genito-urinary: relating to the genitalia and the urinary organs.

Gynaecology: the study of the diseases special to women.

Hepatic: relating to the liver.

Holography: a process of imagery. A diffraction pattern is first generated from the original object, an image of which is subsequently reconstructed by coherent radiation.

Hydatidiform mole: a uterine tumour resulting from the degeneration in early pregnancy of the membrane enveloping the foetus.

Hydramnios: excess amniotic fluid.

Hysteresis: the extent to which the instaneous strain depends upon the previous stress history.

Integration: a process in which the output is equal to the sum of the input, with respect to a third quantity (often time).

Interference: the phenomenon in which two or more waves add together according to their amplitudes and phases.

Intermediate frequency (i.f.): the frequency of the carrier wave of the output from the frequency changer in a superheterodyne receiver.

Isotropic: having a non-directional orientation.

Jitter: small irregularities in the timing of a waveform.

Kinetic energy: energy which a system possesses by virtue of its motion.

Logarithmic amplifier: an amplifier in which the output is proportional to the logarithm of the input.

Malpresentation: unfavourable presentation of the foetus at birth.

Medulla oblongata: the lower part of the brain stem.

Mesentery: a fold of the membrane which lines the abdominal cavity, which connects the digestive tube with the abdominal wall.

Metastases: secondary tumours transferred from a primary tumour by the conveyance of causal agents through blood vessels or lymph channels.

Mitral valve: the atrioventricular valve on the left side of the heart.

Monotonic: a wave in which all the energy occurs at a single frequency.

Neurology: the study of the nervous system.

Obstetrics: relating to midwifery.

Obstructive jaundice: the presence of bile pigments in the blood due to interference with the outflow of bile by mechanical obstruction of the biliary passages.

Occlusion: a closing or shutting up, often of a blood vessel.

Ophthalmology: the study of diseases of the eye.

Penetration: the distance between the target and the transducer. Equal to half the total path length in an echo system.

Pedal artery: the main artery supplying the foot.

Pericardium: the membranous sac which holds the heart.

Phacometry: the measurement of the refractive power of the lens of the eye.

Phonocardiogram: a graphic recording of the sounds associated with the cardiac cycle.

Photomultiplier: a photo-electric cell in which photo-electrons emitted from the cathode are amplified by the production of secondary electrons in an auxiliary electrode assembly.

Piezoelectricity: the coupling between electric and dielectric phenomena.

Placenta: the organ on the wall of the uterus through which the foetus is nourished.

Plasma: the fluid portion of blood.

Polarization: the alignment of charge or magnetic domains.

Polymer: a material consisting of molecules each formed by the combination of several similar molecules.

Popliteal artery: the artery supplying the area behind the knee.

Potential energy: energy which a system possesses by virtue of its configuration.

Potentiometer: a device for the accurate division of an electrical voltage.

Prosthesis: an artificial substitute for a missing part.

Pulmonary valve: the valve between the right ventricle of the heart and the pulmonary artery.

Pulse-stretching: increase in pulse length due, for example, to bandwidth limitation.

Radial mode: the mode of vibration along the radius of a disc.

Radio frequency: the frequency of the carrier wave at the input to an amplifier.

Regurgitation: the backflow of blood through a defective heart valve.

Renal: relating to the kidney.

Resolution: either the minimum distance in space between two point targets at which separate registrations can just be distinguished on the display; or the area or distance which appears to be occupied on the display by a point target in space; or the minimum time interval for two separate events to be distinguished on the display.

Reverberation: the phenomenon of multiple reflection within a closed system.

Scale factor: the ratio of the displayed size of an object to the real size of the object.

Simple harmonic motion: motion in a straight line in which particle acceleration is directed towards a fixed point on the line and is proportional to the distance from the line.

Soft tissue: any aggregate of cells apart from bone and cartilage.

Specular reflection: reflection in which the beam appears, after reflection, to originate at an image of the source in the reflecting surface.

Sputtering: deposition of a material on a surface following disintegration of a cathode in a vacuum.

Steady state: the situation in which conditions are constant, apart from periodic variations.

Stenosis: constriction or narrowing.

Striated muscle: a muscle consisting of cross-striped muscle fibres.

Suppression: the elimination of weak signals by the introduction of a threshold level.

Swept gain: the process by which the gain of a pulse-echo system is controlled with time to compensate for the effects of absorption.

Systole: the period of contraction during which blood is expelled from a chamber of the heart.

Tensor: the magnitude of a vector which defines its direction with reference to some standard direction.

Threshold: the level below which signals are not transmitted through the system.

Thyratron: a gas-filled triode valve.

Time constant: the time in which the output of a system changes by a fraction $\left(1 - \dfrac{1}{e}\right)$ of its ultimate change.

Transcutaneous: across the skin.

Transducer: a device capable of converting one form of energy into another. In ultrasonics, the conversion is usually between electrical and mechanical energies.

Transonic: an area through which ultrasound is transmitted, and from which the echoes fall below the threshold level of the display.

Tricuspid valve: the valve between the right atrium and ventricle.

Tumour: a swelling, benign or malignant.

Ultrasound: mechanical vibrations the frequencies of which lie within the range 20 kHz to 1 GHz (1000 MHz). Most medical applications employ ultrasonic frequencies in the range 1–15 MHz

Ultrasoundcardiogram: a graphic recording of the changing position of a cardiac structure obtained by an ultrasonic technique.

Ventricle: a cavity containing liquid.

Video frequency: the frequency of the signal at the output from the demodulator, possibly extending up to around 10 MHz.

MATHEMATICAL SYMBOLS

Symbol	Quantity	Section
A	Maximum amplitude	1.5
	Radius of curvature	3.2
$A_c(\omega)$	Amplitude of Fourier series cosine term	2.7
$A_s(\omega)$	Amplitude of Fourier series sine term	2.7
A_t	Transducer area	2.9
A_x	Area of transformer core	2.9
$A(\omega)$	Overall amplitude	2.7
$A_0, A_1, \ldots, A_N$	Amplitude of successive cycles in a wave train	2.5
a	Instantaneous particle acceleration	1.1
C	Capacitance	2.9
C_t	Capacitance of transducer	2.9
c	Propagation velocity	1.2, 1.3, 1.5, 1.6, 1.7, 1.8, 1.12, 1.13, 1.16, 5.1, 5.2.a, 5.2.b
c_1	Propagation velocity in first medium	1.8
	Propagation velocity in lens	3.2
c_2	Propagation velocity in second medium	1.8
	Propagation velocity in load	3.2
D_r	Directivity function of receiver	3.1
D_s	Directivity function of source	3.1, 3.4.c
d	Piezoelectric transmitting coefficient	2.2, 2.3
	Distance	4.7.e, 5.1
d_1	First distance from transducer to reflector	4.7.e
d_2	Second distance from transducer to reflector	4.7.e

Symbol	Quantity	Section
E	Energy density	1.5
	Effective value of voltage	4.4.a
e	Instantaneous particle energy	1.5
	Napierian base $= 2{\cdot}718$	2.5, 4.4.c, 4.5.c
e_k	Instantaneous particle kinetic energy	1.5
e_p	Instantaneous particle potential energy	1.5
F	Force due to radiation pressure	1.13
	Position of focus	3.2
	Noise figure	4.4.a
$F(t)$	Instantaneous pulse amplitude	2.7
f	Frequency	1.1, 1.3, 1.5, 1.12, 1.15, 1.16, 1.17, 2.7, 2.8, 2.9, 5.2.a, 5.2.b
f_D	Doppler shift frequency	1.12, 5.2a, 5.2b
f_l	Focal length	3.2
f_r	Apparent frequency	1.12, 5.2.a
f_0	Resonant frequency	2.5, 2.8, 2.9
f_1	Lower frequency limit	2.5, 4.4.a
f_2	Upper frequency limit	2.5, 4.4.a
G	Shear modulus	1.2
	Intensity gain	3.2
g	Piezoelectric receiving coefficient	2.2, 2.3
	Stage gain	4.5.e
g_m	Mutual conductance	4.4.a, 4.4.b
h	Depth of concave surface	3.2
h_{FE}	Common emitter forward current gain	4.4.c
h_{RE}	Common emitter reverse current gain	4.4.c
I	Intensity	1.5, 1.8
	Current	4.4.c
I_{DSS}	Zero-gate-voltage drain current	4.4.c
I_{ES}	Emitter reverse saturation current	4.5.c
I_a	Anode current	4.4.b
I_b	Base current	4.4.c
I_c	Intensity at centre of curvature	3.2
	Collector current	4.5.c
I_i	Incident intensity	1.8
	Intensity at transducer surface	3.2
I_k	Cathode current	4.4.a

Symbol	Quantity	Section
I_r	Reflected intensity	1.8
I_s	Screen grid current	4.4.a
	Reverse saturation current	4.4.c
I_t	Transmitted intensity	1.8
I_x	Axial intensity at distance x from source	3.1
I_0	Maximum axial intensity	3.1
i	Instantaneous current	4.4.e
K	Bulk modulus	1.2
K_a	Adiabatic bulk modulus	1.2
K_i	Isothermal bulk modulus	1.2
k	Wavelength constant	1.11, 3.1
	Electromechanical coupling coefficient	2.2.c
	Boltzman's constant $= 1{\cdot}37 \times 10^{-23}$ joule per deg. K	4.4.a, 4.4.c, 4.5.c
L	Inductance	2.9
l	Thickness	1.11
l_t	Transducer thickness	2.9
l_x	Length of transformer core	2.9
m	Particle mass	1.5
N	Number of oscillations	2.5
	Ultrasonic frequency (MHz)	4.1.b
n	Number of turns	2.9
	Number of stages	4.4.a, 4.5.e
P	Power	1.5, 1.13
	Penetration	3.2
p	Instantaneous particle pressure	1.6, 1.8
p_i	Instantaneous incident particle pressure	1.8
p_r	Instantaneous reflected particle pressure	1.8
p_t	Instantaneous transmitted particle pressure	1.8
p_0	Peak particle pressure	1.8
p_{0i}	Peak incident particle pressure	1.10
p_{0r}	Peak reflected particle pressure	1.10
Q	Quality factor	2.3, 2.5, 2.6.a, 2.8
q	Electronic charge $= 1{\cdot}60 \times 10^{-19}$ coulomb	4.4.c, 4.5.c
R	Resistance	4.4.a, 4.4.e
R_L	Load resistance	4.4.e

Symbol	Quantity	Section
R_p	Equivalent resistance for partition noise	4.4.a
R_s	Equivalent resistance for shot noise	4.4.a
	Source resistance	4.4.e
r	Radius of source	3.1, 3.2
r_D	Dynamic resistance of diode	4.4.c, 4.4.e
r_{DS}	Dynamic drain-to-source resistance	4.4.c
r_T	Dynamic emitter-collector resistance	4.4.c
r_0	Forward diode resistance	4.4.e
SWR	Standing wave ratio	1.10
s	Elastic compliance	2.2.c
s^D	Elastic compliance, constant charge density	2.2.c
s^E	Elastic compliance, constant electric field	2.2.c
T	Wave period	1.3
	Absolute temperature	4.4.a, 4.4.c, 4.5.c
t	Instantaneous time	1.1, 1.2, 1.6, 2.7, 4.7.e
t_{g1}	First gate time in sequence	4.7.e
t_{g2}	Second gate time in sequence	4.7.e
t_m	Time in sequence of mitral valve echo	4.7.e
t_0	Time of initiation of sequence	4.4.d, 4.5.d, 4.7.e
t_1	First time in sequence	4.4.d, 4.5.d
t_2	Second time in sequence	4.4.d, 4.5.d
t_3	Third time in sequence	4.5.d
u	Instantaneous particle displacement amplitude	1.1, 1:2, 1.5
u_0	Peak particle displacement amplitude	1.1, 1.2, 1.5
V	Voltage	4.4.c, 4.4.e
V_{GS}	Gate-to-source voltage	4.4.c
V_P	Gate-to-source voltage cut-off	4.4.c
V_a	Anode voltage	4.4.b
V_{ce}	Collector-emitter voltage	4.4.c
V_e	Emitter-to-base voltage	4.5.c
V_{g1}	Control grid voltage	4.4.b
V_{g2}	Screen grid voltage	4.4.b

Symbol	Quantity	Section
V_i	Peak input voltage to saturate stage	4.5.c
V_{in}	Peak input voltage	4.5.c
V_{out}	Peak output voltage	4.5.c
V_s	Peak output voltage from saturated stage	4.5.e
V_x	Voltage corresponding to x-position	4.7.c
V_y	Voltage corresponding to y-position	4.7.c
v	Instantaneous particle velocity	1.1, 1.6, 1.8
	Instantaneous voltage	4.4.e, 4.7.e
	Flow velocity	5.1
	Velocity of reflector along direction of flow	5.2.a, 5.2.b
v_i	Instantaneous incident particle velocity	1.8
	Velocity of reflector away from source	1.12, 5.2.a
v_{in}	Instantaneous input voltage	4.4.e
v_m	Velocity of medium in direction of propagation	1.12
v_{out}	Instantaneous output voltage	4.4.e
v_r	Instantaneous reflected particle velocity	1.8
	Velocity of receiver away from source	1.12, 5.2.b
v_s	Velocity of source in same direction as v_r	1.12, 5.2.b
v_t	Instantaneous transmitted particle velocity	1.8
v_0	Peak particle velocity	1.5, 1.6, 1.8
v_1	Voltage corresponding to d_1	4.7.e
v_2	Voltage corresponding to d_2	4.7.e
X_t	Reactance of transducer	2.9
x	Distance along direction of propagation	1.2, 3.1
x_{max}	Position of axial maximum	3.1
x'_{max}	Position of last axial maximum	3.1, 3.2
x_{min}	Position of axial minimum	3.1
Y	Young's modulus	1.2
Z	Characteristic impedance	1.7, 2.8

Symbol	Quantity	Section
Z_b	Characteristic impedance of backing medium	2.4, 2.6.a
Z_l	Characteristic impedance of loading medium	2.4, 2.6.a
Z_t	Characteristic impedance of transducer	2.4, 2.6.a
Z_1	Characteristic impedance of first medium	1.8, 1.11
Z_2	Characteristic impedance of second medium	1.8, 1.11
Z_3	Characteristic impedance of third medium	1.11
α	Absorption coefficient	1.5, 1.15, 1.16, 1.17, 4.1.b, 4.4.b
	Gain of adding circuit	4.5.c
	Angle in polar co-ordinates	4.7.c
	Angle between transmitting beam and flow direction	5.2.b
α_n	Normal common base current gain	4.5.c
α_r	Intensity reflection coefficient	1.8
α_t	Intensity transmission coefficient	1.8, 1.11
β	Angle in polar co-ordinates	4.7.c
	Angle between receiving beam and flow direction	5.2.b
β_i	Inverted common emitter current gain	4.4.c
β_n	Normal common emitter current gain	4.4.c
γ	Ratio of specific heat at constant pressure to that at constant volume	1.2
	Angle of attack	5.2.a, 5.2.b
Δ_t	Up and down stream transit time difference	5.1
ϵ	Dielectric constant	2.2.b, 2.9
ϵ^S	Dielectric constant, clamped transducer	2.2.b, 2.2.c
ϵ^T	Dielectric constant, free transducer	2.2.b, 2.2.c

Symbol	Quantity	Section
θ	Semiangle of central lobe	3.1
	Angle from central axis	3.1, 3.2
	Direction of ultrasonic beam relative to fixed axis	4.7.c, 5.1
	Angle between transmitting and receiving beams	5.2.b
θ_i	Angle of incidence	1.8
θ_r	Angle of reflection	1.8
θ_t	Angle of transmission	1.8
λ	Wavelength	1.3, 1.11, 1.17, 3.1, 3.2, 4.1.b
μ	Permeability	2.9
ρ	Mean density	1.2, 1.5, 1.6, 1.7, 1.8
σ	Poisson's ratio	1.2
ϕ	Contact potential	4.4.c
ω	Angular frequency	1.1, 1.2, 1.6, 2.7

AUTHOR INDEX

Numbers in italics are those pages on which references are listed.

A

Abdulla, U., 170, *243*
Alcock, R. N., 127, 130, *238*
Aldridge, E. E., 69, *233*
Alred, R. V., 125, *238*
Ambrose, J., 143, *239*
An, S., 143, 146, 149, *239*
Anderson, R. H., 139, *238*
Andrew, D. S., 225, *251*
Andrews, F. A., 53, *232*
Ardenne, M., von, 186, *245*
Arnold, R. T., 76, *235*
Åsberg, A., 166, *243*
Asperger, Z., 143, 181, *240*, *245*
Atsumi, K., 143, 154, 157, 166, 185, *240*, *242*, *244*, *246*
Avant, W. S., 180, *244*
Aveyard, S., 70, *234*

B

Baker, D. W., 193, 194, 197, 198, 202, 204, 207, *246*, *247*, *248*, *249*
Baldes, E. J., 193, 194, *246*
Ballantine, H. T., 212, *249*
Bang, J., 143, 149, 166, 180, 181, *239*, *243*, *244*
Barnes, N. F., 65, 66, 73, *234*, *235*
Barnes, R. S., 66, *234*
Basauri, L., 225, *251*
Bastir, R., 142, *240*
Bate, A. E., 17, 19, *228*
Baum, G., 157, 166, 187, *241*, *243*, *245*
Bechman, R., 32, *230*
Begui, Z. E., 6, 25, *227*, *228*
Belle, T. S., 60, *233*
Bellinger, J. L., 65, 66, 73, *234*, *235*
Berger, H., 213, *250*
Berkley, C., 188, *246*
Berlincourt, D. A., 29, *230*
Beveridge, H. N., 43, *231*

Beyer, R. T., 27, *229*
Bilotti, A., 113, *237*
Biquard, P., 65, *234*
Blanchard, J. B., 143, 146, 147, *241*
Bleifeld, W., 180, *245*
Bliss, W. R., 157, 164, *242*, *243*
Blitz, J., 9, 18, 37, 76, *227*, *228*, *230*, *235*
Böhme, W., 175, *245*
Boland, J. P., 208, *249*
Bolt, R. H., 18, 20, 25, 36, 55, 69, 212, 224, *228*, *229*, *230*, *232*, *234*, *249*, *250*, *251*
Böni, A., 225, *251*
Borgnis, F. E., 18, *228*
Braak, J. W. G., ter, 148, 180, *239*, *244*
Bradfield, G., 57, *232*
Brady, L. W., 157, 166, *241*, *244*
Breazeale, M. A., 76, *235*
Brinker, R. A., 123, 143, 148, 166, *237*, *239*, *243*
Bronson, N. R., 143, *239*
Brown, C. S., 29, *230*
Brown, T. G., 95, 157, 159, 160, 165, 171, 187, 225, *236*, *241*, *243*, *246*, *251*
Bullen, M. A., 66, 67, 73, 74, 75, 97, 225, *234*, *235*, *236*, *251*
Burtner, R. L., 188, *246*
Burton, C. S., 66, *234*
Buschmann, W., 143, 151, 192, *239*, *246*

C

Cady, W. G., 32, *230*
Callagan, D. A., 207, *249*
Campbell, S., 149, *239*
Carlin, B., 143, 150, *239*
Carome, E. F., 40, *230*
Carstensen, E. L., 23, 24, 25, *228*, *229*
Carter, A. H., 56, *232*
Chandler, C. H., 188, *246*
Chang, C. P., 143, 166, *241*, *244*

Chaston, J., 150, *240*
Chiang, Y. N., 143, 166, *241*, *244*
Chih-Chang, H., 143, 146, 149, *239*
Chou, J. T. Y., 225, *251*
Christie, D. G., 64, 70, *233*, *234*
Cmolik, C., 29, *230*
Coleman, D. J., 143, 150, *239*
Collis, W. J., 213, *250*
Colombati, S., 24, 25, *229*
Cook, E. G., 37, 39, 41, *231*
Crawford, A. E., 29, 33, *230*
Crawford, H. D., 210, *249*
Croney, J., 127, 128, *238*
Cuellar, J., 143, *240*
Curtis, J. C., 225, *251*
Cushman, C. R., 188, *246*

D

Dalton, G. A., 66, 67, 225, *234*, *251*
Damascelli, B., 166, *243*
Darby, R. A., 53, *232*
Davies, J. G., 96, *236*
Davis, K. H., 205, *248*
Day, N. J., 143, 149, *241*
Debye, R., 65, *234*
Deferrari, H. A., 53, *232*
Dehn, J. T., 56, *232*
Diggdon, P., 143, *240*
Donald, I., 95, 143, 149, 160, 166, 170, 171, 225, *236*, *239*, *241*, *243*, *244*, *251*
Dreher, J. J., 217, *250*
Dudrick, S. J., 143, *240*
Duggan, T. C., 143, 149, *241*
Dunn, F., 22, 23, 24, 25, 27, 212, 225, *229*, *249*, *251*
Dunn, H. K., 205, *248*
Dussik, F., 211, *250*
Dussik, K. T., 211, *250*
Dye, W. D., 53, *232*
Dyer, H. J., 224, *251*
Dyson, M., 225, *252*

E

Edler, I., 180, 181, 182, 183, 185, 223, *244*, *245*, *250*
Effert, S., 175, 180, *245*
Ellis, R. M., 193, 194, 198, 210, *246*, *247*, *249*
El-Sum, H. M. A., 217, *250*
Ensminger, D., 68, *234*
Ernst, P. J., 73, *235*

Esche, R., 25, *229*
Eskin, D. J., 143, *240*
Etienne, J., 25, 157, 162, *229*, *241*
Evans, G. C., 157, 166, 180, 181, *241*, *244*, *245*
Evans, K. T., 105, 107, 108, 116, 124, 132, 133, 153, 157, 166, 167, *237*, *238*, *242*, *244*

F

Farn, C. L. S., 64, *233*
Farrall, W. R., 193, 194, *246*
Feigenbaum, H., 143, 180, 183, *239*, *245*
Feigl, P., 208, *249*
Fielder, F. D., 198, 200, 202, 207, *247*, *249*
Fielder, G., 212, *250*
Filipczynski, L., 25, 63, 64, 75, 76, 157, 162, 163, *229*, *233*, *235*, *241*
Fink, J. S., 210, *249*
Firestone, F. A., 77, *236*
Fleming, J. E., 160, 187, *241*, *246*
Follett, D. H., 73, *235*
Ford, R., 143, 148, *239*
Foucault, L., 65, *234*
Fox, F. E., 26, 27, 58, *229*, *233*
Franklin, D. L., 193, 194, 195, 198, 202, 204, 208, 210, *246*, *247*, *248*, *249*
Freeman, M. H., 150, *239*
Freitag, W., 213, 214, *250*
French, L. A., 141, 225, *239*, *251*
Freundlich, H. F., 66, 67, 73, 74, 75, 97, 225, *234*, *235*, *236*, *251*
Frey, P., 16, 55, *228*, *232*
Fritz-Niggli, H., 225, *251*
Frucht, A. H., 6, *227*
Fry, F. J., 225, *251*
Fry, R. B., 73, *235*
Fry, W. J., 22, 24, 25, 73, 212, 225, *229*, *235*, *249*, *251*
Fujimoto, Y., 166, *243*

G

Gabor, D., 187, *246*
Galil, U., 127, *238*
Galt, J. K., 44, *231*
Garg, A. G., 225, *251*
Garrett, W. J., 51, 61, 62, 63, 94, 98, 124, 154, 157, 160, 166, *232*, *233*, *236*, *238*, *242*, *244*
Gauster, W. B., 76, *235*

Gay, M. J., 110, *236*
Gericke, O. R., 48, *231*
Gessert, W. L., 73, *235*
Gimenez, J., 180, 183, *245*
Goldberg, B. B., 143, 180, 181, *240, 245*
Goldman, D. E., 6, 23, 24, 25, 207, *227, 229, 249*
Goldman, R. G., 215, 216, *250*
Gordon, D., 70, 71, 143, 146, 157, 162, 163, *234, 239, 241*
Gottesfeld, K. R., 149, 166, *240, 243*
Gottesfeld, M. D., 171, *243*
Graham, B., 213, *250*
Granato, A., 57, *232*
Greatorex, C. A., 157, *241*
Green, P. S., 195, *247*
Greenspan, M., 4, *227*
Greenwood, I., 157, 166, 187, *241, 243, 245*
Greguss, P., 221, *250*
Griffing, V., 58, *233*
Groniowski, J. T., 75, 76, 157, 162, *235*
Grossman, C. C., 166, *243*
Guntheroth, W. G., 211, *249*
Güttner, W., 142, 212, *240, 250*

H

Hall, A. J., 160, 187, *241, 246*
Halstead, J., 218, *250*
Hanaoka, Y., 196, 206, *247, 248*
Hart, D. J., 157, *241*
Haselberg, K., von, 57, *232*
Haugen, M. C., 193, 194, *246*
Hawley, S. A., 225, *251*
Hayashi, S., 166, *243*
Heller, R. E., 115, *237*
Herrick, J. F., 193, 194, 225, *246, 251*
Hertz, C. H., 59, 157, 175, 181, *233, 241, 245*
Hey, E. B., 180, 183, *245*
Hiedemann, E. A., 68, 73, *234, 235*
Higashino, S., 225, *252*
Hikita, G., 202, 206, *247, 248*
Hill, C. R., 224, *251*
Hirose, M., 166, *243*
Hixon, T. J., 209, *249*
Hodgkinson, W. L., 70, *234*
Hoffman, C. W., 73, *235*
Holm, H. H., 143, 149, 157, 166, 180, 181, *239, 242, 243, 244*
Holmes, J. H., 143, 149, 157, 160, 166, 170, 171, 188, 192, 225, *239, 240, 242, 243, 246, 251*
Horn, C. A., 211, *249*
Horton, C. W., 58, *233*
Howry, D. H., 153, 157, 160, 164, 165, 166, 188, 225, *242, 243, 246, 251*
Hsiang-Huei, W., 143, 146, 149, *239*
Huane, H., 64, *233*
Hueter, T. F., 18, 20, 22, 23, 24, 25, 36, 55, 69, 212, 224, *228, 229, 230, 232, 234, 249, 250, 251*
Hughes, D. E., 225, *251*
Hunter, H. H., 68, *234*

I

Iams, H. A., 188, *246*
Ide, M., 69, *234*
Ireland, H. J. D., 157, *241*
Isard, H. J., 143, 180, 181, *240, 245*
Ishikawa, S., 166, *243*
Ito, K., 143, 166, *241, 243, 244*
Izumi, T., 208, *248*

J

Jacobs, J. E., 213, 214, 215, 217, 219, *250*
Jacobsen, E. H., 37, *231*
Jaffe, B., 29, *230*
Jaffe, H., 29, *230*
James, J. A., 66, 67, 73, 225, *234, 235, 251*
Jansson, F., 143, 150, *239*
Jeppsson, S., 143, 148, *239*
Johnson, J., 180, 183, *245*
Johnson, S., 66, *234*
Johnson, W. L., 204, 207, *248, 249*
Joyner, C. R., 143, 180, 181, 183, *240, 245*

K

Kalmus, H. P., 193, *246*
Kaneko, Z., 197, 198, 208, *247, 248*
Kao, J. Y., 143, 166, *241, 244*
Kaspar'yants, A. A., 64, *233*
Kato, K., 208, *248*
Kaye, G. W. C., 5, 21, *227, 228*
Kazan, B., 138, *238*
Keith, W. W., 43, *231*
Kell, R. C., 29, *230*
Kelsey, C. A., 209, *249*
Kikuchi, Y., 143, 157, 166, *241, 242, 243, 244*

Kimoto, J., 166, *244*
Kimoto, S., 143, 154, 157, 185, *240, 242, 246*
King, D. L., 143, 148, *239*
Kinsler, L. E., 16, 55, *228, 232*
Kingsley, B., 143, 180, 181, *240, 245*
Klinik, E., 213, *250*
Knight, P. R., 143, *240*
Knoll, M., 138, *238*
Koenig, W., 205, *248*
Kohashi, Y., 196, 206, *247, 248*
Kolsky, H., 45, 76, *231, 235*
Koppelmann, J., 69, *234*
Korn, G. A., 118, *237*
Korn, T. M., 118, *237*
Kossoff, G., 10, 21, 22, 46, 47, 48, 51, 61, 62, 63, 64, 74, 86, 94, 98, 124, 127, 128, 129, 130, 143, 146, 154, 157, 160, 166, 173, 211, *227, 228, 229, 231, 232, 233, 235, 236, 238, 240, 242, 244, 245, 249*
Kozma, A., 187, *246*
Krasil'nikov, V. A., 26, 27, *229*
Krause, W. E. E., 157, 166, *242, 244*
Krautkramer, J., 57, *232*
Krueger, H. H. A., 29, *230*
Kruezer, J. L., 220, *250*
Kuno, H., 196, 206, *247, 248*
Kuo-Juei, Y., 143, 146, 149, *239*

L

Laby, T. H., 5, 21, *227, 228*
La Casce, E. O., 14, *228*
Lacy, L. Y., 205, *248*
Land, E. H., 140, *238*
Larmore, L., 217, *250*
Larsen, F. J., 104, *237*
Lattuada, A., 166, *243*
Leary, G. A., 143, 150, *240*
Lehman, J. S., 157, 166, 180, 181, *241, 244, 245*
Lein, J. N., 207, *249*
Leith, E. N., 187, *246*
Leksell, L., 142, *240*
Lele, P. P., 225, *251*
Lester, W. W., 68, *234*
Li, K., 23, 24, 25, *228*
Likoff, W., 143, 180, 181, *240, 245*
Lithander, B., 143, 146, *240*
Litovitz, T. A., 21, *228*

Liu, C. N., 61, 63, 98, 127, 128, 129, 130, 154, *233, 236, 238, 242*
Loomis, A. L., 225, *252*
Lord, A. E., 58, *232*
Lubé, V. M., 197, 199, 202, 204, *247, 248*
Lucas, R., 65, *234*
Ludwig, G. D., 6, 10, 212, *227, 249*
Ludwig, J., 141, *240*
Lumb, R. F., 33, 47, 50, *230, 232*
Lunsford, J. S., 132, *238*
Lutsch, A., 38, *231*
Lutsch, A. G., 27, *229*
Lypacewicz, G., 25, 157, 162, *229, 241*

M

McCarthy, C. F., 166, 170, 223, *244, 250*
McCutcheon, E. P., 204, 208, *248, 249*
Machii, K., 196, 206, *247, 248*
MacKey, J. E., 76, *235*
McKinney, W. M., 60, 186, *233, 247*
McLeod, F. D., 197, 206, *247, 248*
McLeod, R. M., 225, *251*
McRae, D. L., 148, 166, *239, 244*
McSkimin, H. J., 46, 57, *232*
MacVicar, J., 95, 171, 225, *236, 244, 251*
Makow, D. M., 157, 166, *242, 244*
Mapp, E. McD., 208, *249*
Markham, M. F., 46, *231*
Martin, H. J., 213, 214, *250*
Martin, T. B., 113, *237*
Marzullo, S., 29, *230*
Mason, W. P., 29, 31, 32, *230*
Massey, N., 187, *246*
Mathes, R. C., 205, *248*
Meeks, E. L., 76, *235*
Mellen, R. H., 69, *234*
Merkulova, V. M., 45, *231*
Metherell, A. F., 217, 219, *250*
Meyer, E. P., 157, 160, *242*
Micsky, L. I. von, 166, *244*
Miller, L. D., 143, *240*
Millman, J., 36, 96, 124, *230, 236, 238*
Millner, R., 186, *245*
Minifie, F. D., 209, *249*
Mishina, Y., 196, 206, *247, 248*
Mitchell, M., 96, *236*
Miyazawa, R., 143, 166, *241, 243, 244*
Molin, C. E., 157, 166, *242, 244*
Moore, A. D., 110, *236*.

Mori, M., 202, 206, *247, 248*
Moroi, T., 143, 154, 157, 166, 185, *240, 242, 244, 246*
Morris, A. G., 111, *237*
Motomiya, M., 208, *248*
Mraz, S. J., 40, *230*
Mullins, G. L., 211, *249*
Musumeci, R., 166, *243*

N

Nakanishi, K., 202, 206, *247, 248*
Naral, F. C., 58, *233*
Nasser, W. K., 180, *245*
Neal, D., 141, 225, *239, 251*
Newell, J. A., 74, 143, *235, 240*
Nimura, Y., 202, 206, *247, 248*
Nomoto, O., 73, *235*
Northeved, A., 157, *242*
Norwine, A. C., 205, *248*
Nyborg, W. L., 224, *251*

O

Oberhettinger, F., 64, *233*
Ohta, S., 196, 206, *247, 248*
Oka, A., 166, *243*
Oksala, A., 143, *240*
Okujima, M., 69, *234*
Okumura, T., 208, *248*
Olofsson, S., 58, 59, 157, *233, 241*
Omizo, H., 208, *248*
Omoto, R., 143, 154, 157, 166, 185, 186, *240, 242, 243, 244, 246*
O'Neil, H. T., 61, 62, *233*
Ophir, D., 127, *238*
Osawa, N., 225, *252*
Ostrum, B. J., 143, 180, 181, *240, 245*

P

Panian, F. C., 70, *234*
Papadakis, E. P., 38, *232*
Parks, P. E., 40, *230*
Paterson, W. L., 131, *238*
Patrick, M. K., 225, *251*
Pätzold, J., 142, 212, *240, 250*
Peabody, C. O., 143, *240*
Pell, R. L., 143, *240*
Pellam, J. R., 44, *231*
Petersen, R. G., 40, *231*
Petralia, S., 24, 25, *229*
Pfander, F., 6, *227*

Pocock, P., 207, *249*
Pohlman, R., 24, 25, *229*
Pond, J., 225, *251, 252*
Ponomarev, P. V., 37, *231*
Popky, G. L., 208, *249*
Posakony, G. J., 188, 157, 160, *242, 246*
Poynton, F. Y., 213, 214, 215, *250*
Preston, H., 220, *250*
Pridie, R. B., 185, *245*

R

Ramakrishna, B. S., 206, *248*
Ramaswamy, T. K., 206, *248*
Ramsden, D., 143, *240*
Rayleigh, J. W., 15, *228*
Read, A. E. A., 166, 170, 223, *244, 250*
Real, R. R., 157, *242*
Redman, J. D., 187, *246*
Redwood, M., 40, 41, 42, 43, 44, 45, *231*
Reid, J. M., 104, 124, 142, 143, 157, 164, 166, 180, 183, *237, 238, 241, 242, 244, 245*
Reiss, A., 125, *238*
Renger, F., 143, *240*
Rich, C., 212, *250*
Richards, J. R., 6, *227*
Richards, M. J., 150, *240*
Ridenour, L. N., 203, *247*
Robinson, D., 211, *249*
Robinson, D. E., 51, 61, 62, 63, 94, 98, 124, 127, 128, 129, 130, 143, 146, 154, 157, 160, *232, 233, 236, 238, 240, 242,*
Robinson, D. H., 166, *244*
Romanenko, E. V., 69, *234*
Rosen, M., 40, *231*
Ross, F. G. M., 166, 170, 175, 177, 179, 181, 182, 185, 223, *244, 245, 250*
Roth, R. S., 29, *230*
Rowland, T. C., 207, *249*
Ruppel, A. E., 205, *248*
Rushmer, R. F., 193, 194, 197, 198, 202, 204, 207, 208, 210, *246, 247, 248, 249*
Ryan, R. P., 27, *229*

S

Safonov, Yu. D., 197, 199, 202, 204, *247, 248*
Sah, C. T., 111, *237*
Sahl, R., 66, *234*
Salkowski, J., 25, 157, 162, *229, 241*

Saneyoshi, J., 69, *234*
Satomura, S., 197, 198, 202, 204, 206, *247, 248*
Sayers, J. F., 213, 214, 215, *250*
Schellbach, G., 213, 214, *250*
Schentke, K. U., 143, *240*
Schlegal, J. V., 143, *240*
Schlegal, W. A., 195, 198, 202, 204, 208, *247, 248*
Schmitt, H. J., 69, *234*
Schmitt, O. H., 188, *246*
Schultz, R. D., 204, 207, 208, *248, 249*
Schwann, H. P., 23, 24, 25, *228, 229*
Sears, F. W., 65, *234*
Seegall, M. I., 18, *228*
Segal, B. L., 143, 180, 181, *240, 245*
Seki, H., 57, *232*
Sekiguchi, H., 196, 206, *248*
Semennikov, Iu. B., 213, *250*
Serabian, S., 46, *231*
Sette, D., 60, *233*
Severini, A., 166, *243*
Sevin, L. J., 113, *237*
Sharaf, H. F., 53, *232*
Sharpe, C. J., 143, 211, *240, 249*
Shih-Liang, C., 143, 146, 149, *239*
Shih-Yuan, A., 143, 146, 149, *239*
Shikurya, T., 225, *252*
Shimuzu, S., 196, 206, *247, 248*
Shiraishi, J., 208, *248*
Shockley, W., 110, *237*
Sigel, B., 208, *249*
Sjöberg, A., 66, *234*
Skingley, J. A., 110, *236*
Smith, R., 213, *250*
Smyth, C. N., 213, 214, 215, *250*
Smyth, M. G., 157, 225, *241, 252*
Soldner, R. E., 157, 166, *242, 244*
Soller, T., 134, *238*
Soloff, L. A., 180, 183, *245*
Somer, J. C., 163, 164, *242*
Sorsby, A., 150, *240*
Speight, R. G., 143, *240*
Stahle, J., 66, *234*
Starr, M. A., 134, *238*
Stegall, H. F., 197, 198, 202, 207, *247, 249*
Stephens, R. W. B., 17, 19, *228*
Sterke, A. de, 157, 166, *242, 244*
Strandness, D. E., 204, 207, 208, *248, 249*

Struthers, F., 141, *240*
Stutz, D. E., 68, *234*
Sumner, D. S., 204, 207, 208, *248, 249*
Sundén, B., 166, *244*
Sunstein, D. E., 116, *237*

T

Takagi, S. F., 225, *252*
Takagishi, S., 202, 206, *247, 248*
Tamarkin, P., 15, *228*
Tanaka, K., 157, *242*
Tao-Hsin, W., 143, 146, 149, *239*
Tarnóczy, T., 61, *233*
Taub, H., 36, 96, 124, *230, 236, 238*
Taveras, J. A., 123, *237*
Taveras, J. M., 143, 148, 166, *239, 243*
Taylor, A. R., 225, *251*
Taylor, E. S., 149, 171, *240, 243*
Taylor, R., 29, *230*
Theisman, H., 6, *227*
Thomas, L. A., 29, *230*
Thompson, H. E., 149, 171, *240, 243*
Thurstone, F. L., 60, 186, 217, *233, 246, 250*
Tjaden, K., 58, *232*
Tolansky, S., 53, *232*
Töpler, A., 65, *234*
Truell, R., 57, *232*
Tschiegg, C. E., 4, *227*
Tsunemoto, M., 143, 154, 157, 166, 185, *240, 242, 244, 246*
Tucker, D., 225, *251*
Turnbull, T. A., 185, *245*

U

Uchida, R., 143, 154, 157, 166, 185, *240, 242, 243, 244, 246*
Uematsu, K., 166, *243*
Ullrich, O. A., 68, *234*
Upatnieks, J., 187, *246*
Urick, R. J., 6, *227*

V

Valkenburg, H. E. van, 70, *234*
Valley, G. E., 101, 102, 103, 105, 134, *236, 237, 238*
Van der Pauw, L. J., 41, *231*
Ven, C. van der, 157, 166, *242, 244*
Vlieger, M. de, 142, 148, 149, 157, 166, 180, *239, 240, 242, 244*

W

Wagai, T., 143, 157, 166, *241, 242, 243, 244*
Wagner, D. K., 208, *249*
Waldhausen, J. A., 143, 180, 183, *239, 245*
Walker, D. C. B., 33, 47, 50, *230, 232*
Wallace, W. A., 27, *229*
Wallman, H., 101, 102, 103, 105, *236, 237*
Walton, W. P., 187, *246*
Wang, C. E., 143, 166, *241, 244*
Wang, H. F., 143, 166, *241, 244*
Warren, D. G., 76, *215*
Warwick, R., 225, *251*
Washington, A. B. G., 38, *231*
Watson, N. W., 195, 202, 204, 208, *247, 248*
Wells, P. N. T., 6, 66, 67, 70, 73, 74, 75, 83, 91, 94, 97, 105, 107, 108, 116, 124, 132, 133, 153, 154, 157, 159, 166, 167, 170, 175, 177, 179, 181, 182, 185, 196, 223, 225, *227, 234, 235, 236, 237, 238, 242, 244, 245, 247, 250, 251, 252*
Wetterer, E., 194, *246*
White, D. N., 143, 146, 148, *241*
Wilcken, D. E. L., 173, *245*

Wild, J. J., 104, 124, 141, 142, 143, 157, 164, 166, 210, 225, *237, 238, 239, 241, 242, 244, 249, 251*
Willard, G. W., 61, 65, 66, *233, 234*
Williams, A. O., 56, *232*
Willocks, J., 143, 149, *241*
Winters, W. L., 180, 183, *245*
Wolf, P. I., 210, *249*
Wood, A. B., 3, 18, *227, 228*
Wood, M. D., 107, *237*
Wood, R. W., 225, *252*
Wright, W., 157, 160, *242*
Wulff, V. J., 225, *251*
Wyt, L., 211, *250*

Y

Yakiemenkov, L. I., 197, 199, 202, 204, *247, 248*
Yoshida, T., 202, 206, *247, 248*
Yoshitoshi, Y., 196, 206, *247, 248*
Yü, L., 143, 166, *241, 244*

Z

Zaky, A., 143, 180, 183, *239, 245*
Zarembo, L. K., 26, 27, *229*
Ziskin, M., 180, 181, *245*

SUBJECT INDEX

A

A-scan, 78, 80, 81, 151, 178, 186
  from hydatidiform mole, 149
  from localization of brain mid-line,
    146, 147, 148
  from localization of placenta, 149
  of cystic masses, 144, 145
  of diseased liver, 144, 145
  of tumours of breast, 142, 144
  production, 78, 80
A-scope, 81, 123, 141–151, 175, 179,
    183
  comparison with B-scope, 151, 152
  dynamic range, 123, 151
  in ultrasonic diagnosis, 142–151
A-scope in ultrasonic diagnosis
  in estimation of intracranial pressure,
    148
  in examination of eye, 150, 151
  in foetal cephalometry, 149
  in localization of brain mid-line, 146–
    149
  in localization of placenta, 149,
    150
  in measurement of axial length of eye,
    150
  of cystic masses, 144
  of hydatidiform mole, 149
  of liver disease, 144, 146
  of tumours of breast, 142, 144
Absorption coefficient
  for waves of finite amplitude, 26
  of air at S.T.P., 21
  of aluminium, 21
  of Araldite, 21
  of castor oil, 21
  of mercury, 21
  of perspex, 21
  of polythene, 21
  of water, 21, 82, 91

  variation with frequency in diagnosis,
    95, 96
Absorption of ultrasound in biological
    materials, 22–26
  absorption coefficient, 22, 23
  effect of frequency, 23, 24
  effect of material type, 23, 24, 25
  effect of temperature, 23
  in anisotropic tissues, 22
  in blood, 23, 25
  in bone, 23, 24, 25
  in brain, 25
  in fat, 25
  in heart muscle, 25
  in humour of eye, 25
  in kidney, 25
  in lens of eye, 25
  in liver, 25
  in lung tissue, 24, 25
  in medulla oblongata, 25
  in muscle, 25
  in spinal cord, 25
  post-mortem change, 23
Amplifier, linear radio frequency, 103–
    110
  feedback control by neutralization,
    107, 109
  feedback control with cascode circuit,
    109, 110
  gain control by attenuator, 110–116
  gain control by bias adjustment, 104–
    107
  internal feedback, 107, 109, 110
  requirements, 103
  swept gain, 104–107
  transistorized gain controlled band-
    pass, 107
  unilateralization, 107, 108
Amplifier, linear video
  cut-off, 125
  design, 124

differentiation, 124, 125
Amplifier, logarithmic video
  characteristics, 125
  combination with linear amplifier,
    126, 127
  disadvantages, 126
  dynamic range, 131
  dynamic range compression, 127
  five-stage, 130, 131
  in cascade, 127, 128
  negative feedback by transistor, 131,
    132
  non-linear stage response, 128, 129
  swept gain, 126
  transfer characteristic at n stages, 129,
    130
  unbalanced stages, 129
  with Zener diode, 127
Amplifier, radio frequency, 99–103
  demodulation, 118–123
  frequency response width, 103
  gain-bandwidth product, 102
  gain control by attenuator, 110–116
  gain control by bias adjustment, 104–
    110
  noise figure, 102
  noise reduction, 101
  non-linear gain control, 116, 118
  receiver paralysis, 102, 103, 104
  requirements for ultrasonic applica-
    tions, 103
  source of noise, 100, 101
  stagger-tuned, 103
  superheterodyne receiver, 103, 104
  suppression, 122, 123
  swept gain, 104–107, 116, 118
  swept gain function generator, 116–
    118
  transistorized, 101, 107, 109, 110
Amplifier, video
  dynamic range, 123
  requirements, 123
Analogue converter, time-to-voltage,
    175–179
  circuit, 176
  in time-position recording, 175, 179
  operation, 178
  waveforms, 177
Attenuation of waves, 19–24
  by heat conduction, 20
  by hysteretic absorption, 20
  by relaxation, 20
Attenuator
  controlled resistor circuit, 114, 115
  in amplifier gain control, 104, 110–
    116
  positioning in amplifier, 115, 116

B

B-scan, 80, 124, 151, 152, 173, 186
  compound, 152
  production, 80
B-scan, compound, 152
  of diseased liver, 169
  of breast tumours, 167
  of early stage of pregnancy, 172
  of hydatidiform mole, 172
  of multiple pregnancy, 172
  of ovarian cyst, 172
  of placenta, 172
B-scope, 81, 123, 151, 186
  comparison with A-scope, 151, 152
  dynamic range, 123
  resolution, 151
  two-dimensional scanned, 151–155
B-scope, two-dimensional scanned, 151–
    155, 157
  comparison with A-scope, 152
  electrical coupling, 155, 158–162
  electronic scanning, 163, 164
  internal probe, 154
  in ultrasonic diagnosis, 164–171
  mechanical coupling, 162, 163
  mirror system, 154
  multiple reflections, 153
  resolution, 153
  water bath, 153, 154, 155
B-scope, two-dimensional scanned, in
    ultrasonic diagnosis
  localization of placenta, 171
  of breast tumours, 165, 166, 168
  of early pregnancy, 170
  of fibroids, 171
  of hydatidiform mole, 171
  of liver disease, 168, 170
  of multiple pregnancy, 171
  of ovarian cyst, 171

C

C-scope, 185, 186, 213

in atrial septal defect diagnosis, 185, 186

Capacitance
of transducer, 50

Characteristic impedance
of air at S.T.P., 10
of aluminium, 10
of aqueous humour of eye, 10
of Araldite, 10
of blood, 10
of brain, 10
of brass 10
of castor oil, 10
of fat, 10
of human tissue, mean value, 10
of kidney, 10
of lens of eye, 10
of liver, 10
of mercury, 10
of muscle, 10
of perspex, 10
of polythene, 10
of skull bone, 10
of spleen, 10
of vitreous humour of eye, 10
of water, 10

Cathode ray tube, 134–138
brightness-modulated, 137
electromagnetic deflection, 134, 135
electrostatic deflection, 134, 135
information storage, 138–140
in production of A-scan, 80, 123
in production of B-scan, 80, 123, 124
phosphors, 136
post-deflection beam acceleration, 134 135, 136
resolution, 136
screen, 136
spot size, 136, 137
video integration, 137

D

Decibel
definition, 7
power and amplitude ratios, 8
relation to neper, 7, 8

Demodulation
diode network, 118, 119, 120, 122
full-wave, 121
half-wave, 118, 119, 120, 121

Dielectric constant
of transducer, 29

Diode, *pin*
as controlled resistor, 115

Diode, type 1N916
forward characteristics, 111, 112

Doppler effect, 17
in measurement of interface movement, 17

Doppler effect in ultrasonic diagnosis
blood flow studies, 193, 195, 196, 197, 198, 207, 208
cardiology, 206, 207
foetal heart movement, 207, 209
heart valve operation, 206, 207
in study of larynx, 209

Doppler effect, ultrasonic
in measurement of flow velocity, 193, 194–197
in medical diagnosis, 193, 206–209

Doppler flowmeter, ultrasonic, 194, 195
advantages, 195
disadvantages, 196
measurement of blood velocity, 193, 195, 196, 197, 198, 207
nomogram, 196

Doppler frequency shift detector, ultrasonic
receiver design, 200, 201, 203
system, 200, 201, 202
system noise, 203
transducer arrangement, 197, 198
transmitter, 200

Doppler frequency shift, reflected ultrasonic
in velocity measurement, 194–197, 199, 200
signal analysis, 204–206

Doppler signal analysis
by bandpass filter, 204
by ear, 204
by ratemeter, 204
by sound spectroscope, 205, 206

E

Echo amplitude
effect of angle of incidence, 90, 91
effect of interface, 90, 92, 93
effect of pulse bandwidth, 86
effect of target range, 91, 92, 93
in pulse-echo system, 86, 90–93

of anterior mitral valve leaflet, 93
of brain mid-line, 93
of cirrhotic liver, 93
of foetal skull, 93
of hydatidiform mole, 93
of normal liver, 93
of posterior heart surface, 93
of posterior liver surface, 93
of smooth skin in water, 93
of uterine fibroid, 93
Echoencephalography, 142
Elastic compliance
of transducer, 30, 32
Electrocardiogram, 182, 184
Electromechanical coupling coefficient, 30
of transducer, 30, 32
relation to piezoelectric coefficient, 30
Electronic storage tube, 138–140
bistable, 139, 140
direct view, 138, 139
dynamic range, 140
information storage in ultrasonic diagnosis, 138–140
transmission control, 138, 139

F

Fraunhofer zone, 55, 56, 57
Frésnel zone, 55, 56, 57, 58, 82, 85, 92

H

Huygen's principle
in analysis of directivity of transducer, 53, 55

I

Impedance matching, electrical, 49, 50, 51
effect of cable length on tuning, 51
effect on sensitivity, 50
Impedance matching, mechanical, 46–49
effect on bandwidth, 46, 47
Inductance
of transducer, 50

L

Loss
in pulse-echo system, 85

in transducer, 47, 48, 49, 51
in ultrasonic beam focussing, 59

M

Microphone
in observation of ultrasonic field, 69, 70

N

Normal incidence intensity reflection
at interface, 13, 14
of biological media, 13
of non-biological media, 13

O

Oscilloscope photography, 140–141
in ultrasonic diagnosis, 140, 141

P

Phonocardiogram, 182, 184
Phosphor
characteristics, 136
Piezoelectric coefficient, 29, 31
of transducer, 29, 30
relation to electromechanical coupling coefficient, 30
tensor notation, 31
Piezoelectric effect, 28, 29, 30
constants, 29
in ferroelectric materials, 28
in generation of narrow-beam ultrasonic radiation, 30
nature, 28
occurrence, 28
Pulse-echo system
amplifiers, 99–110
calibration, 189, 190, 191
characteristics, 91, 92
dynamic range, 80, 81, 85, 87, 89, 95, 99
echo amplitude, 86, 90, 91, 92, 93
echo attenuation, 80
in lossless medium, 85
lateral resolution, 81, 82, 84, 85, 87, 186
multiple reflection artifacts, 93, 94, 95
non-directional targets, 82
noise, 99, 100
performance, 188–192

precision, 89
principles, 77, 78
range resolution, 87, 89, 90, 99
receiver, 99, 100
relation between dynamic range and resolution, 81, 82, 85
resolution, 89, 90
sensitivity, 188
signal processing circuit, 79, 80
signal-to-noise ratio, 99, 102
swept gain, 82, 85, 87, 90, 95, 104–107, 132, 134
swept gain generator triggering by first echo, 132, 133, 134
system diagram, 79
threshold, 87
time-position recording, 171–179
timing circuits, 96, 97
transmitter circuit, 97, 98, 99
trigger pulse, 132, 133, 134
in ultrasonic field investigation, 70–72
Pulse-echo system, echo amplitude
effect of angle of incidence, 90, 91
effect of bandwidth, 86
effect of interface, 90, 92, 93
effect of target range, 91, 92, 93
Pulse-echo system, resolution
effect of demodulation, 89
effect of receiver bandwidth, 89, 90
Pulse frequency spectrum, 43–46, 49, 85, 86, 89, 90
modification by receiver frequency response, 85

Q

Q-factor, 35, 36
effect on transducer frequency characteristics, 35, 36
effect on transducer electrical performance, 36, 37

R

Reactance
of transducer, 49
Receiver
noise energy, 100
recovery time, 102, 103, 104
source of noise, 100
Resolution, 81–85, 87, 89, 90, 99, 186

S

Schlieren system
for observation of ultrasonic field, 65–69
image analysis, 68
image observation, 66, 68
principle, 65, 66, 67
sensitivity, 65
Semiconductor
current-voltage relation at pn junction, 110, 111
Suppression, 82, 122 123
Swept gain, 82, 85, 87, 90, 99, 104–107, 132, 134

T

Three-dimensional scan, 186–188
Time-position recording
analogue converter, 173–179
calibration of system, 179
in ultrasonic diagnosis, 179–185
methods, 173, 174
photographic recording, 173
square-wave pulse recording, 175
strip-chart recording, 173
Time-position recording in ultrasonic diagnosis, 179–185
of abdominal aortic aneurism, 180, 181
of foetal heart movement, 181
of heart valve movements, 183
of intracranial pulsations, 180
of mitral valve abnormalities, 181–183, 184, 185
of pericardial effusion, 183, 185
Timing circuit, 96, 97
delay generator, 96
rate generator, 96
time-base generator, 96, 97
Transducer, 28–52
as receiver, 33, 34, 38, 41, 47, 50, 57
as transmitter, 33, 47, 50, 57
attenuation of beam, 57
bandwidth, 48, 49, 89, 90
barium titanate, 28, 41
beam energy in side lobes, 56, 57
beam focussing, 58–63
beam uniformity, 55, 56, 57
beamwidth, 62, 63
capacitance, 50
curved, 61, 62, 186

damping, 39, 40
dielectric constant, 29
directivity function, 56, 57
dynamic range, 51, 52, 81, 99
elastic compliance, 30, 32
electrical impedance matching, 49, 50, 51
electromagnetic, 75, 76
electromechanical coupling coefficient, 30, 32
electromechanical properties, 32
electrostatic, 75, 76
excitation, 37, 38, 39, 40, 97, 98, 99
Fraunhofer zone, 55, 56, 57, 63
frequency characteristic, 35, 37
Frésnel zone, 55, 56, 57, 58, 82, 85, 92
fundamental resonant frequency, 34, 35, 37
generation of short pulses, 37, 38, 39
generation of single stress waves, 39, 40, 41
geometrical diffraction, 57, 58
inductance, 50
in the steady state, 53–58
in ultrasonic diagnosis, 30–33
lead titanate zirconate, 29, 31, 32, 33, 49, 51
lithium sulphate, 33
loop gain, 47, 50
loss reduction, 47, 49, 51
maximum efficiency, 35
mechanical impedance matching, 46, 47, 48, 49
nature, 28
non-uniformity of vibration, 53
piezoelectric coefficient, 29, 30
pulse response, 41, 42
PZT, 32, 33, 35, 47
Q-factor, 32, 35, 36, 37, 38, 49
quartz, 31, 32, 33, 35
reactance, 49
relation between dynamic range and resolution, 82
resolution, 81, 82, 83, 87
resonance, 33, 34, 35, 49
resonant frequency, 50
sensitivity, 34, 35, 57
stress wave analysis, 41, 43
thickness expanding type, 31
treatment as cophasally vibrating piston, 53, 55, 57

Transistor
as controlled resistor, 111, 112, 113
field-effect, 113
in amplifier, 101, 107, 109, 110
metal-oxide semiconductor, 113
non-unilateral, 107
Transmitter
blocking oscillator, 98
for fast rise-time pulse, 98
gated sine wave oscillator, 99
shock-exciting, 97, 98

U

Ultrasonic beam
alteration of directivity, 58
beamwidth, 62, 63
focussed, 58–63, 85
highly focussed, 186
power measurement, 73–76
resolution, 59, 63, 82, 83, 84, 85
Ultrasonic beam focussing, 58–63, 186
by lenses, 59, 60, 61
by reflectors, 58, 59, 60
by use of curved transducer, 61, 62
loss, 59
methods, 58, 59
optimization, 62, 63
Ultrasonic beam power
measurement by calorimetry, 73
measurement by radiation pressure, 74, 75
Ultrasonic diagnosis
choice of frequency, 95
hazards, 223–226
importance of frequency spectrum, 44
information storage, 138–141
narrow radiation beams, 30
using a highly focussed beam, 186
using electrically scanned transmission, 213–217
using holography, 217–221
using mechanically scanned transmission, 211–213
using the A-scope, 142–151
using the B-scope, two-dimensional scanned, 164–171
using the Doppler effect, 206–209
using three-dimensional scan, 186–188
using time-position recording, 179–185

using unscanned transmission, 210–213

Ultrasonic energy
transmission, 1

Ultrasonic field
directivity, 58, 63
Fraunhofer zone, 55, 56, 57, 63
Frésnel zone, 55, 56, 57, 58, 82, 85
observation, 65–73
parameters, 222, 223
steady state, 53, 55, 56, 57, 63, 64
transient conditions, 63, 64

Ultrasonic field investigation
absolute intensity distribution, 73
by dyes, 73
by image system, 73
by microphones, 69, 70
by phosphors, 73
by pulse-echo, 70, 71, 72
by schlieren method, 65–69
by shadowgraph, 73
by stroboscope, 73
by temperature-sensitive chromotrophic compounds, 73
intensity distribution plot, 69, 72

Ultrasonic holography
advantages, 217
difficulties, 219, 220
distortion, 219
glare, 220, 221
system, 218

Ultrasonic intensity, 7
half-power distance, 9
units, 7

Ultrasonic pulse
absolute intensity, 75
effect of absorption on frequency spectrum, 45, 46
frequency spectrum, 43–46, 49, 85
generation, 37, 38, 39, 49, 97–99
in interface depth measurement, 77, 78
power, 73–76, 97, 98
very fast rise time, 98
very short, 39, 40, 41

Ultrasonic radiation
generation of narrow beam, 30
tissue penetration, 95

Ultrasonic signal path, performance
effect of beam shape, 189
effect of frequency, 188
effect of overall dynamic range, 190, 191
effect of overall paralysis time, 192
effect of overall voltage transfer function, 47, 48, 189
effect of pulse amplitude and shape, 188, 189
effect of pulse repetition frequency, 189
effect of receiver bandwidth, 189
effect of receiver gain, 189
effect of signal processing arrangement, 190
effect of swept gain rate, 189, 190
effect of transducer diameter, 189

Ultrasonic transmission techniques, electrically scanned
sensitivity, 214
system, 213, 214, 215, 216

Ultrasonic transmission techniques, mechanically scanned
in brain scanning, 212
to measure bone mass, 213

Ultrasonic transmission techniques, unscanned
to assess fracture union in bone, 211
to measure change in mesenteric blood volume, 211

Ultrasound
absorption in biological materials, 22–26
attenuation of wave, 19–22
biophysical effect, cavitation, 223, 224
biophysical effect, thermal, 223
velocity in biological materials, 5

Ultrasoundcardiogram, 182, 183, 184

W

Waves
acceleration, 2
amplitude, 1
analysis of amplitude distribution, 43, 44
attenuation, 19
characteristic impedance, 9
Doppler effect, 17
energy, 7
finite amplitude, 26
frequency, 1, 5
intensity, 7

non-linear effects, 26
non-planar, 19
particle pressure, 9
phase, 2
power, 7
radiation pressure, 18
reflection at plane surfaces, 10–14
reflection at rough interfaces, 14, 15
refraction at plane surfaces, 10–14
spherical, 19
standing, 15
static pressure, 18
transmission through layers, 16
velocity, 2
velocity of propagation, 2, 3
wavelength, 5
Wave motion
 modes, 1
Wave propagation velocity, 3, 4, 5
 dependence on bulk modulus, 3, 4
 dependence on density, 3
 dependence on elasticity, 3
 dependence on shear modulus, 3, 4
 dependence on wave frequency, 5

of air at S.T.P., 5
of aluminium, 5
of aqueous humour of eye, 6
of blood, 6
of brain, 6
of brass, 5
of castor oil, 5
of eye lens, 6
of fat, 6
of human tissue, mean value, 6
of kidney, 6
of liver, 6
of mercury, 5
of muscle, 6
of perspex, 5
of polythene, 5
of skull bone, 6
of spleen, 6
of vitreous humour of eye, 6
of water, 5
relation with Young's modulus, 4
variation with temperature, 4
Wavelength
 relation with frequency, 5